1-2-3 JOY!

1-2-3 JOY!

EASY, NATURAL WEIGHT LOSS THAT IS SCIENTIFIC, PROVEN, DRUG-FREE & FUN

LAUREL MELLIN, PHD

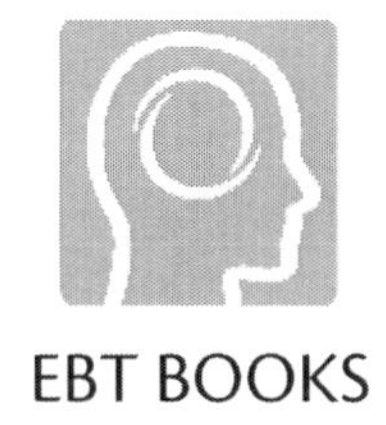

EBT BOOKS

Emotional Brain Training (EBT) is a science-based approach to health, using techniques based on neurophysiology and emotional neuroplasticity that are designed to promote stress resilience and raise the brain's set point. Like any skills training program, EBT is not without risk and may be unsafe or ineffective for some people. If you have any psychological or medical problems, consult with your physician and other health professionals before beginning this program. Using the method with the support of the program's mobile app is recommended. Participating in coaching and small group training facilitated by Certified EBT Providers is also recommended. The health outcomes associated with self-study use of EBT are not known. The author, The Solution Foundation (a non-profit corporation), and EBT, Inc. (a California corporation) disclaim all liability for any adverse effects that may result from the use or application of the information contained in this book. The characters discussed in this publication are composites of several individuals, and the names of all individuals have been changed to maintain anonymity.

The nutritional recommendations included in this publication are not a substitute for a consultation with a physician and registered dietitian. If possible, consult with a registered dietitian who is a Certified EBT Provider.

1-2-3 JOY!
Easy, Natural Weight Loss that is
Scientific, Proven, Drug-free & Fun

Printed in the United States of America.

Editors: Michele Blanchard Welling and Frannie Wilson. Design Consultant: Mel Truit. InDesign: Amnet. Cover Photograph: Jamie Rain, Lunchbreak Headshots. Production: Michael McClure. Technology: Dev Singh and Andrea Singh. Technology design: Joe Mellin. Graphics: Joyce Davis. Provider coordinator: Cassidy McCorkle. Creative advisor: Walt Rose. Manager: Kelly McGrath.

ISBN: 978-1-893265-14-1
Author: Laurel Mellin, PhD
Published by: EBT Books,
a division of EBT, Inc.
138 Woodland Avenue, San Anselmo, CA 94960
WEBSITE: www.ebt.org
BLOG: www.brainbasedhealth.org
E-MAIL: support@ebt.org

The EBT Spiral Up Community

We invite you to visit EBT.ORG for information about joining. The membership fee is $1 to start, which includes: the Spiral Up! mobile app, daily live drop-in sessions with a Certified EBT Provider, and the complete EBT 1-2-3 JOY Program.

To EBT master trainers and leaders:
Walt, Charlie, Igor, Lynda, Lindsey, Dev, Michael,
Kelly, Michele, Dave, Judy, Deanne, Frannie,
Barbara, Arinn, Bill, Angie, Edie, Sherry, Anna,
Robin, Molly, Cassidy, Valerie, and Eve, and
those who orchestrated sharing EBT with the world:
Jaime, Vern, Bruce, Jeffery, Jason, Mel,
Grace, Mark, Vicki, and Eric

Also by Laurel Mellin

The Stress Solution
What's my number?
The EBT Handbook
The Stress Eating Solution
The Stress Overload Solution
Spiral Up!
Wired for Joy
The 3-Day Solution Plan
The Pathway
The Solution
Shapedown

Contents

Introduction

A New Paradigm

Step 1: Clear Stress

Step 2: Boost Rewards

Step 3: Change Habits

Profound and Lasting Results

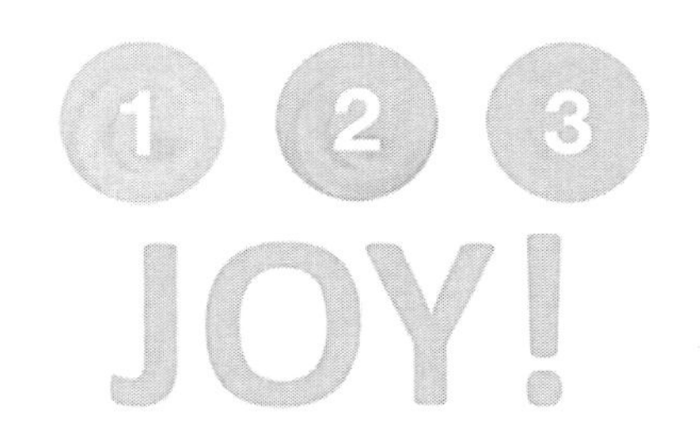

Introduction

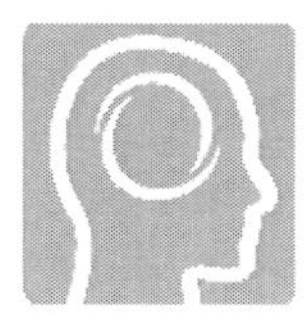

Easy, Natural Weight Loss

Amy, a real estate broker, said she had started gaining weight a decade before when she entered perimenopause. Then the pandemic hit, which stymied her business, and she put on another 20 pounds. Amy was desperate to control her weight and was on the brink of taking weight-loss drugs. Then her sister suggested using EBT as a natural alternative.

Amy told me, "I've tried everything, but it is so hard for me to lose weight."

Right away I knew that I could help her.

I said, "Amy, weight loss is only hard if you are going up against the chemicals that drive overeating and weight gain. They are activated when you are stressed. You don't need weight-loss drugs. Instead, you can use EBT and start switching off those chemicals naturally. Your brain will automatically activate chemicals that make it easy to eat healthy, lose weight, and keep it off."

She said, "Change myself chemically without drugs? How do I do that?"

"You take your stress seriously. Whenever you feel stressed or have a craving, you take a couple of minutes, and use your emotions in an innovative way."

She said, "I've been to therapy and it didn't help my weight."

I said, "EBT is not a psychological method. It uses emotions to change your biochemistry. You turn stress into joy, and when you are in joy, all your chemicals improve, including the ones that drive overeating and weight gain."

"So, I don't count grams of protein?"

"No, you count 'Joy Points,' moments of self-created, biologically impactful, intensely positive emotions."

Amy started laughing. "I was so depressed about having to lose weight because I can't stand another diet and I don't want to take any more drugs. Then, you tell me that the weight-loss strategy is to create joy. How come I didn't find out about EBT 10 years ago?"

The method, Emotional Brain Training (EBT) is a new paradigm in weight loss that is based on neuroscience. The conceptual basis of the method, Emotional Plasticity Theory, that by changing our brain circuits we improve our health, is based on the most respected neuroscience research available today. Yet that research is largely buried in neuroscience journals. Most health professionals treating obesity are not aware of this science or how it is applied in EBT, so this book is designed for anyone who struggles with food and weight and for the health professionals who treat them.

I said, "Adjusting food matters, but it makes sense to switch off the chemicals that drive overeating first so that you only change what you eat when doing so is a nurturing act. Typically, that is about a month or two into using the program, depending upon how often you use the tools, when your appetite is suppressed and you are naturally drawn to making a few strategic improvements in your diet."

Amy could use weight-loss drugs if she wanted to, but why go to the expense and put artificial chemicals into her body if she did not need to? Injections are not a solution to obesity as when the injections stop, so does the weight loss. Her brain could start altering her chemical drives to overeat and gain weight without drugs and natural solutions are safer and more lasting than artificial ones.

EBT is based on the observation that stress is the root cause of all the imbalances that cause weight gain, either directly or indirectly. Most weight-loss drugs provide a synthetic chemical that mimics GLP-1, a peptide that impacts appetite and also affects some of the stress-induced imbalances in cortisol, dopamine, and insulin. They work at the chemical level, relying on external sources of chemicals and therefore, promoting dependency.

EBT works by switching off the brain's stress response. It shuts off the brain circuits that not only cause not only these chemicals to go rogue but also cause the thinking brain to function poorly and inadvertently activate unhealthy moods, thoughts, and behaviors. The method goes "upstream" from where weight-loss drugs intervene to impact the brain at a more fundamental level, changing our entire biochemistry for the better naturally. EBT trains the brain to deliver these chemical effects, offering an internal solution that promotes independence.

I said to Amy, "With EBT, you read the state of your emotional brain, as that is where the circuits of the stress response are stored. You pay attention to your emotions because they inform you about what is going on physiologically in your body. When you feel a glow in your body, a lightness, or a tingle, those are "signs of joy" that mean you have been successful in switching off the chemicals that cause cravings, chronic hunger, lethargy, and weight gain."

Amy responded, "So I need to be emotionally aware?"

I said, "Precisely, so you are motivated to use the tools more often. The more you use them, the more the brain automatically activates these pathways. The brain rewires itself based on what feels good."

Evolution gave us a brain that naturally switches off negative emotions and activates positive ones. The most sustainable positive emotions come from an awareness of the deeper meanings of life, which is why we do things to protect the young, vulnerable, and elderly and care about the world we leave to the next generation. Purpose is powerful in the brain and the emotional brain (the "stress brain") is the seat of the soul. Early in developing EBT, I saw participants becoming more purpose-driven and spiritual as they used the tools over time. I didn't know then that the tools were connecting thoughts of higher purpose in the thinking brain to the reward centers in the emotional brain, creating access to awareness of purpose and moments of transcendence.

I said to Amy, "The emotional brain is the seat of the soul, and joy is a spiritual state, so, chances are as you use these skills you'll notice a spiritual deepening."

In that optimal state of joy, it is common to experience the other "elevated emotions" that are a response to moral beauty and include love, compassion, gratitude, hope, forgiveness, and awe. In that state, we can readily identify our higher purpose for all that we do, including the choice to eat healthy and release extra weight. This awareness is then chemically beneficial, boosting dopamine and endorphins naturally, which swamp the stress so we can eat healthy and lose weight.

Raising awareness that chemicals drive obesity

The development of weight-loss drugs came about because diets did not switch off the chemicals that drive overeating. Although it makes sense that changing what we eat changes weight, only lasting weight loss improves health. Short-term changes do not, and research shows that by six months to a year after starting diet-based programs, any weight lost has been regained.

The good news about weight-loss drugs is that they have raised public awareness that obesity is caused by chemicals. However, most people do not know that their brain is perfectly capable of changing the wires that activate these chemicals without drugs.

The primary purpose of this book is to map out the science and practice of EBT. It is to show you why and how your brain can change so it provides you with more of the natural chemicals that promote healthy eating and weight loss. For most people, the EBT Program is all they need to lose weight and keep it off, however, the method is compatible with all other strategies as its mechanism of action is to improve overall physiology and rewire errant circuits that cause chronic diseases like obesity and mental health problems. If you want to combine it with other strategies, you can.

However, even if you combine EBT with other methods, there is no substitute for learning how to control the wires in your own emotional brain and the chemicals that they unleash. Nobody can take better care of us than we can, as stress can be activated anytime and anywhere. As most health problems are symptoms of untreated stress, EBT provides a foundation for all of healthcare. Once you have the skills, you have them for life and have more control over your mood, thoughts, behaviors, relationships, productivity, and overall health.

The other purpose of this book is to enhance your confidence in the goodness of life. In developing the method over time, the elegance of the design of life, that we have an emotional brain that is so open to change, has continued to bring me to awe. Stress is defined as when the organism has to work harder to stay healthy and that wear and tear exacts a price. Chronic stress is like having a slow leak in the tire of your car. If you don't take care of it, at some point, you have a flat. Any genetic vulnerability, errant brain pathway caused by trauma, or borderline bad habit becomes more extreme with stress, and if unattended it causes a "flat tire" or health problem. Medical care bypasses treating stress in favor of fixing the flat tire by pumping it up with medications, procedures, and devices, rather than fixing the leak.

EBT fixes that leak. We're stressed because information overload, our toxic environment, the speed of change, and our shrinking resources overpower the capacity of the brain to think our way out of problems and clear our stress. We live in the age of the emotional brain, as with this stress level, the brain automatically puts emotional processing in charge, which is perfect. If we process negative emotions back to positive feelings, the stress response shuts off. Each switch ("spiral up") accomplishes the two most important objectives in healthcare: self-regulation (resiliency) and reconsolidation (rewiring). The tools of the method rapidly switch off stress, as emotions work faster and more effectively than thoughts. Also, each rapid resiliency experience changes the brain, making small but important improvements in errant circuits encoded in trauma that activate stress., What's more, the tools can help us cope with and even change our genes through the route of epigenetics. Essentially, these tools offer a neuroscientific solution for life.

I asked Amy, "What's the most important thing you learned from our session?"

She said, "That my weight is not my fault, and there is something I can do about it."

A scientific approach to weight loss

Obesity rates have quadrupled in the last 40 years despite no change in the genetics of the population. In the graph below, obesity, which is widely regarded as a "stress symptom," increases in lock-step with rising stress levels. Although the food environment has also become more toxic during the last 40 years, our job in healthcare is to be sure that people have the skills to "stress-protect" themselves from the environment. Based on national data, our current methods of processing stress appear to have fallen short by 1990.

As stress increased, we bypassed treating the emotional brain and instead used drugs, surgery, and diets to treat obesity, but like most "workarounds," it was not successful. These methods have not solved our nation's obesity epidemic; in fact, it has only become worse.

Nickie, a college student who came to EBT because her mother had used it to lose weight, said, "I think of my problem as my hand. It reaches for cookies, but the real problem is a wire in my brain that makes me want the cookies to start with."

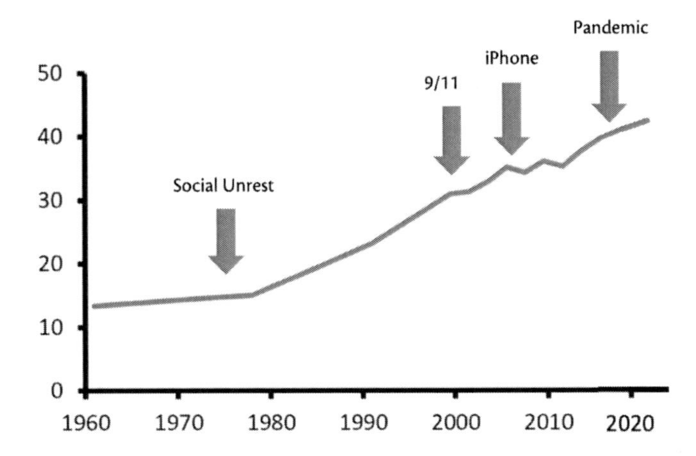

Adult obesity from NHANES and NHES through September 2023

We have solved other health problems by becoming more sophisticated in our treatments. By making a shift away from treating the symptom of overeating, and instead treating the root cause, I believe we can empower many people to lose weight and keep it off. By making these life-changing skills of EBT widely available, we can turn around the obesity epidemic as well as the epidemics of other chronic diseases and mental health problems caused by stress. It is time.

Treat stress to turn around the obesity crisis

EBT will give you a direct way to engage your emotional brain with a new goal – to rewire your emotional brain and turn off the biochemical drives that cause overeating and weight gain. You will be apt to see changes right from the start. Just use it before you eat and notice that you want the food less. You eat healthier naturally. To make lasting changes in the brain takes one year. Most people see important changes within a few months and report that family members and friends say, "What changed? You are so vibrant, full of joy, with a new zest for life." These changes become deeper and more rewarding the longer you use EBT and the more rigorously you apply it.

You might wonder why you haven't heard of EBT. The method has largely been hidden away for the last 15 years while we studied and refined the skills to make them faster and more effective. Although about 500,000 people have used EBT, we have not publicized it in recent years. Then, in June of 2022, two participants in the EBT program whose lives had been transformed by using the tools endowed EBT with resources to bring the method to the world. This book and our new "Emotional Health for All" website and campaign have followed. Their gift came at the perfect time, right when stress-induced health problems, including obesity, were reaching crisis proportions. EBT is here to help.

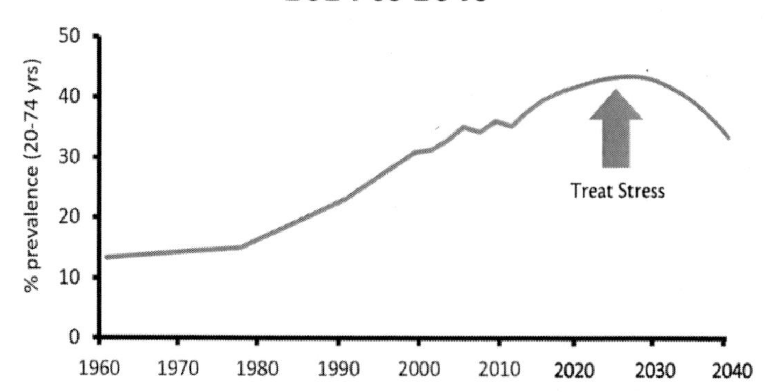

Data from NHANES and NHES through September 2023.
Estimates for 2040 by author if stress overload is treated effectively.

The obesity rate has increased rapidly, and our goal at EBT is to turn it around rapidly, cutting the obesity rate in half within two decades. In the graphic above, see the turning point this year. That may seem unlikely – a real moonshot – but already one government initiative has supported the widespread dissemination of EBT starting in January 2024. Given that stress is causing or exacerbating most public health problems, more may come. Please do not underestimate the combination of the power of the human brain when unencumbered by raging stress chemicals and the current motivation to stop cravings and weight gain. If EBT catches on, who knows what could happen?

Using the new paradigm personally

The entire EBT team joins me in welcoming you to discover how these magical skills can work for you. Use our app before eating. Feel a slight shift in your body and realize that you have just switched off stress chemicals, and you are eating a little bit healthier naturally. Use it before an important work meeting, prior to social situations, or whenever you want an instant dopamine boost. Feel the difference! Keep using EBT until you find that the drive to overeat has faded, and you naturally eat healthy, lose weight, and keep it off.

It all starts with you. Imagine that on the day you were born, you had all the inherent strength, goodness, and wisdom you would ever need to lose weight and keep it off. All you required were the skills to access it. EBT will give you the skills. All you do is "spiral up" and switch off the stress response. When you do, the emotional brain circuits that have promoted cravings, hunger, lethargy, and weight gain begin to change.

Celebrate that all you have to do is start right where you are and follow the 1-2-3 JOY Program. Do not diet. Instead, 1) clear stress so the chemicals that drive overeating quiet down, and 2) boost rewards so you don't need the dopamine surge from processed foods. Then, 3) make subtle adjustments in your eating and they are natural, nurturing, and sustainable. You are in joy.

This approach plays by the rules of the emotional brain, the most powerful processor on the planet. Use it to discover that you have far more power than you know and can easily stop overeating and release extra weight. Releasing weight is not a chore, but a way to take care of yourself, all while making it fun and creating more joy in your life.

The EBT method is magical, scientific, and ready for you. All you must do is begin . . .

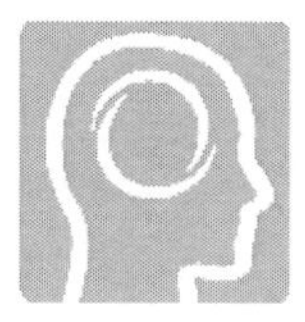

Engage the Emotional Brain

It seems rather complicated. We want to eat healthy, so we track our diet, analyze what we eat and question why we ate those cookies after lunch. Based on neuroscience, how do we most efficiently change our eating?

It's pretty easy. Stop thinking, except for asking one question: What's my number? That is your stress level or brain state.

To find out, turn your attention to your body where you experience the activations of your emotional brain. That's it! You have now engaged your emotional brain, which is the controller of the chemical cascade that controls food intake.

Moments ago, I was facilitating a daily intensive course in EBT. The group begins with each person taking a minute or two to describe an "amazing learning," something that excited them when using the skills or a new tool they learned in the course. Kathleen, who was completing her second intensive, spoke up.

She said, "My amazing learning is that I love EBT. Whenever I overeat, I do not think. I use the skills. I find out what was driving me to stuff myself with food, and when I finish using them, I feel this electricity all over, and I feel great."

I was happy she said that because everyone else in the group was new to EBT, so it was a great chance to talk about the unconscious mind and physiology. Kathleen felt that tingle because she had changed the chemicals and electricity in every cell of her body. She had engaged her emotional brain.

The emotional brain as the grand unifier

The emotional brain is the storehouse of unconscious memories, all our life experiences. We cannot find those memories by thinking, as the circuits are emotional. It's only through the avenue of emotions that we change these circuits.

Stress activates emotions, and by processing negative emotions back to positive ones, we clear stress. The objective is to use the tools until you experience a moment of joy, which means a slight tingle, feeling present and rewarded, a glow, or a lightness of being. Even a nanosecond of joy is the best medicine as it turns off the stress response.

Harnessing the power of emotions

Neuroscientist Antonio Damasio's work on emotions is important to understanding EBT in two ways. One is that he described the link between emotions and physiology in his landmark book, *Looking for Spinoza: Joy, Sorrow, and the Feeling Brain.* First, he noted that optimal physiology was not signified by the absence of stress, but by the presence of joy. Our entire physiology is humming along at its best when we feel a tingle or glow in our body associated with that joy.

The other breakthrough of his work is that emotions are the "entity" that we can process to rapidly change our physiology: molecules, cells, organs, and organ systems. Dr. Damasio proposed the Nesting Principle, that chemicals and electricity are transported through the bloodstream, and neural circuits signal the brain for metabolic regulation, basic reflexes, behaviors, pain and pleasure, biological drives, and our motivation, all appearing as emotions that are read by the thinking brain as feelings. These feelings are a synthesis of our entire physiology.

Where does stress fit in? The stress activation of the sympathetic nervous system is associated with negative emotions, and the parasympathetic nervous system of relaxation is associated with positive emotions. By processing negative feelings until they turn into positive ones, we change our physiology for the better and switch off the stress response.

How do we control our eating, weight, and stress? We process extreme, negative emotions in times of high stress in a highly effective way. What follows is the story of the conceptual basis of EBT and how the 5-Point System of Emotional and Behavioral Regulation was designed to accomplish that.

The EBT 5-Point System

As spiritual beings who are attached to physical bodies that are assaulted daily by stressful stimuli in modern life, we are always in the business of processing emotions. But where do they come from? They come from the activation of neuronal Stress Circuits ("wires") stored in our brain's amygdala, the first response of which is to launch a simple, fast, emotional message to get our attention that a threat is being perceived. This emotional experience varies in intensity, duration, and importance and turns the black/white world of thoughts into Kodachrome. Everything important in life – beauty, connection, spirituality, love, meaning, passion, and most notably, survival – comes from these wires.

Although we perceive this emotional blast as realistic to the present moment, it does not originate from just one wire but the echoes of our past, all mixed together in the wonderful, confusing experience we call life. Not only is our present the product of which diverse wires are activated from our memories, but the situation becomes more complicated once the activation lands us in a particular brain state.

Based on state-specific memory, other memories that have been encoded at the same level of stress are "hot" or "online" when a wire is activated, and those from other stress levels are "cold" or "offline," making each activation a separate life experience. The online wires coactivate with our initial response. Combined with our physiology, we are in essence "different people" with each activation and brain state. And this happens without our permission or awareness that this is a wire, while we truly believe it is based on our current reality. If the initial response is unwanted (for example, we have the urge to eat the entire apple pie or a desire to unleash our full, uncensored wrath on someone who betrayed us), we must "pounce" on that wire and switch it off or our troubles begin.

Chaos happens when more equally dysfunctional wires join the "emotional brain party." They are not well-mannered, and they recruit others to join in, all of the same negative ilk. This is not a problem when a beautiful or joyful wire is activated and we're in rapture, wanting to amplify and extend our bliss. Depending on the coactivated wires, we could experience a spectacular gala of hope, love, and joy or, if a neural "glitch" is activated, a real brawl with police on the way and the neighbors banging on our door. All of this happens in a flash and is beyond our control unless we have a way to switch off the initial activation. We can always bring it to mind on a later date ("cognitively activate the circuit") and clear it with the same emotional processing tools, but it is likely to then be a bigger, more dominant circuit and require more repetitions of the spiral-up procedure to clear it.

Stress Level

There are 5 different levels of stress in the brain.

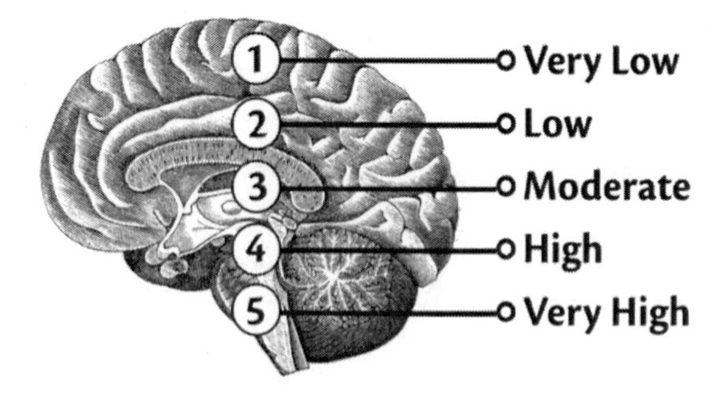

How can we organize all this? We do it by numbering our brain states on a one to five scale. The actual number of brain states is not really known. However, based on observed phenomena in EBT, which are consistent with the work of Bruce Perry when he investigated the effects of trauma, there are five distinct brain states. That's the number we settled on because we only require five emotional resilience tools, one for each brain state, to stress-protect ourselves and take charge of our unconscious mind. Why make it more complicated than needed?

In a hierarchical fashion, each brain state puts a different brain area in charge, the one that provides the greatest chances of survival. In high stress, the lower, faster, more primitive, and more extreme brain region – the emotional brain – is dominant.

Imagine meeting up with a lion on your way to a stream to get water. If you could instantly access extreme emotions to yell and scream or run like mad to the nearest cave, it would increase your chances of surviving and ultimately passing along your genes. The higher, slower, more evolved region of the brain – the thinking brain – takes charge when we are in low stress. Whispering sweet nothings into the ear of a potential love partner wins their affection better than the brash and extreme responses wielded by the emotional brain. The abstract thoughts, poetic choices of words, and delicate planning – all functions of this top-down thinking brain – are just what we need to succeed and thrive in that situation.

Brain Areas in Charge

A different brain area is in charge at each level.

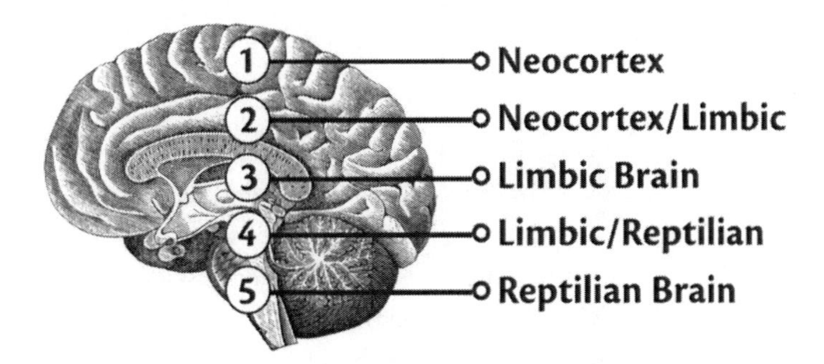

Despite our best intentions, in stress the emotional brain outmuscles the thinking brain, and it happens in a flash. The sensible food plans formulated in a great session with a registered dietitian one day are inaccessible and irrelevant the next day when you are swamped with a work deadline, a child's emotional meltdown, or a splitting headache. Survival drives supplant our best-laid plans.

How do we control our brain state? It's a rude awakening for those who like to be in complete control (everybody?), but to gain control, we must release control. As much as "zoning out" with thinking is a national pastime, the most effective strategy is to assign the thinking brain the task of staying attuned to the emotions and sensations in the body. This is where the activations of the emotional brain express themselves. That attention to emotions is biologically based, as emotions are not primarily psychological but biological. They are the essential substrate for knowing our most important needs and fueling our passion to follow through and meet those needs. Emotions, not thoughts, are our pathway to optimal health and quality of life.

Thinking Brain Effectiveness

Executive functioning varies by stress level. Funtioning falters at levels 3, 4, and 5.

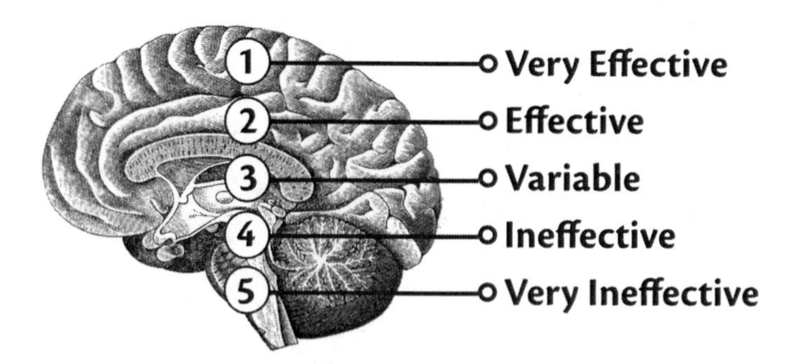

The effectiveness of our beloved thinking brain varies with stress level. This is important because if we rely on cognitive control (positive thinking, mindful awareness, acceptance therapy, or analysis), it works well at low-stress levels, but "drops the ball" in higher stress levels. In higher stress, the thinking brain is not effective, and the emotions activated by stress are much more difficult to process. We will hit a blockade of stressed emotions. The mind shuts off and we relinquish control to the emotional brain, which can use distractions, unhealthy habits, and stressed emotional states to cope.

The fact that the thinking brain functions poorly under stress makes sense based on evolutionary biology when we had to run from a lion. But this becomes a challenge and has negative consequences in modern life. Our human genome evolved when stress was primarily physical, which was much simpler. You either had to fight, flee, or freeze. Who needs the thinking brain to be highly effective in such situations?

However, in modern life most stress is psychological, and any overwhelming experience that is not emotionally processed becomes a liability. Suppressed emotions, expectations, and response drives go unedited by common sense as the thinking brain is on holiday during stress, and then these drives and expectations are stored in the least plastic and most inaccessible areas of the emotional brain. We call these faulty wires "glitches." We are now stuck with them, and they can be reactivated throughout our lives, unless we stress activate them, clear the suppressed emotions, update their ridiculous expectations, and finally update the wires themselves – this is the work of EBT.

We store a large number of these faulty circuits. The key to untangling them is to notice when we are stressed and use that moment of "checking in" as a wake-up call, not to judge ourselves but to process our emotions proactively. Unfortunately, this can become confusing because our approach to our emotions varies by brain state. Let's see how EBT can help with that.

Types of Emotions

A different type of emotion is generated at each level.

Emotions become distorted at levels 3, 4, and 5.

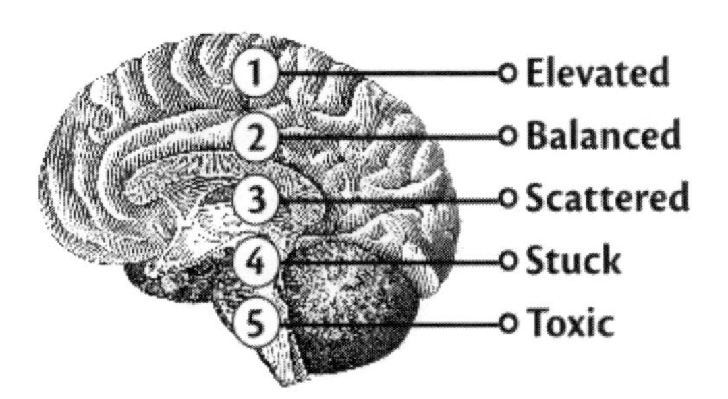

At levels 1 and 2, we can trust our emotions. They tell us what we need. However, in levels 3, 4, and 5, provided the stress is not caused by a physical threat (no lions chasing us), we cannot trust our emotions. They are scattered, stuck, toxic, and really hard to process. Think of them as "smokescreens." We need to clear the air and break down the emotional barriers they create by processing our stress back to level 1 or 2 where we can again trust our emotions to point to our true needs. At levels 3, 4, and 5, we are chronically hungry, fielding cravings, and only satisfied if we can get our hands on sugary, fatty, yummy foods.

At levels 1 and 2, we feel satisfied and are aware of our more subtle needs, like being tired, tense, lonely, sad, or sick, and we can meet those needs without calories. We read our hunger signals accurately, and the brain does not generate biochemically-driven hunger as we have plenty of fat stores and we know that we are really not going to starve.

That shift from trusting our emotions completely in lower stress to recognizing that the emotional messages in higher stress are either unclear or completely haywire because a glitch activated them is essential. Learning when to trust and when not to trust, and also to pause and use EBT to spiral up, can change our functioning and health on the spot. Without that discernment, we might trust those emotions and act on them, with later regret, or become stressed about our stressed state ("secondary stress") and waste time and energy feeling bad.

Part of the EBT training is to recognize when a glitch is activated and take action immediately. Learn to switch off the glitch and reestablish your natural state of joy. Your brain wants you to be in joy, but only you can reach for the EBT app and make it a reality. Emotions do not process themselves. You must do the work.

The EBT Skills

Each type of emotion requires a different processing method.

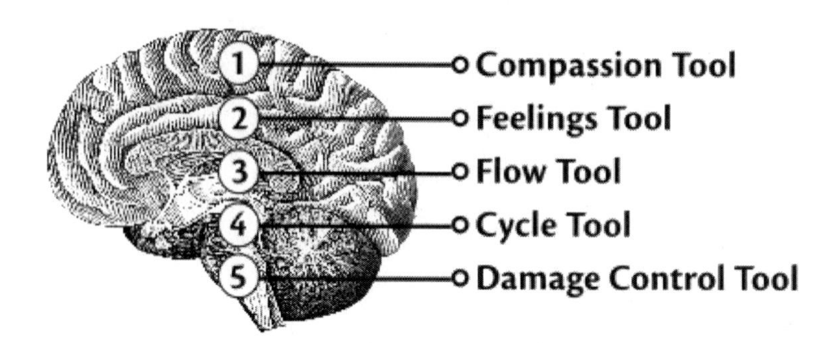

The tools of EBT are designed to respond to the physiological challenges and opportunities at each level of stress. The strategy is to keep the thinking brain online and return it to optimal functioning, then process the emotions and plan a behavior change, ending up at Brain State 1. This set of skills gives us security because we are always in one of five brain states, and there is always a state-specific skill that, in a key-in-lock fashion, raises or enhances our state.

Brain States and Quality of Life

Stress Level	Thoughts	Emotions	Behavior	Relationships	Health
1	Abstract	Elevated	Optimal	Intimate	Excellent
2	Concrete	Balanced	Healthy	Companionable	Good
3	Rigid	Scattered	Moderate	Social	Fair
4	Reactive	Stuck	Unhealthy	Detached/ Needy	Poor
5	Irrational	Toxic	Extremely Unhealthy	Disengaged/ Merged	Very Poor

Emotional skills work quickly! You do not need to worry about being sure you are using the right tool. If one tool doesn't take you to joy, just try another until you get to Brain State 1. Use these skills before eating to make it easier to eat healthy. Use the same tools to rewire the circuits that drive overeating for more lasting results.

With these ideas in mind, the best way to learn EBT is by using it. The next step is to start spiraling up in your daily life and developing an EBT Practice . . .

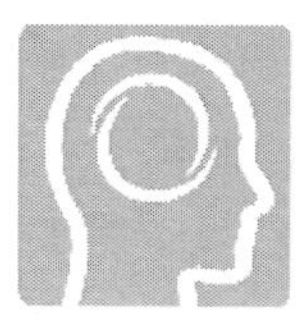

Keep it Simple: Create Joy

The most exciting part of EBT is its simplicity: your brain can create joy. In that "joy state," the neural pathways that promote brilliant choices and healthy drives – including eating and weight loss – spontaneously open up and welcome us to use them. Even better, we are only limited in our greatness by our willingness to use these tools. We can create that joy state anytime, anywhere.

The strategy is to keep creating joy through your EBT Practice until you find that you have freedom from stress eating and easy, natural weight loss. The emphasis in EBT is on "easy and natural" as opposed to thinking brain programs that force change. These cognitive programs often require you to track what you eat. That's necessary because they do not shut off the biochemical drives of the emotional brain.

EBT goes to the source of the problem – circuits in the emotional brain – and switches off these wires. Immediately, the drive can ease, and, over time, can rewire the circuits for lasting results.

You have evidence that you have rewired a circuit when you leave food on your plate – it doesn't interest you anymore. You notice that your pants are getting loose, and although you will celebrate that, most of your attention will go toward your next adventure and making your dreams come true. You have so much more time now because you are relying on your emotional brain to tell you what to eat, when, and why. You can also feel free to overeat now and then, but you do it intentionally as you are now more important than your food or your weight.

It is an exciting time: a new paradigm in weight loss

Being overweight has become a global epidemic, with an economic impact of obesity that could reach $4.32 trillion annually by 2035 if current trends continue. This is equivalent to around three percent of global GDP — or as much as a year of economic growth — the same impact COVID-19 had in 2020.

In the US, over the past two decades, obesity rates have climbed for all population groups. Obesity rates in children have more than tripled since the mid-1970s, and in 2022, 22 states had an adult obesity rate at or above 35 percent, up from 19 states the prior year. Compare this to a decade ago, when no state had an adult obesity rate at or above 35 percent.

With obesity rates so catastrophic and weight-loss drugs and surgery not addressing the root cause of the problem, the brain, the time is perfect for this paradigm change. Training the brain for resilience and optimal natural biochemistry, emotions, thoughts, and behaviors is an idea whose time has come. Give people the power to control their own brain circuits, then add on medications and surgery as needed.

One fall day several years ago, I visited neuroscientist Michael Merzenich in his San Francisco offices to tape a talk for an elective on EBT for medical students. Professor of OB/GYN Patty Robertson, pediatrician Carol Miller, EBT clinical director Lynda Frassetto, and EBT scientific director Igor Mitrovic coordinated the course and presented talks. All the students were in their first year of medical school and learning how to diagnose and treat problems with medications (chemicals) and procedures.

Dr. Merzenich's presentation was brief and to the point. He said that if there is truly a solution to a health problem, it will not be by using chemicals but by training the brain for resilience. He said, "The brain basically has to train itself out of its problems to the best of its ability. Only in that way can the training be complete and natural enough to sustain the benefits to confer strong resilience to any future relapse or problems that will come."

When people rewire their circuits, the chemical impact can be broad-spectrum, more like the health elixir that I remember reading about in second grade — Ponce de Leon, with his tales of sacred, restorative waters — except we are activating the chemicals of homeostasis, the healing elixir that evolved over the eons.

With the new paradigm of empowering people to rewire their own brains and have the potential to enhance their brain's emotional architecture and improve their own chemicals, we can change healthcare. Instead of treating their symptoms, each person can measurably and meaningfully improve their own biochemistry without drugs.

That is sustainable, as there are no side effects except joy, and once the skills are learned, people can use them for life to activate surges of health-promoting chemicals. The chemicals in weight-loss drugs do not treat a biochemical deficiency of glucagon-like-peptide 1 (GLP-1) but use it to sustain potency as an agonist that mimics the natural hormone. Like all artificial chemical treatments, the body responds with downregulation – it will change how the hormone is naturally made and metabolized in the body to return to a more normal level of functioning. When that happens, more of that chemical is needed to have the same impact, and in time, the drug can stop working altogether and/or rewire itself to drive a substitute addiction.

Diane, a patient who was referred to EBT by an endocrinologist, had lost 25 pounds on weight-loss drugs but still felt unhappy and lethargic.

She told me, "I stopped overeating by taking the drug, so the symptom of feeling hungry is better. I still have diarrhea, nausea, and depression, and I've substituted spending and drinking wine for overeating."

Diane's desperation is warranted. How many of us binge night after night, and weight cycle until we are completely exhausted and looking for any way out? That's why using weight-loss medications can offer a bridge for some people. Still, the downsides of the drugs are "wearing out," substitute addictions, missed skills training, and loss of joy.

Our desperation to lose weight has led to the wholesale approval of bariatric surgery, even for the young. In facilitating an EBT program for weight-loss surgery patients who had regained weight they had lost, one participant, Juanita, said, "Surgery changed my stomach, but my stomach was not the problem. If the program didn't change my brain, what's the use?"

These surgeries – gastric bypass, sleeve gastrectomy, and duodenal switch – create anatomical changes in the stomach or small intestine. That impacts appetite, satiety, and a myriad of metabolic chemicals to discourage overeating and weight. However, when the intervention does not address the root cause and is designed to fix something that is not broken, people suffer. There must be a better way. Here it is . . .

The EBT 1-2-3 JOY Program

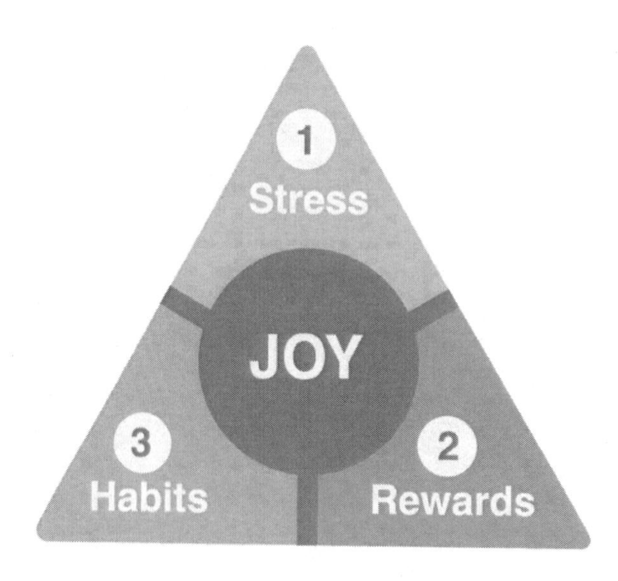

The EBT Program starts with learning how to use the 5-Point System to engage the emotional brain. It's easy and fun, and it works. However, the real value of EBT is the way it gives you power to rewire the past for lasting and profound changes. You can use EBT to rewire the maladaptive pathways (also called Stress Circuits or "glitches") that cause you problems. Select a problem, and rewire it. As they are just wires, you can learn how to use the tools to roust out these circuits and rewire them using the method in more powerful ways. When you do, changes in your behavior will occur spontaneously. The evidence you have rewired a circuit is that the drive stops. It ceases! Your natural response changes effortlessly.

These Stress Circuits impact three brain areas: the amygdala, the nucleus accumbens, and the hypothalamus. The first step is to rewire the amygdala, the stress center, as stress negatively impacts all domains of life. The second step is to boost reward. Finally (and only when doing so is a nurturing act), the third step is to make brain-savvy changes in our eating habits. Behavior change is natural and easier when stress is at bay and we feel fully rewarded, so that food is just food, and we can change what we eat without feeling deprived.

Step 1. Clear Stress

Your amygdala may be a little touchy right now, a bit reactive. This is the area of the brain where Stress Glitches ("threat detection errors") encoded during momentary fight-or-flight responses reside and tell you that you are unsafe. The first step in the program is to rewire the glitches that cause you to perceive stress when there is no real threat. Begin by learning how to zap cravings and create joy anytime, anywhere, then rewire four circuits that drive overeating and weight gain: the Food, Mood, Love, and Body Circuits.

Step 2. Boost Reward

Your nucleus accumbens is the brain area that delivers dopamine based on the salient nature and reward of things. The nucleus accumbens needs a retrofit because there are some Reward Glitches ("reward detection errors") that focus on getting big blasts of dopamine from highly palatable foods and cause us to underappreciate healthy foods that give us normal doses of dopamine. The second step in EBT is to train your brain to find healthy sources of natural pleasure to decrease your reliance on ultra-processed food and make you feel rewarded.

Step 3. Change Habits

The hypothalamus is the habit center of the brain. Once you have cleared stress and boosted your reward, you will be more aware that the way you are eating is making you hungry, lethargic, and obese. The problem is that you have some Habit Glitches ("metabolic adaptation errors"). These glitches have trained your brain and body to store the calories you eat as fat, resulting in missing the energy and optimism you need to live a happy, healthy life. You learn to make a few adjustments in your diet, so you eat real food without any sense of anxiety or deprivation.

Naturally moving through the three steps

All of EBT is arranged to mimic how people change naturally. Over and over again, I have watched participants who forced themselves to diet fail. Then they blamed themselves, gave up trying to control their eating, or used methods that were higher risk and more expensive.

This is why we say, "If it's not fun, it's not EBT." But this is not happiness training. It is a treatment program that is designed to follow the steps that bring more success and better health outcomes. Here is Phoebe's story:

I met Phoebe when she dropped in for a Spiral Up Group I was facilitating. She had lost her husband due to an automobile accident two years before and had buried herself in her work as a preschool teacher. She said that her weight and eating had never been "perfect," but she packed on pounds as she comforted herself with food in the evenings.

Phoebe said, "I am hiding from the world. I know I haven't grieved the death of my husband, but I'm completely stuck. I am a preschool teacher and I love my work, but I need to make a new life for myself. I don't know where to turn, and a friend recommended EBT. She used it and it worked for her."

We mapped out a plan for her to join a weekly premium group so she could make Connections between sessions (five minutes by telephone to use the skills). These Connections assist with more weight loss and better overall improvements in health. She enrolled.

Once she settled in, she worked the program. She showed up at the group, sometimes rushed from a long school conference, sometimes aggravated about a relationship with a friend who was too demanding, and a few times she did Cycles ("spiraled up") about food or weight. She did the coursework and Connections.

Freedom from eating and weight issues

Then, almost a year after she joined the group, I once again called in to facilitate her group. A new member had joined, and I explained the program to her:

"We overeat for three reasons: stress, reward, and hunger. We have bypassed the emotional brain, but it controls our eating and weight. Start by learning to spiral up and clear stress. Next, add more joy to your life but only when you sense that the drive to overeat has switched off and you feel some excitement and joy about releasing weight. Only then will you want to change what you eat because it feels like a nurturing act. Finally, raise the set point of your brain for lasting results. Food and weight stop being issues in your life."

Phoebe spoke up, "Laurel, that's what happened to me."

I asked, "What did you do?"

Phoebe said, somewhat indignantly, "I did just what you told me to do." Then, she said "I spiraled up and cleared stress and rewired the four major circuits: my Food, Mood, Love, and Body Circuits. I was determined to clear them. I really smashed them."

By crushing these four circuits, the set point of the brain goes up and the stress drives fade. The freedom EBT can bring begins . . .

Phoebe went on. "It took me two months to finally clear my Food Circuit, but I did it! Then I cleared my Mood Circuit – overthinking everything – and my Love Circuit – I stopped over-pleasing people. Last, I faced and obliterated my harsh judgments in my Body Circuit. I was relentless. I didn't stop clearing them until the drives were dead. I stopped those drives that had been stressing me out my whole life."

She was clearly jubilant.

Phoebe continued, "Then I started clearing away the emotional clutter about my husband, all the things I "should" have done, and came to peace about that. I started to enjoy releasing extra weight. It was liberating and I found that eating real food – more fat, protein, and fiber – worked for me. It's not a diet. I am free to eat whatever I want, but my body wants healthier foods."

I knew she was on target for success because she had soundly rewired the four major circuits, which is essential. Also, she had developed a habit of learning one new EBT skill each day, so she was completing the program and making Connections with others in the group for a lot of support. All of us have emotional clutter – unprocessed emotions that silently activate stress and cravings – and she had cleared hers.

I asked, "How did that work for you?"

Phoebe said in a calm but proud voice, "I've lost 60 pounds."

Several people in the group gasped. Even the other members who had been in the same group with her for months had no idea she had lost so much weight.

I was surprised as well. In EBT, we don't monitor food and weight because the best predictor of lasting weight loss is to rewire the root cause – the circuits – so eating real food comes naturally.

Phoebe continued, "I stopped wanting the extra food, and the weight has been coming off naturally. I haven't done spiral ups on food and weight during the group for a long time because I rewired those circuits early in the program. They don't bother me anymore. My focus is on creating joy. I've never been happier, healthier, and more at peace. I have a new life."

Phoebe's experience using EBT was markedly different than using drugs, surgery, or diet programs. She stopped struggling. Instead, she focused on connecting with her body and noticing if she was stressed. If she was, she used EBT to return to her natural state of joy.

Changes in her food and weight followed because each time she spiraled up to feel better in the moment, her brain got better. What had seemed like a burden – losing weight – became a blessing, as to resolve her issues with food and weight, she learned skills that would change the trajectory of her life. Instead of living with a brain that triggered her to reach outside herself for ways to feel better, her brain automatically activated drives to find paradise and purpose inside.

Phoebe experienced monumental shifts in her inner life from EBT, just what I have seen thousands of others experience over my 40 years of clinical practice. She not only stopped her suffering caused by disconnecting from herself and connecting with food. Phoebe discovered how to connect to her inherent strength, goodness, and wisdom . . . and find paradise inside for the first time in her life.

How can this be so much fun?

A big surprise for many new members is that EBT is celebratory – we have the power to rewire! – and fun. About 10 years ago, a nurse practitioner was talking about what she liked about EBT. She said, "When I went to therapy, it was so sad and dreary. In EBT, we celebrate our power to rewire the past. We prevail over our circuits. It's a blast!"

The next week, when I called into my Monday evening telegroup, I heard Bonnie, a particularly creative group member say, "This isn't a group. It's a party. We are crushing circuits and gaining freedom!"

The sessions are deep, gritty, exciting, and fun. Every session includes the EBT Provider coaching a volunteer from the group to use the skills to spiral up, first expressing what's bothering them, spiraling up to joy, typically locating an unconscious expectation, and getting an "aha" moment, too.

As the emotional brain has no walls, the brains of the other members in the group catch the joy and the experience of listening changes them, too. Everyone leaves the session feeling inspired and in joy.

The Spiral Up! app

Our new app is user-friendly. We have shaped the tools to respond to the three different needs of participants. You choose option 1, 2, or 3.

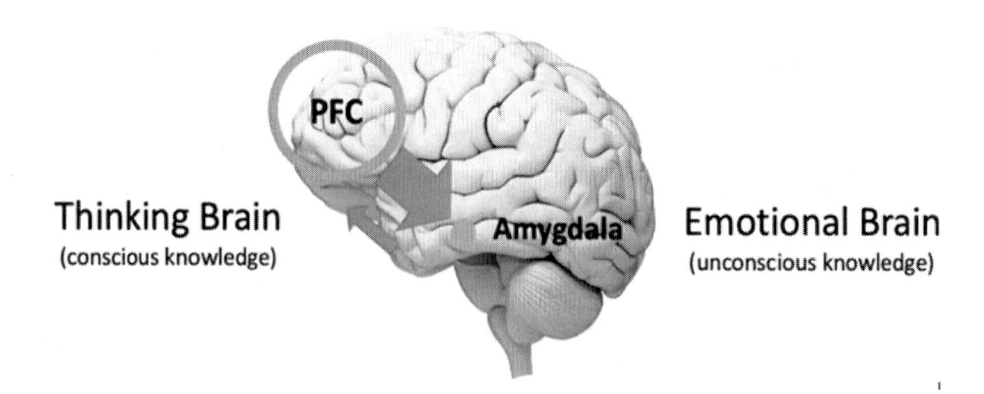

If you want to do something quick, like zap a craving or get an instant boost of joy, select #1, as it only takes a minute or so and is very effective. You can even use it at work, because it does not require that you feel your feelings. It works based on sensations, not emotions.

If you want to feel your feelings and connect a little deeper with yourself, select #2. In about two minutes, you will feel a surge of dopamine and endorphins.

Last, the most satisfying and powerful use of EBT is with precision, switching off and rewiring circuits encoded in trauma. If that is your desire, select #3, for deep work. It takes three minutes or so and targets the circuits that therapists and psychiatrists go after. This pathway essentially delivers neuroscience-based self-therapy.

Your choice: Use EBT solo or in community

You can use EBT quietly and alone with the Spiral Up! mobile app. However, the emotional brain is the social brain, and the work goes deeper in the brain and brings more positive emotions when we use it with another person being a warm presence: a good listener. Research on EBT conducted at the University of Kentucky showed that the number of Connections a participant made in group programs was the best predictor of weight loss.

To access the full program, visit EBT.ORG. Membership includes a mobile app, a video program for learning one new skill each day, and daily, live, drop-in Spiral Up Groups with Certified EBT Providers. Drop in for a weekly, live Zoom webinar, Spiral Up with Dr. Laurel and other Master Trainers for a riveting session. You can start your membership for only $1. After the trial period, continue at whatever service level is right for you until food and weight are no longer issues in your life and you have an abundance of all seven of the higher-order rewards.

We offer daily 30-minute Spiral Up Groups with all memberships for general support. They do not include Connections. The premium weekly groups (30-minute or 60-minute) offer a private EBT Provider, the same eight people to work together, and one-touch Connections between sessions. People love these groups. The average stay in a group is one year, and the private, confidential Connections offering instant support are now averaging eight per week per participant. The groups are a fantastic value.

What if you are a loner, and want to do this on your own? Honor your need and go it alone. In time, you may be curious about groups and Connections, but go at your own pace. Six months ago, Joyce dropped into a Spiral Up Group I was facilitating. She was just listening. Three months ago, I substituted for another provider and facilitated that group again. Joyce volunteered to do a Cycle and did a great job. I asked if she had Connection Buddies among her family members and friends, and she said she did not. Then last week, she joined an intensive daily course.

I asked her, "What happened?"

She said, "I was curious, and ready for more!"

The desire to connect with others in using EBT, whether it is a spouse, family member, or friend – or an EBT group – tends to grow on people.

Welcome to EBT! Enjoy your journey. Tell us how you feel and what you need and keep spiraling up. Day by day, your resiliency pathways will become stronger and fire more automatically. Keep spiraling up and moving through the program, until you have freedom from stress eating, natural, lasting weight loss, and all seven rewards of a purposeful life. Thank you for choosing EBT.

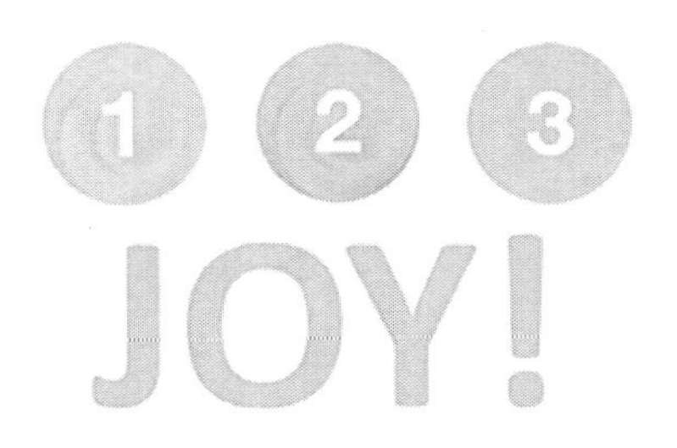

A New Paradigm

1

Where It All Begins: One Misbehaving Wire

After turning the knob of the screen door, I stepped into the kitchen. It was a 1960s kitchen with a lime green Formica table and aluminum-tubed vinyl chairs.

I was home. That day, at age 11, the emotional wind had been knocked out of me. Another girl at school had bullied me right after I found out that I had amassed only three votes in my run for vice president of our 6th-grade class, one of which was mine.

A time of ice cream trucks and simple lives

As a child, I lived in an era of mothers staying home, sewing, and vacuuming. Fathers kept to a 40-hour week, arriving home with a flourish of greetings from children and a sit-down dinner of meat, potatoes, and green beans. Food was structured into three meals with an afterschool snack: a piece of fruit.

Sure, we had treats, but only now and then. A favorite time for my brother Steve and me was when the ice cream truck would travel down our street on summer evenings, the driver ringing a bell and all the neighborhood children flocking to his vehicle. At the sound of the bell, my mother would parcel out 25 cents each to Steve and me, plenty for us to order a rainbow missile or ice cream sandwich.

On this particular afternoon, however, there were no happy flourishes going on. I was devastated, and my emotions were jumbled up. As I look back now, I was at Brain State 5, in hyperarousal with a mixture of shame, self-loathing, and panic. I had no idea what to do with my feelings.

In a perfect world, I would have talked to my mother. I could hear her in the back bedroom vacuuming, but what would I say to her? I was not at a connected Brain State 1 or 2, where

I could express my feelings, but in a full-blown stress response, Brain State 5, where I had no words. I did not know what to do except to burst into tears or fly into a rage, which were not the norm at our house.

Just then, as my world was crashing in on me, I spotted a rectangle of cellophane-covered cinnamon rolls lying on the counter, the kind with thick white icing. Instantly, I grabbed the package, ripped it open, and devoured three. I have no memory of eating them, which is typical of Brain State 5 because in that state we are either numb with no feelings, emotionally very low, or in the rapture of a false high. The next thing I remember was this strange sensation in my fingers. They were sticky from the icing, and I didn't feel just full. I felt stuffed – and scared.

I heard the vacuum cleaner shut off, so I knew my mother would be coming to the kitchen soon and that I had done something wrong.

It was not about me. It was that wire!

Until that moment, food had never been *that* important to me, but starting on that day, my relationship with food shifted because my brain had encoded a Food Circuit to help me deal with the stress I was feeling.

That's how our emotional brains work. The wire I had encoded was a particular kind called a Survival Circuit. In EBT, these are wires we discover and clear during the first three months of the program. These wires hurt us the most because they cause us to abandon ourselves, unplug from our inner wisdom and love, and repeat a self-harming response reflexively.

According to neuroscience, these Survival Circuits are "false associations" between a natural survival drive, like safety (an unconditioned stimulus), and whatever other circuits happen to be activated at the same time, like eating sugary food.

Most learning is associative, small circuits locking together, but what makes these circuits so important to rewire is that they lock together a fight-or-flight drive meant to enable us to escape being eaten by a hungry lion with a response that does not work, and even, instead of saving us, damages us.

Without our permission or awareness, the brain over-remembers that wire because it enabled us to survive a traumatic experience and it automatically tags our response as a keeper. In fact, it stores that faulty wire in the most primitive area of the brain and, to be sure that when it is activated again, it unleashes such a monumental bolt of stress chemicals that it puts our prefrontal cortex (thinking brain) out of commission. That way the wire instantly comes to our rescue and is protected from allowing conscious control to rewire it – until the discovery of EBT.

A new science: Emotional brain literacy

EBT gives us the power to take charge of these circuits, so they stop controlling us. What if we don't know about how the emotional brain operates or what to do about it? What if we do not know how to reframe the lightning bolt of stress chemicals as the activation of a wire? And once reframed, what if we do not know that by using a few simple skills, we could shut off the wire? We would feel out of control, as once activated, we "are" that circuit. After the encoding of my Food Circuit, when it was activated again, I became that 11-year-old who was ashamed, lonely, scared – and hungry – all because of an errant wire (a "glitch"). With EBT, we don't have to live that way anymore. Most overeating is caused by Survival Circuits. Karen, who had weight cycled since high school told me, "I wake up in the morning and tell myself that I am not going to binge eat that day. I am firmly committed to stopping all sugar. Then at around 3:00 p.m., this little 'ping' in my brain goes off, and that's the end of it. I don't care what I 'should' do. I'm going to get that food no matter what. It's like I have no choice. I have to get cookies, candy, or something sweet or I am going to die."

That's why we are a "different person" when in a stressed state. If Karen had seen that "ping" as a physical entity, a wire, she could have heeded the message, processed the toxic emotions, and in a minute or two, been at Brain State 1.

With her thinking brain's filter of "is this reasonable?" she would have laughed and said, "That's ridiculous. I'm not hungry. I don't need that." Even more importantly, by processing her emotions on the spot, she would shut off the biochemical drives to overeat. This procedure – notice the sensation, reframe it as a faulty wire, and use emotions to switch it off – is the ultimate whole-brain solution. That action reinstates her cognitive functioning and causes the biochemical drives to shut off. If Karen learned that one procedure, she would stop weight cycling, cease feeling out of control of her eating, lose weight, and keep it off.

Food wires? They are really easy to identify

The good news for those of us who have food wires is that we have observable evidence of those wires: we overeat. However, many Survival Circuits are harder to pinpoint because that overreaction or unwanted response triggers socially-acceptable maladaptive behaviors like overworking, social media addiction, gambling, and overspending as well as negative moods, difficult relationships, and attitudes toward our bodies.

These wires are particularly damaging to smart, accomplished, thinking-oriented people because they are accustomed to gaining control in any situation. However, these wires do not listen to planning, deciding, and analyzing, so even all the efforts of our thinking brain to stop repeating the pattern fall flat.

The telltale sign of a Survival Circuit activation is our saying to ourselves, often for decades: "Why did I do that?" and, most particularly, "Why do I do what I do when I know I shouldn't do it?" The answer to those questions is: It's a wire. They are "brain glitches" that create a biochemically-driven and exceptionally strong urge to repeat the same response in the future as if our life depended on it.

When I encoded my Food Circuit, I could have reactivated the memory before going to sleep that night, as my hippocampus would have stored it in long-term memory. If I had been able to do that, my brain state would have been higher, and my prefrontal cortex fully capable of spiraling up through my emotions and clearing that glitch. However, this was back in the pre-neuroscience era, when we didn't know people had the power to do that.

Our wires travel with us everywhere we go

I was stuck with this wire, and I mean stuck, as my brain could activate it without my awareness or approval at school, visiting friends, or even sitting in my room alone trying to be calm. If that happened, a charge would appear in my body and cause an authoritative drive that I had to get sugary, fatty, highly-rewarding food – no matter what.

There is no "source attribution" or body sense of a warning sign that a circuit is activated. In the moment, it feels like an immediate threat that is undeniable and overwhelmingly real.

The saddest part of my new situation was that the circuit did not solve my original problem: stress. I was stressed, so I ate, and now, instead of offloading the stress, I got more stressed. It saddled me with a brain-based glitch, a liability, that stressed me more.

I don't mean that I had more psychological stress, but more physiological stress. In normal physiology, creating stress happens when an organism engages extra internal resources to maintain normal function. Every time my Food Circuit was activated, my entire being went into overdrive, both on a subcellular and cellular level, including all my organs and organ systems, all the way up to impacting me as a whole organism.

What type of wire: Spiral Up or Spiral Down?

Stress isn't all bad. Short bursts of stress that allow healing states ("homeostasis") to repair the damage done can actually boost resilience. They spiral us up to a higher brain state. The stressed states tend to become stuck on and chronic ("allostatic"), spiraling us down into chronic stress and amplifying wear and tear to the body.

We become less and less able to bounce back from stressful situations, and our brain adapts by reframing "being stressed out" as our new habit, establishing a default state or set point in stress. At that point, more glitches are encoded, and chronic stress becomes comfortable to us, so our previously natural state of joy feels rather uncomfortable.

Then, even if we win the lottery, our joy would be short-lived because within one to two years the brain's set point in stress would have us recreate misery. Stress is now our safe place, what makes our brain "happy." Stress activates endorphins and dopamine and easily becomes its own addiction.

All I wanted when my Food Circuit was created was to feel better, but I was penalized as I didn't have the skills to access my brain's optimal resiliency pathways, which are emotional, and process my toxic feelings back to joy. I had acquired a faulty circuit that added to my stress, rather than relieving it. I interpreted my drive as a psychological problem (e.g., "emotional overeating") or a character defect (e.g., "no willpower"), as I had no plausible option based on the physiology available to me.

All I knew at that time was that I felt out of control and had sugar cravings that I buckled under. It happened often so my body was laying down extra fat and my legs were blossoming "dimples." I wasn't sure what was happening to me, but I didn't care. I just wanted to eat.

These Survival Circuits alter us chemically. As long as we have them in our brains, we are "chemically affected." They give off a torrent of stress chemicals that drive us and attach us to responses that give a huge wallop of dopamine. When my Food Circuit was activated, sensible activities like reading a book or playing my piano were not on my radar. They wouldn't give me the biochemical fix I needed. Nor would eating an apple, let alone munching on broccoli or carrots.

If I could have found another way to get the strong chemical impact – becoming violent and taking a bat to the furniture in my room, stealing vodka from my parents' liquor cabinet, or finding a way to get drugs from my friends – I probably would have been helped. My parents may have taken me to a therapist who would listen to what was bothering me.

If I had chosen a socially-acceptable way to bypass my toxic feelings, like becoming a super athlete, getting straight "As," or making my appearance perfect, I would have been rewarded for these things, at least initially. Only later would the physiologic stress of the bypass of my emotional brain be apparent, typically showing up as health issues or relationship problems.

The #1 Survival Circuit nationwide: Food

The most common emotional bypass solution is food, and the weight gain that follows. Not only do overeating and holding on to extra weight exacerbate stress, but they will never be a rallying call to help us learn how to process emotions and set limits with ourselves and the world, as standard treatments do not enhance our emotional evolution. Instead, they admonish us to change our behavior to make our bodies stop gaining weight. The wires in our emotional brain do not even come up in the equation, so we do not address the source of our drives.

My weight gain was particularly painful because my family was oriented towards perfect appearance, and my growing pudginess was not only visible but open for discussion. One day, my mother confided in me that Dad had noticed that my knees were fat. Instantly, my mind went blank. I felt like I was no longer safe, even in my own home.

I couldn't escape the wire, as it was activated several times daily, because we all have to eat, and just the thought of food could call up that wire. What would I do when that happened? As I was always bypassing my emotional brain, I developed a "thinking too much" wire and would start thinking about what I was going to eat later, and what I had just eaten, and charting my day based on how "well" I had done with my eating – did I "blow it" or not? This just made my Food Circuit stronger, more dominant, and more damaging to my quality of life. Also, my brain encoded a Body Circuit, a drive to judge my body so I had internalized the original insult that was encoded by my Food Circuit, which was being bullied by a girl at school, and now I was bullying myself.

My mother, who did not have a Food Wire, was worried about me, and suggested a 1200-calorie diet. That was the standard treatment for weight at the time. She even said she'd go on a diet with me, so I agreed. Together we measured food and tracked our program, but my Food Wire had a way of making me creative, and I found ways to get around the system. My mother lost three pounds, and I gained three.

The emotional bypass and those diet rules

In the next year or two, I decided to learn more about nutrition. At the time, food that was low in fat was thought to be healthy. I went through a meringue phase, making cookies on Friday nights when my parents were at parties with their friends. Meringues were a rational choice. Egg whites had only seven calories each, and sugar was low fat, so I whipped up a bowl of five egg whites and a half cup of sugar and spooned puffy white blobs on cookie sheets, baking them until golden. Within an hour, I had eaten them all.

As we had not yet discovered interoceptive awareness (the ability to tune into sensations in our body), I didn't have the genuine emotional skills at that time to connect with my body and accurately read my sensations and emotions. I had no reliable, internal compass for measuring hunger and satiety. I couldn't integrate all the necessary factors – hunger, the meaning of food, how quickly it could deliver what I needed, the stress relief that follows the reward, and most of all, the higher purpose for eating. The only option I had was to go "neocortical" and use my thinking brain to try to figure it out.

I did not know that each of us is five different eaters, a different one in each of our brain states, but the only one that hits the mark of responsiveness is Brain State 1 where we eat for purpose. As I didn't know how to get to Brain State 1, I'd overeat, undereat, or in some other way miss the mark of giving myself what I truly needed. In the other brain states, I'd be apt to use food to meet my emotional survival needs, even though food cannot meet them effectively, which is why I'd continue to overeat.

The other eating drives are pleasure (Brain State 2), comfort (Brain State 3), love (Brain State 4), and safety (Brain State 5). Stress causes tunnel vision. For example, in Brain State 2, it is my job to give myself pleasure in many ways – but in stress, I would instead make a beeline for my Food Circuit, and rather than being satisfied with a subtle high from healthy food, I would need a blast of pleasure chemicals from sugary, fatty foods. One cookie would not do. I would "need" a bunch of them.

The 5 Eating Drives

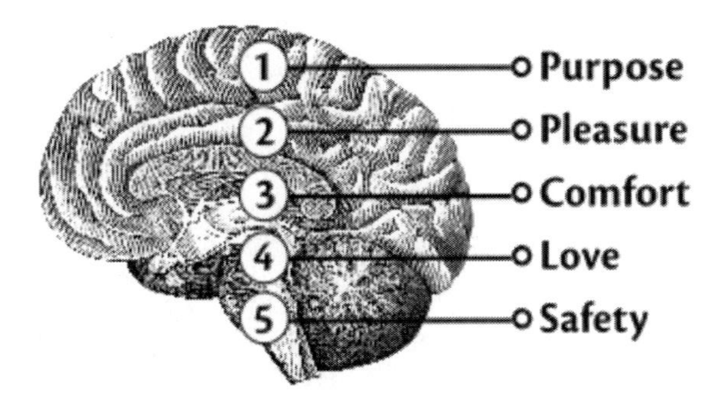

It is always possible to try to take the edge off the need by stuffing myself with artificial food, or food of any kind in extreme amounts. Think of the consequences to my body and brain of loading myself up with food when I am not hungry. I would never put other chemicals in my body, like drinking water when I was not thirsty or draining my father's bottle of Johnny Walker Red Label. However, I thought nothing of ingesting chemicals from food.

Keep it simple: Spiral Up!

All I needed to do was stop suppressing my emotions and use the magical resiliency pathways in my brain to spiral up to Brain State 1, and my problems would be solved. Two things would happen. One, I would not have to go up against fight-or-flight wires to eat healthy and release extra weight. Two, I would be the recipient of surges of beneficial biochemicals activated by purpose. They would further quash my stress by supercharging me to do anything hard with ease, and even joy. However, I was in the stress ditch and did not have the slightest idea how to get out of it.

We all have some of these wires, and they vary in strength and with the nature of the drive. Say a wire is encoded at Brain State 5 where safety is at stake, the drive is the strongest. At Brain State 4, the brain is unable to connect the prefrontal cortex to the emotional brain, so we yearn for connection, to find love. The drive is slightly weaker than Brain State 5. At Brain State 3, all we are looking for is comfort, to have a sense of well-being. At Brain State 2, we feel safe, loved, and comforted, but the brain's reward centers are not activated. The brain is reward-driven, but if our wires point to food as the only suitable pathway to pleasure, we overeat.

Only the Brain State 1 wires bring about truly rational behavior and naturally adaptive choices. In that state, all our primitive needs (pleasure, comfort, love, and safety) are met. The stress chemicals are cleared, and the reward chemicals are flowing. Although we have a scaffold of knowledge about how food impacts us, at Brain State 1 we automatically activate "wise wires." We do not need rigid rules about eating. Instead, we listen to our bodies and are present to our sensations. Each bite is intentional, and the moment we feel satisfied, eating the next bite is not attractive, so we stop. It is not hard, as our response is governed by the unconscious mind, the emotional brain, which is exceedingly convincing.

At Brain State 1, the time warp caused by stress no longer blocks our access to the chemical reward surges activated by a higher purpose. In stress, we do not care about a potential food hangover tomorrow. We just want what we want when we want it, without regard to how it will impact us or others in the longer term. Instead, the reward chemicals activated by the conscious mind from wires of eating for Freedom, Vibrancy, Integrity, or another higher purpose quiet our drives for sugary, fatty, artificial, and self-damaging foods. And these wires of eating for higher purpose continue to be activated and become stronger with repeated experiences.

That natural, internal dopamine surge, in combination with the feeling of being grounded in our body, aware of any sensations of satiety, and a healthy fear of the negative consequences of overeating, gives us the effortless power to eat healthy. We do not obsess about our food, force ourselves to be perfect on our diets, or second-guess what we should have eaten. Food is not an issue in our lives. We are at peace in our relationship with ourselves and food.

I certainly wasn't running a Brain State 1 wire ("1 Circuit"). It was more like a 4 Circuit or, at times when I was binge eating, a 5 Circuit. The wire's message was that I had to have food to feel safety, pleasure, comfort, or love. Because of that, my thinking brain was clear – I *deserved* to have my needs met. I needed that food.

The problem is that when we do not pause and take a minute or two to emotionally process the faulty message from a wire and dismantle it, food has its way with us. We believe the message and act on it. We eat, and we pay the price for our emotional bypass in three ways:

- **Our true needs go unmet** – The most impactful result of an emotional bypass is that our actual need goes unmet. Anesthetizing yourself or somehow canceling out the urgent desire can't meet that need. No donut matches the need for a hug. The more my unmet needs piled up, the more stressed I became, and the more stress triggered my Food Circuit.
- **The brain delivers an afterburn** – We feel bad afterward when we try to meet our true needs with an artificial reward. I felt bad after my Food Circuit was triggered. Our genetic code delivers a "bad feeling" in our body when we do not meet our deepest needs in a key-in-lock fashion. It might be a food hangover, a slight uneasiness, or shame. We could be "food shaming" ourselves. However, the real source of our afterburn is often grieving that the food did not meet our needs, and now, what do we do? We think we know what we are doing, but it does not work. The brain spirals down

with stress-induced negative beliefs such as "there is something wrong with me," "I have no power," or, quite often, "I am bad."

- **The circuit becomes stronger and more vicious** – We continue to let our glitches, those "stupid wires," win. I had activated a glitch, and therefore made it stronger. The wire delivered a fight-or-flight drive to connect to an ineffective substitute: food. Remember that these wires are encoded through no fault of our own, but they disconnect us from our inherent strength, goodness, and wisdom. This is self-sabotage in action. The next time the wire is triggered, it will be stronger, more dominant, and better equipped to disconnect our brain, taking our thinking brain offline, and putting us on autopilot. We become victims of that wire.

As much as following food rules gives us the illusion of safety, all food rules are inherently unresponsive to our needs. Our need is to get to Brain State 1 where we can accurately assess what we truly need.

Without the strategy to put your brain state first, and get to One before eating, all the rules become self-harming. For example, a common rule is to eat when hungry. However, when in stress, it's impossible to know if you need food, because stress disconnects the thinking brain and the emotional brain and only through the pathway of the emotional brain can we read our sensations of hunger and satiety. What's more, the biochemical imbalances of stress activate drives to stress eat, reward eat, and eat because of hunger that is chronic and self-created.

If I continued to let my Food Circuit rule me, it would wipe out my connection to my body. It's only through the connection to our emotional brain, which is optimal at Brain State 1, that we have the necessary interoceptive awareness. Eating mindfully, slowing down our food intake, and being aware of our hunger and satiety is good advice, but nobody can do it when a 5 Circuit is raging.

It is only possible to make the sophisticated calculations needed to decide on the next bite if we can access sensory information. Most of the time, I would have been apt to restrain myself from eating some delectable tidbits I really wanted at the moment, then later let loose with all that pent-up deprivation and binge eat. As one faulty wire activates another, following that I would probably blame the world for tempting me with access to potential high-addiction foods (as if I think it is the world's job to be my internal parent and take care of my food intake). Alternatively, I could shame myself for not having been perfect in my eating and end up feeling stressed out, blocking my joy for hours or days on end.

Small changes matter: The impact of one circuit

Imagine, one bad day at school resulted in one errant "cinnamon roll" circuit that continued to cause me stress and block my joy. Everyone has these glitches, and a problem only arises if we try to change the behavior without addressing the emotional root cause or don't try to rewire them at all. The brain adapts by encoding and strengthening more of these wires, which over time impact our most crucial health index: our set point.

The brain's set point is the brain state it defaults to naturally. We boomerang back to whatever is our most common brain state. The brain is extremely adaptable, so if one has had traumatic events in childhood or stress overload comes in adulthood, the brain adapts by favoring stress. It shrugs and says, "Okay, if we are going to live in stress, I'll just expect it – and even prefer to stay in that state." Although the joy state (Brain State 1) is the physiologically "safe state," our brain always tries to adapt to the hand it is dealt. It lowers the set point based on our most prevalent brain state. Once we are locked into chronic stress, our brain tags that stressed brain state as safe, and sees stress as our new "joy." We become addicted to stress. This is why in the early phases of EBT, joy feels . . . well . . . a little weird, even scary. This experience is normal, and it will pass as you continue your EBT work.

All areas of life take a hit when the set point goes into the stress zone. Our functioning is rooted in physiology, so in stress, our emotions, thoughts, behaviors, spirituality, relationships, creativity, and productivity all go downhill. We may have a particular problem that bothers us, but if our set point is in stress, all domains of life suffer.

What's happening to my set point?

At the time of the encoding of my Food Circuit, my set point was about 2, but soon went down to 3, then 4. That period of time is a blur for me now. However, I do remember feeling increasingly uncomfortable in social situations and so depressed that I became overly attached to my first boyfriend, as if his nurturing would make up for the lack of safety I felt inside. In my freshman year of high school, I did not study at all, and my grades showed it. Given my ongoing emotional bypass, when I stopped underachieving, I switched to overachieving, a pattern that continued, even when I graduated from UC Berkeley in three years.

Brain States and Food

Stress Level	Impulse Control	Hunger Awareness	Decision Making	Motivation to Eat	Relationship with Food
1	Exceptional	Exceptional	Exceptional	Purpose	Very Healthy
2	Good	Good	Good	Pleasure	Healthy
3	Fair	Fair	Fair	Comfort	Moderate
4	Poor	Poor	Poor	Love	Unhealthy
5	Very Poor	Very Poor	Very Poor	Safety	Addictive

However, on any given day I was much more sensitive about my dysfunction with eating than I was to my scholastic achievements. I could not control my eating. It is no wonder, because stress causes our natural resilience to go on holiday. The table below shows how it is easy in Brain State 1 to take charge of eating, but in brain states of stress, impulse control, hunger awareness, decision-making, and motivation to eat all disappear and the set point supports overeating. No wonder I could not snap out of it. My brain wasn't functioning well enough for me to eat healthy, and my relationship with food became even more complicated and dysfunctional.

Although all these functional factors about stress and food are important, the biggest loss to me was in the damaged relationship between my thinking brain (the internal parent) and my emotional brain (the little kid inside me). The thinking brain is the loving parent with reasonable limits and processes the emotions generated by the little kid in the emotional brain. With my stress chemicals surging – cortisol is the "judgment chemical" – I became a really bad parent to myself. The seeds of my discontent were already in place before my Food Wire encoded itself, but now I had real evidence that I was bad – just look at how I ate. This caused my discontent to grow even more.

One wire leads to encoding another

Quite early on, by about age 14 or 15, my brain had encoded other wires. Most of us have four major circuits that cause overeating and block weight loss. Besides the Food Wire, relationship issues can come up and encode a Love Circuit. Often, we find a particular mood that becomes our emotional home base when stressed and then becomes a string of neurons in our brain called a Mood Circuit.

Last, the brain often encodes a damaging way of relating to our body called a Body Circuit. Sometimes, it tells us to be judgmental about or obsessed with our appearance, looking for perfection. Other times, that wire causes us to use body size as armor to protect us against our inner demons or the outside world. I had all four of the major circuits.

My dieting habit quickly transitioned to disordered eating. I vividly remember babysitting for the next-door neighbor one evening. After putting the children to sleep, I went into their TV room and sank into an oversized, overstuffed chair, only to glimpse my reflection in the sliding glass door. I looked so fat! Instantly, I was depressed. And there was no chance I would process my self-damaging feelings, as my emotional bypass was still in full force. Instead, I sprang out of the chair, went to the kitchen, and rummaged through the cupboards until I found a box of chocolate chip cookies, and I ate them all. Then, realizing that I would be found out, I was in a panic. What would my neighbors think of me?

This Food Wire had caused me to become addicted to sugar and judge my body mercilessly. Of course, I sank into depression, because my brain had learned to shut off joy and go straight to negativity. I could not unpack my emotions and connect to the deepest, most loving part of myself, so I was overly dependent on the validation of others. If my neighbor found out that I stole those cookies and judged me, how would I survive?

That one wire had not only lowered my set point and taken a wrecking ball to my relationship with food, but also harmed the most essential aspect of my life: my connection to the deepest part of myself.

No second guessing: It's all perfect

What would have happened if I had known on that day at age 11 how to engage my emotional brain instead of bypassing it? I may have processed my emotions at the time or even reached out to my mother and talked about all my feelings, even the socially unacceptable ones. Instead, I had encoded the wire, started overeating, and then began judging myself. What if I had realized that it was just a wire, and I could rewire it?

I will never know, but I believe the emotional brain takes care of us, and "everything is perfect." The adversity in our life gives us just the pain we need to learn, change, and grow in just the way that makes our life complete. Those 20 years of struggling with my Food Wire, then dismantling it and the various circuits it generated, led me to know and love myself more. Those moments of feeling like it is all over, that there is no hope, but then somehow staying present to our emotions make us empathetic, and ultimately heal us.

At face value, it appears that I "wasted" so much time struggling with food and weight, but most days I see my Food Wire as a blessing. It gave me just what I needed: the empathy and passion to develop EBT.

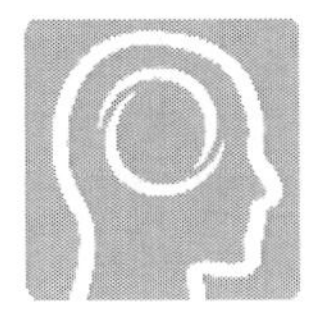

2

From Counting Calories to Collecting Joy Points

It all began because of the generosity of the man who became the first father of EBT, Charles Irwin.

A UCSF professor of pediatrics, Dr. Irwin is an internationally acclaimed leader in adolescent interdisciplinary health. He needed to recruit a nutrition faculty member for his grant, training leaders in adolescent medicine. I happened upon the listing while at my first post-graduate position, teaching education theory to dietitians.

As I was only 28 at the time, the interview process was particularly daunting. It was in the age of women wearing suits with skirts, jackets, silk blouses, and heels to work, and definitely to interviews.

The interview process involved 10 private sessions with big names in medicine, including Melvin Grumbach, whose research discovered the hormonal basis for growth hormone and the hypothalamic-pituitary axis ("HPA Axis"). The HPA Axis includes the hypothalamus and pituitary gland in the emotional brain, as well as the adrenal glands on top of the kidneys. This system controls stress, eating, weight, immune responses, moods, emotions, and just about everything important to our health and quality of life. It is the HPA Axis that is switched off by the skills of EBT.

Dr. Grumbach's office had three-foot-high stacks of journals on every square inch of surface. Growing up, I was always chastised (for good reason) for being messy, so I felt instant affection for this man – and liberated. His massive corner office was even more cluttered than my bedroom. Authenticity, with an underbelly of vulnerability, is inherently attractive to humans.

After completing all the interviews, I heard nothing for weeks. Finally, driven by desperation and sure I had nothing to lose, I called Dr. Irwin. He answered the phone and was friendly and enthusiastic, inviting me back for another interview and, soon after that, giving me the job.

I quickly realized this position was as close to heaven as I could get: an interdisciplinary team at the forefront of a new approach to healthcare. At the time, nutrition was still on the edge of the medical spectrum, the least valued discipline on the team. The grant required the team to have a nutrition faculty member on board, and my role was to give lectures on nutrition and adolescent development. Other than that, it was a time for me to learn. I had already been immersed in developing cognitively-based programs for obesity since my previous position. Now, I could continue that work with the opportunity to learn from brilliant clinicians while conducting research.

It was the late '70s when the idea of group process was new. As the grant was innovative, we did a lot of interesting things – we went together on retreats, sat together in hot tubs, and mapped out how we would change the future of adolescent healthcare. The innovation we were designing centered around the biopsychosocial model of care, the precursor of today's integrative medicine. I learned psychosocial development, family systems theory, research methods, clinical care, and patient management conferencing. I was a virtual sponge for this new information.

Three months into the position, I discovered I was pregnant with my daughter. I had lost my first child seven years before at 29 weeks gestation, when I was warned that I would never be able to carry a baby to term. So, when I had signs of an impending loss of my second pregnancy at three months, I went on bedrest and did so with Dr. Irwin's blessings. He even encouraged me, saying that being a parent would make me a better clinician. I relaxed into my pregnancy, but also kept busy while lying in bed. I propped up a wooden tray on a pillow, centered a Selectric typewriter on it, and wrote my first book.

Chaos in the world of obesity

By the early '80s, two fields that would impact the science of obesity – nutrition science (what we eat) and psychiatry (why we eat) – were in dynamic phases of development. However, in the way they pertain to obesity, they were in chaos.

A group of nutritionists from UC Berkeley postulated that obesity was a "culture-bound syndrome." They were following the "Fat Acceptance Movement," which began in 1967 when 500 people came together in New York City's Central Park to protest bias against fat people. The premise of this organization ("the GRAIN group") was that the cause of obesity was the psychological stress inflicted on obese people because of societal judgment of body size.

At about the same time, interest in how weight takes a toll on women was soaring. Psychotherapist Susie Orbach presented grand rounds at UCSF, a primary lecture at the university, and spoke about her book, *Fat is a Feminist Issue,* which charted the lengths to which women have gone in attempts to appeal to men. I recall sitting in the front row with Marion Nestle, dean of the medical school, my mentor, and a leader in nutrition on the campus. We were soaking in every word she said, as they all rang true. Since then, Marion has chaired the nutrition department at New York University and become one of the original food activists in America, writing about the effects of politics on what we eat and, therefore, on our health.

Both of these movements influenced my thinking about obesity. At the time, cognitive behavioral treatment coupled with nutrition education was the standard of care for obesity, but I sensed that they were not enough.

I was steeped in learning the biopsychosocial and family systems approach for the Adolescent Health Training program and decided to create a computer program that teased apart the many contributors to a particular adolescent's obesity.

The resulting instrument, called the Youth Evaluation Scale (YES), was used widely in the initial EBT Program for children and adolescents and was later adopted by the Canadian Health Department and distributed throughout Canada.

The experience of developing YES helped me understand the importance of specific contributors to obesity: body image, roles from childhood that we play out in adulthood, assessing periods of weight gain to give direction to trauma rewiring, and more. Yet, years later when the logical next step in adapting EBT to the healthcare needs of adults was to develop a YES for adults, I decided to let that go. By then, we understood that we needed to do one thing: help people spiral up so many times that they raise their set point, most problems fade, and they can resolve the ones that remain with grace and ease.

Confusion about the root cause

The calorie counting I learned as a teenager had long since been displaced in clinical care by "behaviorism." The theoretical basis of behavioral therapy is conditioning, and it was practical, but it did not address the emotional or physiological root cause of most problems. The initial weight-loss program I developed mirrored that style, which was to identify maladaptive behaviors and change what triggered them ("antecedents") and followed them ("consequences"). Psychological and physiological factors were not discussed, just behavior.

Although this approach was appealing, the results were disappointing, even when changing thoughts was integrated into a program – Cognitive Behavioral Therapy (CBT). Although CBT remains the standard of care for obesity today, research has shown that it falls short in two ways: 1) it only changes the specific behavior targeted and does not generalize and 2) the change is only short-term. As being overweight for only a few weeks of research cannot predict future morbidity and mortality and the rationale for treating the condition is to promote long-term change, CBT is fundamentally flawed.

Yet CBT remains the standard of care, even though it is 100 percent neo-cortically based, while eating and the emotional brain control weight. When this treatment goes on long enough (treating the wrong brain), It's no wonder that people become desperate enough to seek medications and surgery for quick weight loss. They are miserable, and the healthcare system is not giving them options that alleviate their suffering. What's more, health professionals also pay a price. How stressful to go to work each day and tell 70 percent of your patients to eat less and exercise more, even though you know they won't do it? Then, you manage the health problems that trickle down from their untreated obesity. The current care model is hard on everyone.

Emotions as substrates for resilience

Early on in my training, I thought of emotions as psychological, not as entities that people could process to change their biochemistry. The idea of spiraling up as medicine was three decades away. I began treating adolescents with anorexia nervosa and bulimia in the clinic and eventually co-directed the adolescent eating disorder clinic, so I spent more time at Langley Porter Psychiatric Institute (LPPI). I began looking beyond behavioral treatments, as my early results in using them were mediocre at best. A couple of patients did well, but most did not, and I never did see a patient's face light up with joy because of treatment.

I began looking for a new approach and found myself trying to solve problems by sifting through the stacks of journals in the medical library, reviewing the literature. This was before we used faxes, word processing, or the internet, and still in the age of Xerox machines and microfiche. I was paging through four-inch-thick volumes of *Index Medicus*, the key to the labyrinth of studies published with the validation of proper research methods and appearing in peer-reviewed journals. I was desperate. Then, one day I hit paydirt, discovering a study published in 1942. My first reading gave me hope.

Baylor psychoanalyst Hilde Bruch and her colleague Grace Touraine studied the family systems of 40 obese children. All of them displayed a pattern that did not align with currently accepted thinking on responsive parenting. As parent-child interaction encodes patterns of effective self-regulation and secure attachment, something was missing. Instead of high nurturing and high limits, parenting styles fell short.

In Bruch and Touraine's study, all but one family displayed patterns of both permissiveness and deprivation. Of the remainder, five showed a parenting style of deprivation only, and four of permissiveness only. Deprivation and permissiveness styles are associated with trauma and self-regulatory failure. Children are apt to become wired for stress rather than wired for joy. Their feelings often become allostatic, forming an emotional wall that neither they can tear down, nor others can penetrate. Without the skills to clear those toxic emotions, what do children do? Often, they seek comfort, safety, or love from food. They did not have the skills to nurture themselves or create the boundaries – effective limits – to feel comfortable, safe, and loved.

In my youthful zeal at that time, the application of the research seemed simple enough: create a nurturing skill for emotional processing that both the child and parents can use and a limit-setting skill for parents, so that the children receive both an experience of emotional connection and nurturing and the safety of consistent expectations and limit-setting. Later, these two skills would be integrated into tools to change emotional and behavioral regulation: spiraling up. However, in the beginning, the skills were discrete and very simple.

Piloting the use of emotions as medicine

We began piloting the program at UCSF, and I was cautiously optimistic, but somewhat guarded as more research was needed. Then, one evening, the mother of a 10-year-old girl with brown, curly hair caught up with me in the hall outside my office just before the start of a session. Her daughter had a history of stealing money from her mother's purse to buy sweets and would hide the food under her bed.

The mother was exasperated. She asked, "What is happening? Since starting in this program, my daughter doesn't care about the food anymore. Instead, she wants to go outside and play! I'm very happy about it, but I don't understand."

I had no brain-based scientific answer to her question. I was hooked. I sensed that I would be a "bad person" if I didn't devote myself to discovering why this had occurred for her and how to replicate it so others could experience the same. Although I devoted myself to finding an answer, it would be 30 years before neuroscience research led to the development of Emotional Plasticity Theory, the basis for EBT.

When that happened, further progress occurred rapidly both in obesity treatment and understanding the basis of disordered eating. We conducted a study to investigate the ages at which disordered eating could be observed, with 494 girls in San Francisco, aged nine to 18. We found that by age 10, 80 percent had already been on weight-loss diets.

Another study, funded by the Division of Maternal and Child Health, evaluated the impact of teaching emotional connection tools within a behavioral program to obese adolescents. Based on data collected at five locations in Northern California, these adolescents demonstrated a broad spectrum of improvements in weight, depression, and weight-related behavior at both three-month and one-year follow-ups. The most important observation was that weight loss persisted after treatment ended. This suggested that we might be addressing the root cause.

We also observed that demand was growing for the skills used in the study. Parents of obese children and adolescents were asking, "Why do I have to have an obese child to be eligible to learn these skills?" and, "Do I have to develop a weight problem to be eligible to learn these skills?"

At that point, I could not continue to develop the study method and do justice to my work within Charles Irwin's adolescent health training program. I cut back my hours. A remarkable nutritionist, Lucy Adams, took over most of my responsibilities. For several months I was in limbo, wondering if I should remain with the University and if my choice to focus on this method would sabotage my ability to have a more significant impact on healthcare.

At the same time, Marion Nestle, biologist and nutritionist, received a significant grant that seemed to drop into her lap. A Chinese businessman gave her funding to develop a center for training medical students in nutrition. She hired me part-time. This grant was housed in the Department of Family and Community Medicine, giving me a new academic home that I maintained continuously until I retired from the faculty in 2021. This new position was the bridge I needed to study why these emotional tools had impacted that little girl in the pilot program and to adapt them to treat adult obesity. It was my hope that in time these tools could prevent and treat all stress-related health problems.

The emotional brain bypass – how did it happen?

My new position allowed me to focus on refining new EBT tools to help people feel better and see results faster. At that time, I didn't yet think about how EBT fit into the history of medicine or how it could integrate the work of bench scientists and clinicians on a larger scale.

Until the 20th century, infectious diseases would decimate populations. For example, the 1889-1890 pandemic, often called the Asian flu or Russian flu, killed 0.07 percent of the world's population (by comparison, COVID-19 killed 0.009 percent of the population.) That led to the important development of microbiology and bacteriology and the acceptance of germ theory in 1910. This now provided a biological target and facilitated the use of sterilization techniques and antibiotics for treatment.

People began to live longer, long enough to develop chronic diseases. The focus of medicine turned away from saving lives to managing chronic diseases. However, as there was no biological entity to target, modern medicine evolved to use diagnostic tools, procedures, medications, and devices to manage chronic disease. As a result, we now have over 24,000 drugs, 10,000 diseases, and more than 35,000 laboratory tests. The Diagnostic and Statistical Manual of Mental Health (DSM-5) includes 265 diagnoses. Despite these developments, health in the US is at an all-time low, with crises in chronic disease, healthcare costs, mental health, and life expectancy.

As a young faculty member, I sensed a problem as our behavioral health programs were not working, and we needed therapeutic tools to treat obesity, as it was not a psychiatric disorder. We needed something in between, a more integrated approach. What methods could connect the body and the brain?

Meanwhile, mental health was becoming more divided. In the middle of the 19th century, neurology and psychiatry diverged, splitting the mind and body therapeutically. This led to diminishing the power we have to use the mind to control physiology, as physiology is ultimately controlled by circuits in the emotional brain.

Sigmund Freud theorized that errant pathways in the unconscious mind caused most emotional and behavioral problems, and these patterns were often established early in life. However, brain imaging was not available at the time, so he could not prove his beliefs. Freud then continued to develop psychoanalytic theories and treatments based on free association and analysis of unconscious material through dreams to discover the psychological effects of repression, among others, that were not researchable nor scalable. Currently, neuroscientists use fMRIs to validate these theories.

Behaviorism soon came into favor. The behaviorists offered what seemed like a sensible alternative to dreams and mining the unconscious memory system: change aberrant behaviors by manipulating their antecedents and consequences. The history of this includes the researchers Watson, Pavlov, and Beck. John B. Watson launched behavioral methods in 1913, and research on the behavioral model led to a wide variety of behavioral principles. Ivan Pavlov founded classical conditioning based on the famous experiment in which he observed that dogs naturally salivated when presented with food, an unconditioned stimulus. He repeatedly paired a neutral stimulus, such as a bell, with the food, and the dogs eventually began to associate the bell with the arrival of food. In the 1960s and 1970s, Aaron Beck applied behavioral strategies to cognitive changes, becoming the father of Cognitive Behavioral Therapy (CBT).

CBT has dominated clinical care for the last 60 years, but this approach bypasses the emotional brain. This impairs the ability of therapy to impact our physiology and increases vulnerability to continued stress, particularly with patients who have experienced trauma and the increasing environmental stress overload shared globally.

In the past 10 years, researchers have begun to take notice of this. Candace Raio and colleagues at New York University's Emotional Brain Institute questioned the utility of cognitive control of stress. They wondered if cognitive control was the treatment of choice while epidemics of stress-induced health problems were on the rise and if it was really effective in switching off the stress response.

These researchers designed a study to attempt to answer that question. Study participants were trained in the most effective cognitive treatment – reappraisal – and randomly assigned to test its effectiveness in low or moderate stress levels.

In low stress, cognitive control switched off the stress chemical cortisol, just as they intended. However, for subjects in the moderate stress condition, the technique failed. Cortisol levels initially stayed high and the stressed state was persistent, mirroring just what we all want to avoid: chronic stress.

Cognitive control could not switch off the stress response, but Claire Weekes, an Australian physician, was also working on the same problem and proposed a novel idea. Critical of both the psychoanalytical approach and the attempts by behaviorists to "desensitize behaviors through relaxation and breathing techniques," she proposed that the stress response was a two-step process. The first step was a rapid, subcortical emotional blast, followed by a neocortical processing phase. Her approach was to stop the "secondary stress" of the study participants, proposing that patients were afraid of fear itself and recommending the use of acceptance, being able to feel fear and safety at the same time. Joseph LeDoux, director of NYU's Emotional Brain Institute, also supported this observation. Their theories were consistent with the tools of EBT.

Dr. Weekes' use of acceptance of fear was instrumental in the rise of the contextual approach to behaviorism that began in the 1980s, which involved changing one's relationship to emotions, thoughts, and behaviors. Her work supported the acceptance of mindfulness-based and acceptance-based therapies. This approach has merit, particularly for those with low stress. However, now that stress is ubiquitous, it may not be best suited to negotiating the stress of modern life. Based on clinical reports from mindfulness instructors, acceptance may take 30 minutes or more to shut off stress when it is high. Based on evolution, emotions are designed to process stress more rapidly than cognitive control. Also, once stress overload becomes locked in, chronic stress and its markers may be more challenging to treat.

EBT was designed to integrate stress science into clinical methods and has been refined to minimize the amount of time needed to turn off stress. There have also been a number of studies done to verify the efficacy of EBT. One study of EBT participants was conducted, showing that the average time to switch off the stress response using EBT tools was 2.68 minutes. In addition, a University of Kentucky researcher, Kelly Webber, conducted a trial comparing EBT to an acceptance-based method (intuitive eating) in obese adults. All of the physiologic-based variables – weight loss, systolic blood pressure, diastolic blood pressure, perceived stress, and food addiction – showed statistically significant improvements for the EBT group. In contrast, none of them showed significant improvement with the acceptance-based method.

Viewing stress in an entirely new way

Stress research is slow and tedious. However, between 1990 and 2010, five breakthroughs in neuroscience were brewing that would change how we think about stress. As stress is the underlying predictor of health, this also influences how we think about healthcare.

Peter Sterling, a neuroscientist from the University of Pennsylvania, made the first of these breakthroughs. Before his work, only homeostasis was recognized in physiology. Homeostasis is the process of remaining stable (*homeo*) by staying the same (*stasis*) and is a self-correcting, negative feedback loop promoting health. In his book, *What Is Health?* Peter Sterling defines health as homeostasis because it activates "the control systems optimized over billions of years" to promote health.

However, Dr. Sterling's greatest contribution to science occurred in 1981, while studying the slums in Cleveland after the 1966 riots. This historical phenomenon caused significant episodes of stress overload that impacted the entire community, resulting in high rates of strokes and other stress-related diseases. These findings led him to promote the concept of allostasis, defined as creating change in the body to adapt to a new environment while maintaining the same level of function. This compromises our physiology and damages our health as it causes metabolic adaptation errors, a change in the way our body uses energy. His work resulted in ending the separation of mind and body as it relates to physiologic health, as this allostatic overload state creates a "positive feedback loop" between the brain and body that has no "shut-off valve." Dr. Sterling, along with other researchers, then went on to prove that every cell of the body is biologically connected to the brain. What happens psychologically in the mind appears in the body, and what shows up in the body feeds back on the brain, impacting our psychology.

The second breakthrough in neuroscience came from the research of Bruce McEwen of Rockefeller University, who coined the term allostatic load (the wear and tear on the body and brain). In the graphic below, he shows the many factors contributing to the perceived threat and physiologic response of allostasis. For each episode of allostasis, there is a price to pay – the encoding and strengthening of faulty circuits and the allostatic load, which becomes the principal source of stress over time.

Dr. McEwen's work has been applied to EBT, as the method is aimed at reversing allostatic load. There is an age-related decline in our physiologic reserve, or how well our organs can bounce back from illnesses and manage to keep us alive. The bigger the load of Stress Circuits we have (dominance of allostatic wires and emotional clutter compared to homeostatic wires) and wear and tear from episodes of stress, the greater the chance we have of disease and death. Allostatic load is the overriding physiologic indicator of health.

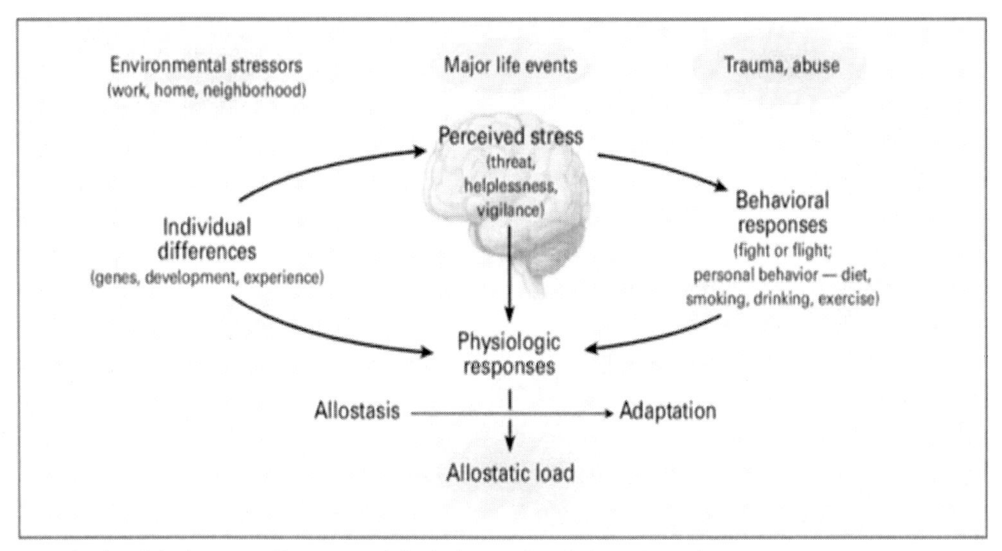

Central role of the brain in allostasis and the behavioral and physiological response to stressors. McEwen, B.S. (1998) *New England Journal of Medicine*, 338, 171–179.

Wear and tear is hard to reverse. If we are able to go to the source, which is the circuits that either prevent stress overload (homeostatic) or promote and exacerbate it (allostatic), we have a more direct route to controlling our health and quality of life. Preventing the encoding of allostatic circuits ("glitches") and rewiring those that the brain has already stored is the conceptual basis for EBT, which aims to reverse allostatic load and achieve our optimal set point: One.

As eradicating allostatic circuits to raise the set point is the strategy of EBT, the method requires a way to weaken and erase these wires. This requires reliance on neuroplasticity, the changing of neural networks in response to the environment, which is the third neuroscience breakthrough.

In 1949, neuroplasticity was propelled forward when Donald Hebb, a Canadian psychologist, proposed the Hebbian theory that changes in the brain are use-dependent and neurons that fire simultaneously strengthen the synaptic connection between them. This is also called use-dependent plasticity. Hebb's rule, "neurons that fire together, wire together," remains a core principle of neuroplasticity.

His breakthrough, however, did not stimulate widespread interest at the time, as the widely-held belief was that adults' brains were fixed, immutable, and no longer capable of changing. Neuroplasticity was thought to occur only in children.

Neuroscientist Michael Merzenich was not convinced. He had conducted research on adult monkeys in his postdoctoral studies at the University of Wisconsin-Madison that suggested their brains could still change. In 1971, at UCSF, he reconnected with one of his postdoctoral associates, Jon Kaas of Vanderbilt University, who was experimenting with owl monkeys. Together, they tested whether the brains of adult monkeys changed with experience. They cut a nerve in one of the monkeys' hands, leaving them with no feeling on the thumb side. The researchers knew that if the monkeys' brains were hardwired and not changed by experience, soon there would be a "black hole" in their brains where they used to receive input via the severed thumb-to-brain nerve.

There was no black hole when they examined the monkeys' brains several months later. The brain area lit up with activity and had already found a new calling – processing the input from the pinky finger side instead.

Their research showed that use-dependent neuroplasticity was possible in adult monkeys, which recruited other scientists to join in. By the end of the century, the plasticity of the adult human brain was widely accepted.

Then, in the early part of 2000, a book entitled *A General Theory of Love* was published, describing a new science of human emotions and biological psychiatry, understanding emotional disorders based on the biological function of the nervous system. It was written by three UCSF psychiatrists, Fari Amini, Richard Lannon, and Thomas Lewis, and proposed that nervous systems are affected by those closest to us and synchronize with them. They maintained that the various forms of psychotherapy are effective to the degree to which the therapist is able to emotionally connect to the patient and modify their wiring (through "limbic revision").

Already, several studies had been conducted on EBT that showed promising long-term results. I thought perhaps this was the underlying mechanism for its effectiveness that we had been searching for. We were relying on both self-attunement and regulation (spiraling up solo) and dyadic attunement and regulation (spiraling up with a provider and with peers). The method seemed to be applying the neuroplasticity approach described in this new book.

I read the book on a plane trip from New York to San Francisco. More than excited, I immediately bundled up a copy of my first book, the research on EBT, and sent it to all three authors. I told them their work helped me think about the method in a new way.

For three weeks, I heard nothing. Then, early one evening, moments after a group I was facilitating concluded, the phone rang. It was Fari Amini.

The first thing he said was, "Where do you live?"

I told him my address.

He said, "You could live anywhere in the world, but you live one mile from me, and you have discovered a public health way to rewire the limbic brain."

Although we knew that the brain could change and we could target circuits, we did not know if memories could be erased. The fourth breakthrough in neuroscience came from a study published by NYU researchers in 2010 that compared methods of erasing fear memories. They encoded a fear memory in participants and then used standard accepted techniques to extinguish it. The variable in this study was whether the memory had been stress activated prior to being extinguished. If it was not stress activated, the memory returned at two follow-up evaluations: three days and one year later.

This finding was consistent with a large body of literature that supported the need to return to the same level of stress that was present when the memory was encoded. This makes the synaptic connections between neurons fluid. That fluidity supports reconsolidation, or the updating and rewiring, of the circuit, which allows the replacement of the previous version of the wire with a homeostatic one.

To rewire memories requires stress activating them first, followed by the process of keeping the thinking brain online through the strong allostatic emotions, long enough to present the brain with an opposing experience, which updates the wire. In EBT, this is accomplished by seeing stress as a good thing, as it is a "moment of opportunity" to rewire and to use "Precision EBT," specific techniques that do the deep work to rewire trauma.

Gaining more time for research

Throughout all these neuroscience breakthroughs, I continued developing EBT. Although challenging at times, we had the wind at our back, including support from Oprah Winfrey. I was in New York City at a conference when I received a phone call from one of her producers inviting me to fly to her studio in Chicago and do a live program the next day. A quote of mine had somehow landed on her desk, which gave EBT new momentum.

Oprah invited me to be a guest three times, but the second time was the most memorable when she held up my first book to her audience of 20 million and said, "This is The Solution."

Her support gave the EBT clinical and research teams new resources to dig deeper into the potential power of the skills. We were learning that the reptilian brain is adept at finding ways to sabotage high-octane resilience. Rousting them out and fine-tuning the method to outsmart the reptile has taken 10 years. To this day, I thank Oprah for allowing us that extra support so we could research rewiring trauma to make it something people now do as part of their daily lives.

The third program Oprah produced that featured EBT, then called The Solution, publicized *The Pathway*, my book that applied EBT to the common excesses of modern life. It became a bestseller that led to a massive breakthrough for EBT in ways that supported the scientific merit of the method.

A chance announcement made the difference

An advertisement about *The Pathway* found its way to the desk of Dr. Marta Margeta, a UCSF scientist. She was worried about her husband, Dr. Igor Mitrovic, a neuroscientist and physiologist, and also a UCSF Professor. He was stressed. It was showing up in his relationship with his son, and Dr. Margeta bought my book as a birthday present for him. When it arrived, he was so stressed that she gave it to him immediately, noting, "The author is on the faculty at UCSF."

Dr. Mitrovic read the book and tried spiraling up, and to his surprise, it worked. Immediately, he joined an EBT group and began moving through the courses. Once he was settled in his weekly group, he picked up the phone and contacted me.

We chatted for several minutes, then Dr. Mitrovic asked, "How did you figure this out?"

I laughed and said, "That's a long story," as discovering that process had taken 25 years of research. Besides, we would have plenty of time to discuss it because we immediately struck up a friendship and began collaborating.

With Igor's expertise in both physiology and neuroscience and his being an active participant in the groups, he brought the method to the next level of rigor. His research is the fifth scientific breakthrough of neuroscience and made the other four applicable to healthcare, as well as self-care.

His work gave us a new "germ" – a biological target for treating stress-induced health problems – because he proposed a connection between brain circuits and physiologic brain states. To overcome infectious diseases, we must target the germs responsible for them. To overcome diseases of chronic stress, we must target allostatic circuits. We can now bring psychology and medicine together with a new biological basis, with EBT providing a neural basis for both.

Igor's biggest scientific contribution occurred in April 2007. We had been teaching a course on EBT to medical students for several years, and one night Igor gave a lecture on EBT and reward pathways. I listened to him map out how joy wasn't optional, that taking back the reward centers of the brain hijacked by stress required access to elevated emotional states, commonly referred to in neuroscience as joy.

The next morning, I woke at 4 a.m., in mourning as my mother, who had a long history of respiratory problems and repeated episodes of intubation in our local hospital, was failing. The room was cold. I felt bone-chillingly alone and depressed, and I reflexively started using the EBT tools. Shockingly, they did not work. I realized I was in the trauma range, a full-blown stress response.

With memories from Igor's talk the previous evening still activating and awareness of how the stress tools that I was using were not enough, I had a realization.

The brain's emotional resiliency pathways did not amount to a three-point system, the model we were using at the time. It was a five-point system. The goal of the entire process must be joy, and it needed a stress overload trauma state. The EBT 5-Point System of Emotional and Behavioral Regulation was born.

A couple of days later, Igor Mitrovic met in his office with Lynda Frassetto and Lindsey Fish, two of the four originators of the method, to talk about conducting further research. Igor was frustrated as he was still trying to figure out why EBT worked. He used EBT personally, so he knew the "body feel" and physiologic changes that occur by spiraling up, but he needed to integrate it with neuroscience and physiology. Suddenly, he had a flash of insight. He said, "EBT is rewiring the stress response!" Immediately, he began drawing on his whiteboard.

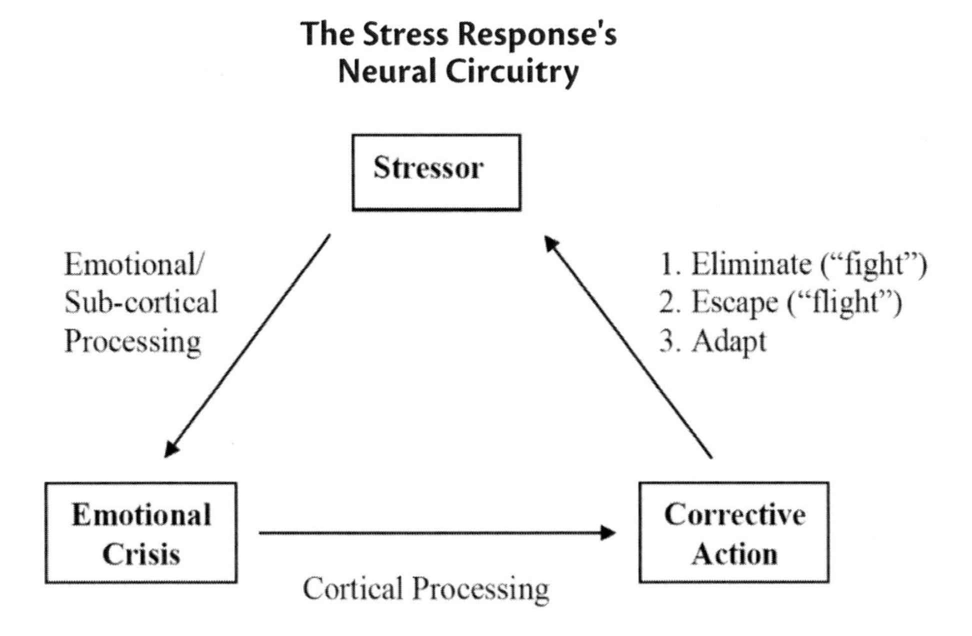

Fish, L., Mellin, L., Mitrovic, I, (2008) Developmental Skills Training: The Neurobiology of Brain Retraining for Promotion of Adaptive Behaviors and State of Well-Being. *Institute for Health Solutions.*

First, he drew a pristine isosceles triangle like the one above on the board. He explained that there are three stages to the stress response: the emotional crisis, which is followed by cognitive processing to identify how to respond to the stressor, and finally, the corrective action or behavior. In essence, the three stages involve a rapid emotional reaction, after which unconscious expectations drive biochemical surges to make a corrective action that decreases stress and promotes reward. The three stages are emotions, expectations, and responses.

That "pristine" triangle represented the stress response in homeostasis: balanced, self-correcting, and health-promoting. Then he erased the pristine triangle and drew one that amounted to a scribble of lines of disparate sizes becoming more and more extreme and out of control. The "loony" triangle represented allostasis: unbalanced, with no "shut-off valves," and health-damaging.

A New Paradigm in Healthcare

These two discoveries – the connection between wires and brain states and the elucidation of the five resiliency pathways in the emotional brain – enabled us to apply all the other scientific breakthroughs in a scalable method. Psychotherapy was effective perhaps because of the emotional connection and neural revision orchestrated by the provider's own emotional resilience.

With the 5-Point System codifying optimal resiliency pathways, therapy could be more scalable, and extended for use in peer support and the connection with a provider who was not necessarily conducting "psychotherapy," but correcting the errant resiliency process encoded early in life and using the same resiliency process with more emotional acuity and repetition to rewire faulty pathways. As the target was not just any memories but the circuits that control human physiology, we could use the power of the prefrontal cortex to direct the precise formulation of emotional processing needed to rewire the faulty pathways that Freud originally proposed as the cause of emotional and behavioral problems.

The difference now was that the intervention was codified and simplified based on the tools I initially taught children. The process lent itself to what the brain needed when rewiring primitive circuits, something people could learn to do the same way repeatedly, so that when stress was activated, and their thinking brain was compromised, they could always rely on the same process. The same tools are applied for self-regulation, and for reconsolidation, activating the health-damaging pathway and cajoling it by using the same optimal resiliency procedure into a health-promoting pathway.

We began to disseminate the method through books and our portal, and in 2011, Igor Mitrovic, Lynda Frassetto, Lindsey Fish, and I co-authored a paper entitled "Rewiring the Stress Response: A New Paradigm in Healthcare." We proposed that the new "germ" or biological target for healthcare was the allostatic circuit. The self-regulatory tools of the 5-Point System produced both optimal self-regulation, going beyond cognitive, mindfulness, and awareness methods, and for rewiring, as positive neuroplasticity occurs with each switch from allostatic to homeostatic wires, from stress to joy.

What began as struggling with a Food Circuit of my own, for which my mother had guided me to count calories, was now a neuroscientific method. For the treatment of obesity, we would no longer be forcing behavior change. Instead, we would go to the modifiable source of the problem: our wires. Instead of asking ourselves to go up against the fight-or-flight response and win, we targeted the source of the biochemical drives, using the skills in an effort to shut them off. Behavior change could become easier and more lasting. The treatment of obesity was now physiologically based. Instead of counting calories, setting doses for injections, or recording medication use, we would count how many times we spiraled up from stress to joy. We would collect Joy Points.

However excited we were, we were far from done. It would take us more than a decade to fine-tune the skills for real-world circumstances, such as being triggered at the supermarket, using the method while at work, and using EBT for couples counseling. We needed a way to make rewiring trauma circuits simple and fun and to expand the use of Joy Points to fit individual preferences, such as sensory pleasure, happy memories, or even bringing up a nurturing inner voice.

In 2022, I integrated all these refinements into "The 23 Steps of Resiliency" and a process of using EBT in counseling called "The Resiliency Pathway." This made it easier for a broad range of interdisciplinary providers to replicate optimal resilience training and rewiring.

For decades, I sensed that EBT needed that next level of precision, so I focused on research rather than dissemination. However, the improvements appeared to have an impact. Participants embraced the more precise techniques, and I saw astonishing results in the groups I facilitated. The turning point for me was when one participant, Mary Sue, used Precision EBT to break her Food Circuit.

What bothered Mary Sue the most was that she couldn't stop her after dinner eating, a circuit that had been encoded when she was eight years old. She was the oldest of four children, and given the chaos in her parents' marriage, she not only did not receive nurturing, but the limits set for her were harsh. She had to shop for the family and attend to the needs of her siblings. Mary Sue enrolled in a daily intensive group, determined to clear her Food Circuit.

She used the Spiral Up #3, which is designed for the most important wires, the trauma circuits, specifically, the Stop A Trigger Tool. The challenge in coaching her through the process was that her evening eating was caused by a 5 Circuit, the best kind. The emotional brain tries to sabotage each of the 23 steps. Each time that she veered away from using the tools "precisely," I gently guided her back to staying on her brain's optimal resiliency pathway.

Finally, she discovered her circuit – and was rather stunned.

The words were: "I get my love from having food in my mouth." Finding the precise words took three tries, but finally, she generated these words, and they rang true. Finding the words that match the unconscious mind's message is essential for "breaking" the circuit.

I asked Mary Sue if saying those words made her feel nauseated (also called the "ick factor"). This is the sign the words express the message of the 5 Circuit.

She said, "Absolutely."

During the group session the next day, Mary Sue updated the group about her progress.

She was in awe, and said, "Last night after dinner, I did not eat. I had no desire. It was like there was nothing to plug into. The desire was just gone. It was at first kind of shocking, then it felt great."

At the next day's session, the spontaneous change in her behavior persisted.

She said, "The changes in my eating held. I must have crushed the circuit."

I asked, "What's that like for you?"

She said, "I feel kind of like an explorer in a new land. At lunch yesterday, I was hungry, and the thought that came into my mind was: 'a deviled egg would be good.' That's completely out of character for me."

Mary Sue had "broken" her circuit. Often after discovering the wire, it takes more rewiring to clear the circuit. We are dealing with the complex and multilayered unconscious mind, and just need to keep using the tools until the unwanted drive vanishes. However, the formula appears to give people far more leverage in rewiring, as by staying with the precise use of the skills, often participants "hit" the wire and see changes immediately.

I was jubilant because of what she said next, which was: "I feel at peace with food and with myself."

Despite all this progress, we still had one more scientific breakthrough to integrate into EBT. This last one provides a more complete framework for why we overeat and how to overcome it, what came to be called the "Stress Triangle."

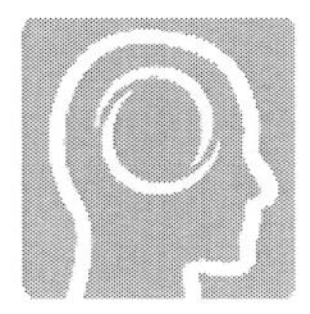

3

The Emotional Brain: The Grand Controller of Eating and Weight

Jessica was happily married and loved her job as a project manager for a small tech company. She had majored in chemistry in college, later taught herself to program, and then landed a job in tech using her analytical talents.

Then she became a mother. Now juggling work and parenting a rambunctious seven-year-old son with special needs and identical twin daughters aged four, she was stressed.

I asked Jessica what brought her to EBT.

She said, "I'm 35 pounds overweight, and I have prediabetes. I need to get my eating under control, and I need to lose weight. I'm not sure how processing emotions can help."

I said, "Moving through your emotions is biologically determined to be the most effective way to clear stress."

Jessica said, "What do you mean 'moving through your emotions?'"

I said, "When we are stressed, emotions become blocked ('allostatic'). The drive to fight, flee, or freeze takes over. The chemicals that drive overeating are persistently activated. EBT is an innovative skill set for breaking through that emotional blockade and turning blocked emotions into flowing ('homeostatic') feelings that take you from stress to joy and switch off the stress response. That can alter the chemicals that control eating and weight: specifically, insulin, cortisol, and dopamine."

Jessica stated matter-of-factly, "That sounds good. I like that."

I said, "It's natural and available to all people. There are no drugs that can hit all three of these chemicals without causing addiction or serious side effects."

She asked, "I can't imagine how emotions impact chemicals."

"The missing link is circuits. Circuits activate the Stress Triangle, which is beyond our conscious control and impacts all three."

She asked, "How do you control something that is not conscious?"

"Emotions. The center of unconscious memories is in the emotional brain. That brain does not respond to thoughts, as when it is activated, the thinking brain is so toxified by stress that It's almost impossible to stay aware of your feelings. If you use your emotions effectively throughout the day, healing chemicals flow."

Jessica was a good candidate for EBT because she was analytical and disciplined. She would need to expand her capacity to process her emotions and become quite analytical about the circuits in her emotional brain.

She said, "I don't have time to do that. I have three kids, so I'm way outnumbered."

I said, "You are always in control. On the app, you touch 1, 2, or 3, so you control how you use it. If you have no time, touch on #1, as it only takes about a minute. Also, use #1 to ease hunger and zap cravings before each meal or snack."

"So, it will help me in my daily life?"

"Yes."

Jessica responded, "I like that."

I said, "It does take a behavior change."

She responded, "I thought this wasn't a diet program."

"The behavior change is to take your joy seriously. If you are not in joy, reach for the app and spiral up. Get your joy back. That shuts off the Stress Triangle."

Jessica said, "I don't want to be happy all the time. My life is full of intense work and heavy-duty mothering."

"Joy is not happiness. It's far more than that. It's a supreme connection to the deepest part of yourself."

Jessica said, "So if you feel joy, you know you've changed yourself chemically. Okay, I like that."

Going to the root cause

Targeting the Stress Triangle makes sense. Currently, more than 100 factors contributing to obesity have been documented. How do you intervene with that many factors? That's enough to make anyone say, "Okay, I give up!"

Scientists are reductionists. They investigate the smallest aspects of a problem to assemble a bigger picture over time. However, that approach may have caused researchers to miss the forest for the trees.

That was not the case for A. Janet Tomiyama, PhD, professor of psychology and director of the Dieting, Stress, and Health (DiSH) lab at the University of California, Los Angeles. She authored a review of obesity and stress in *the Annual Review of Psychology*, documenting the multiple pathways that connect stress and obesity and the failure of both weight loss and dietary strategies to produce lasting results. Dr. Tomiyama concluded, "The most logical intervention target would be stress itself."

As the grand controller of physiology, as well as eating and weight, is the emotional brain, the stress brain, we stand a better chance of interventional success by targeting that grand controller rather than chasing after 100+ causes of the problem.

The question is, how do you accomplish that? My UCSF collaborators, Igor Mitrovic, Lynda Frassetto, Lindsey Fish, and I had already developed a conceptual basis for EBT of rewiring the stress response by using the concepts of neurophysiology and neuroplasticity. However, with my children now raised, I had time to finish a health psychology doctorate, giving me five years to piece together the research to support the theory. Already, 12 studies had supported the method's efficacy and my dissertation added another.

The timing could not have been better. As a young faculty member in Charles Irwin's adolescent health training program, I enrolled in the UCSF health psychology doctoral program, something I could handle alongside my faculty job. I was 33, only to discover that I was expecting my son Joe. Given my high-risk pregnancy history, I withdrew from the program. As an example of the perfection of the emotional brain that provides us with just what we need when we need it, even if it is not what we want, had I not been pregnant, EBT would not have been born. I would have completed my dissertation before the decade of the emotional brain and would have been drawn to stay with the pre-neuroscience paradigm. As it turned out, during my doctoral studies 30 years later, the literature was flooded with groundbreaking studies on the plasticity of the emotional brain, giving me more evidence of the perfection of the brain – and life.

In the early days of EBT becoming brain based, we did not establish a theory. We just applied the sciences of neuroplasticity and neurophysiology. However, my doctoral studies were in health psychology, and psychology is based on theory. I reached out to my collaborators as we needed to construct a theory for EBT. So, Drs. Mitrovic, Frassetto, and I huddled in Igor's office one afternoon. As per usual, medical students kept knocking on his office door, seeking his nurturing and advice. (For more information, see Dr. Mitrovic's Last Lecture: *UCSF Neurobiologist Shares Personal Journey, Life Lessons* in which he shares his EBT experience and his need to love and inspire.)

We rapidly mapped out the science-based postulates of Emotional Plasticity Theory. They are: 1) all living beings have survival drives; 2) emotional memory evolved to improve survival; 3) emotional memories can be adaptive or maladaptive; and 4) positive plasticity of emotional memories improves health.

These postulates gave us a framework as by optimizing overall physiology, we stand a better chance of hitting more of the 100+ causes of obesity by using emotional plasticity to change their biochemical and electrical core. Still, we sensed that something was missing to deliver a more hand-in-glove treatment for overeating and obesity, and I believe Robert Lustig and Michele Meitus-Snyder have identified it.

In their 2008 article *Childhood Obesity: Adrift in the Limbic Triangle*, they proposed a new way to think about the complex chemical cascade orchestrated by three primitive structures in the emotional brain. Their focus was to impact childhood obesity more effectively. It was through my early work with pediatric obesity and my later work at the UCSF Center for Health and Community that I had a connection with them. A few years after I transitioned to the Department of Family and Community Medicine, putting my pediatric obesity work on hold to focus on adult applications of EBT, Dr. Lustig, a pediatric endocrinologist, developed a new pediatric obesity clinic at UCSF.

This contribution came to public attention when one of Dr. Lustig's medical lectures, *Sugar: The Bitter Truth*, went viral. Since then, he has continued to become an international authority on metabolic health and a champion for eating real food. His books on obesity (*Fat Chance*) and metabolic disease (*Metabolica*) include many relevant details that are beyond the scope of this book and serve as sound resources.

Dr. Meitus-Snyder is a pediatric cardiologist, and we were officemates for a year at the Center for Health and Community at UCSF. Not long after that, she affiliated with Children's National Hospital in Washington, DC, and she is still a co-investigator on long-standing bicoastal research with colleagues at the UC Benioff Children's Hospital.

What they outlined in their original review was how, in a stressed world with an endless supply of sugary, fatty treats, this limbic triangle of primitive brain structures spews biochemicals, fueling overeating and weight gain that our hunter-gatherer brain is not designed to deal with. Our genetic makeup guards against weight loss, but "throws care to the wind" when it comes to shutting off weight gain. When activated by stress, the impact of this triangle is so debilitating that the scientists used the metaphor of the Bermuda Triangle to describe it. As you may know, this is a region in the western part of the Atlantic Ocean where aircraft and ships are said to have disappeared under mysterious circumstances, and according to Drs. Lustig and Meitus-Snyder:

> "It should not be surprising that dieting alone
> results in almost universal recidivism.
> In other words, once you enter the limbic triangle,
> it is virtually impossible to get out unassisted."

It's a new world: switch off the triangle

Once we recognize that these drives are biochemical, trying to lose weight or eat healthy with that spigot of disempowering chemicals switched on doesn't make sense. The EBT strategy is to change the wires in the emotional brain that control the spigot of the limbic triangle and rewire them as circuits that promote an empowering chemical cascade, healthy eating, and weight.

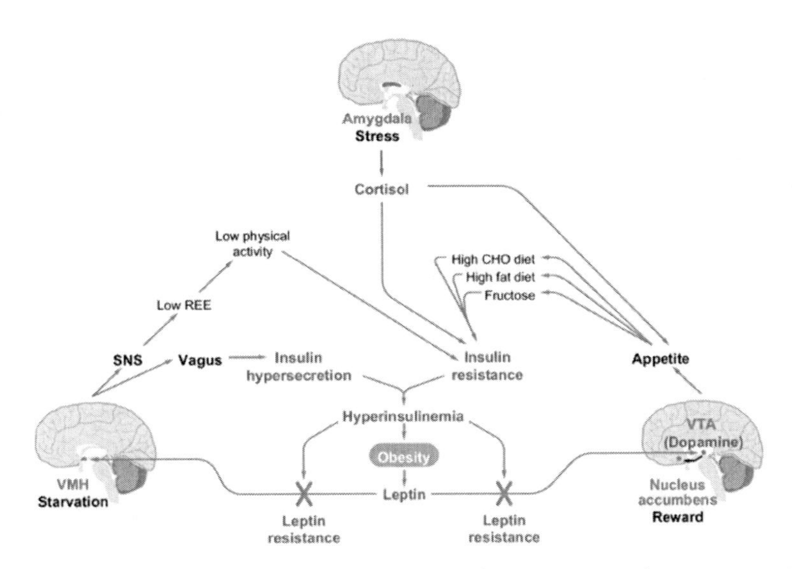

The Limbic Triangle. The original graphic with permission from Mietus-Snyder, M. L. & Lustig, R. H. (2008). Childhood obesity: adrift in the "limbic triangle." *Annual Review of Medicine*, 59:147-62.

This triangle adds an essential element to EBT. First, drug therapies tend to be narrow, whereas the triangle is expansive. Second, we know that controlling the limbic triangle depends on a high-functioning prefrontal cortex. When the triangle is activated, the thinking brain goes "offline," becoming incapable of switching off the stress triangle so we can push away from the table, saying "no" to cupcakes and chocolate. Within this framework, we can see that the problem is the brain-launching chemicals that drive overeating and weight gain. It's a brain problem that we all share.

The three neuroendocrine centers within the primitive core of the brain evolved to promote survival and thrived in the hunter-gatherer lifestyle, but now we're in deep trouble. Imagine our thin ancestors, undernourished from periods of famine or food shortages, stopping off at a stream to fill a water basket. What if instead they were confronted with rows of candy bars, burgers dripping with bacon fat, or images of perfectly toned bodies with rippling six-packs, without having the dial-up options of Peloton and a fitness instructor saying: "Train smart. Train hard. Have fun!"

What would they do? They'd binge eat, judge their bodies, and get depressed. They'd activate their triangle, which would launch biochemical drives. They would have a gap between their hunter-gatherer brain and feeling healthy and in control, given the multiple daily assaults caused by our modern life.

The primitive brain does not evolve rapidly, so we now have a gap between the brain we need to be healthy and happy in modern life and the hunter-gatherer brain we're stuck with. Our prefrontal cortex helps, but the role of EBT is to upgrade the brain's resilience software and fill that gap.

The desire to gain control

I rarely speak with participants about the potential health risks of their eating and weight. They already have formed an opinion about the mental and physical risks of overeating and being overweight, and besides, I'm a staunch believer that people have the right to eat and weigh what they choose. However, most people identify their problem not as excess weight but as feeling out of control. That was the case for Jessica.

She said, "After the kids go to bed, I tell myself to listen to an audiotape book or take a nice, long bath. Instead, I go straight to the kitchen and get myself something rewarding. A banana won't do. I want crunchy, sweet, salty, something ultra-rewarding. I can't control myself."

"Your stress triangle is the problem, not you."

"I get a craving – and I go on automatic – I eat."

"You're going up against the emotional wires that tell you that it is not safe to eat or weigh differently than you do, and the stress of that blocks you from the surges of dopamine and endorphins from higher purpose. You have strong biochemical drives, and that Stress Triangle has blocked your joy of releasing weight."

Jessica said, "I don't even think about weight."

I responded, "That's caused by biochemistry. It's not your fault."

"What do I do about it?"

"You use EBT. When a craving arises, use it to switch off the triangle and change your biochemistry. Stress causes the brain to encode glitches – mixed-up wires – in the triangle, which sets it off. Your triangle has some glitches in it that you can fix with EBT. That will give you control."

"Fix the glitches?"

"Exactly."

Part of a larger movement to innovate

With the broader use of a new generation of weight-loss drugs, more people appreciate that overeating and weight gain are biochemically driven.

The underpinnings of obesity, specifically stress, were the focus of UCSF's Consortium for Obesity Assessment, Study, and Treatment (COAST), formed 15 years ago by Elissa Epel and Nancy Adler, both psychologists who have studied EBT. Drs. Lustig, Meitus-Snyder, and I were affiliated with COAST. The mission was to reduce the prevalence and adverse consequences of obesity, particularly due to stress. The discussions were passionate, with visiting professors presenting regularly at meetings for medical staff, usually attended by about 30 researchers and post-docs – always creating a buzz.

Three of the professors who presented had major influences on EBT. One was Bruce McEwen, the scientist who coined the term allostatic load and changed how we think about stress. Stress is cumulative, and our stress load adds up over time, becoming the primary cause of our stress. I can always explain why circumstances stress me – my husband had surgery, I feel a cold coming on, or there is so much violence in the world – but science doesn't support that. People going through the pandemic whose brains were allostatic from adverse childhood experiences ended up with PTSD at a much higher rate than those who did not. The situational stress lands on top of a pile-up of unprocessed past stress ("high allostatic load") and adds fuel to the fire!

Dr. McEwen, who has since passed away, was a big-hearted man who was intrigued with EBT. We had a long lunch in a small restaurant in Laurel Village in San Francisco near the university, followed by more lunches in the dining room at Rockefeller University in New York City, where he orchestrated collaborations on EBT research with Cornell Weill Medicine's Mary Charlson and Janey Peters. This led to conducting a study of cardiac angioplasty patients and EBT, a relationship that continued as we studied EBT in treating obesity in pregnant inner-city women.

One of the highlights of our discussions was that using EBT could reverse allostatic load, which caused the age-related decline in the set point. EBT directly hits the very circuits that cause or exacerbate allostatic load, which predicts morbidity and mortality. In the 1990s, cardiologist Dean Ornish showed that structured, meaningful lifestyle changes could reverse heart disease. However, using a structured and vigorous approach to rewiring the allostatic circuit to reverse allostatic load can have an even more far-reaching impact on our physical and mental health epidemics.

Dr. McEwen passed away during the pandemic, but as EBT becomes more widely disseminated, more researchers will want to study it. I hope to continue to show that EBT reverses allostatic load, as a way to build on the more than 700 research papers he published on this topic during his career.

The second professor whose pioneering research influenced EBT was Leonard Epstein. A pediatrician and behavioral medicine researcher at the University of Buffalo, he conducted a family-based obesity program that resulted in findings that the children in the study sustained weight loss at a 10-year follow-up. This finding was unheard of at the time and went on to be published in the prestigious *Journal of the American Medical Association*. His study fascinated me because he reinforced the importance of the child and parent connection with shared goals and rewards. I also believed that the operative mechanism for change was connection, so his research gave me more confidence in relying on emotional connection, not dietary prescriptions, to produce lasting results with eating and weight.

Mary Dallman was the third professor with research influencing EBT. A neuroendocrinologist, she was the woman who coined the term "comfort eating." In her lab at UCSF, Dr. Dallman discovered the biological basis for eating highly palatable foods: at first, they dampen the stress response. Even though in the longer term, they pack on pounds and increase stress, their short-term calming effect made them seem "medicinal."

Dr. Dallman passed away recently, but we shared many long "coffees" together in the campus café. She updated me about her latest stress research and cautioned me about how confusing stress definitions were – stress, stressor, stresses – and advised me to lay out the definitions clearly.

In one of our last meetings, we were crossing the street, and with a twinkle in her eye, she said, "As bench scientists, we make discoveries about stress. But you are the only one who has applied them, and you even have the right name as you train the emotional brain."

With that, Dr. Dallman charged off on her way to her laboratory on the 12th floor of the clinical sciences building, with her characteristic determination to discover the truth about how the world works based on science.

The findings from the COAST research and conferences were at their height between 2007 and 2017 and have since been integrated into a national consortium for obesity research. However, because of the devotion of Nancy Adler and Elissa Epel during that decade, the creative energy of COAST researchers propelled EBT forward.

Since 2008, scientific support for the limbic triangle as the chief controller of food and weight has continued to mount. Even the new weight-loss drugs have heightened public awareness that both are driven by biochemistry. As of this writing, the significance of the triangle continues to be documented. My colleagues Dr. Lynda Frassetto, a clinical medicine professor, one of the originators of EBT, and EBT Director of Clinical Research; Dr. Michele Welling, Medical Director of EBT; Dr. Igor Mitrovic, Scientific Director of EBT; and I are collaborating with Drs. Lustig and Meitus-Snyder to integrate the most recent literature into this model with the goal of broadening the use of the Stress Triangle for treating chronic diseases and mental health problems.

To better understand the Stress Triangle, let's take a quick look at the major biochemical players in obesity and overeating. In the next chapter, we'll examine the biological errors ("glitches") caused by stress that block the joy of weight loss and the natural drive to eat healthy for higher purpose.

The three brain structures of the triangle

The target of EBT is the brain because it is the central controller of our lives. The prefrontal cortex is our point of entry into changing everything in the brain and body, and the goal is resilience, or getting out of the stress ditch. The nerves from the brain to the body (efferent) and from the body to the brain (afferent), and the structures within the Stress Triangle itself are all negatively impacted by stress. The storehouse of the Stress Circuits that launch stress overload resides in the part of the Limbic Triangle called the amygdala, so we begin our story there.

The Stress Center

Brain Structure: Amygdala
Primary Chemical: Cortisol

When Jessica goes home after the session, the twins might be quarreling, her son might be having a meltdown, and someone from her tech company may call with an emergency. A wire from her amygdala is launched, eventually leading to a release of cortisol from the adrenal glands. Cortisol is a glucocorticoid hormone that has widespread impacts on the body and brain.

The immediate impact of the secretion of cortisol is to decrease energy intake by triggering the release of glucose from the liver for a quick energy boost. But chronic activation and release of cortisol are associated with overeating, especially high-energy-density "comfort foods." Insulin levels increase to clear the resulting high glucose levels, and the combination of repeated exposure to elevated cortisol, high glucose levels, and corresponding high levels of insulin promote insulin resistance.

When we develop insulin resistance, the cells of the body don't respond normally to insulin, so glucose remains high because it can't enter the cells easily, building up in the bloodstream. This can eventually lead to the downregulation of insulin receptors to try to adapt to the higher level, causing insulin to build up in our bloodstream. Weight gain from ultra-processed foods, which is driven by cortisol, further promotes insulin resistance as fat cells are not responsive to insulin. Calories end up being stored in the fat cells of the belly, which further increases health problems, including heart disease, diabetes, fatty liver disease, some types of cancer, and risk for sudden death. Over time, the pancreas responds by releasing even more insulin (hyperinsulinemia), causing type 2 diabetes. Insulin resistance impacts 70 percent of obese people. In short, insulin makes us fat, more insulin makes us fatter, and insulin resistance makes us even more overweight and unhealthy.

What can Jessica do? She's stressed. She knows she shouldn't eat chips, candy, and (in a pinch) breakfast cereal, but she can't help it because she feels like she is starving. Yes, she ate lunch, but it was an ice cream cone, a Diet Coke, and then some beef jerky while driving in the car. That should have been enough, but it wasn't. What is going on?

An excellent demonstration by Robert Lustig can answer that question. I was joined at a childhood obesity conference in San Francisco by Robert Lustig and Andrea Garber, a nutrition researcher specializing in pediatric obesity. A large meal with oversized white roll sandwiches was included, and Dr. Lustig presented while the attendees ate.

He coached them to wait and notice how they felt 20 minutes after eating, as given the food they consumed the pancreas would over-release insulin and they would self-create hunger. In effect, they would not be eating because their fat cells needed food, but because their elevated insulin levels shuttled what they did eat into fat cells, leaving them with a starvation response. The food itself was literally making them hungry. About 20 minutes later, he checked in with the 200 people in the room. Most raised their hands, having self-created hunger due to the processed food they ate.

As comfort food eating becomes chronic, we inadvertently starve ourselves, causing weight gain, "hangry" (anger + hunger), and lethargy. At a training session for Certified EBT Providers, Robert Lustig presented a recorded session. He gave an example of what happens when the chronic intake of processed foods causes insulin resistance, followed by pumped-up blood insulin levels.

Dr. Lustig said, "Look at Laurel. She eats 2000 calories, she burns 2000 calories, she feels good. Does she gain weight, lose weight, or stay the same? She stays the same. No problem."

He went on to propose that he put an IV in my arm and inject extra insulin every time I eat. That would simulate what would happen if I continued to eat processed foods that led to hyperinsulinemia. Even if I ate 2000 calories daily, because of the extra insulin I would be exposed to, 500 of them would be swept into my fat cells before I had a chance to burn them. I would then be 500 calories heavier. I would only have 1500 calories left to burn even though my body wants 2000 calories because that is where I feel good.

Instead, I would be in starvation mode, feeling lethargic, having no energy to do anything, not wanting to exercise, and feeling ravenous. So, in a world of free access to food, I would eat 500 calories more each day, so now I'd be eating a total of 2500 calories, already 1000 calories heavier, and so it would go.

Our bodies turn into machines that starve us and make us fat because of the combination of eating ultra-processed foods, being stressed out, and carrying extra weight. We are told that we should eat real food and lose weight, but our biochemistry makes us crave carbs, we feel so exhausted we can't get off the couch, and we gain weight.

Jessica said, "That's just what my physician told me: stop eating carbohydrates and exercise so that you lose weight."

Dr. Lustig states, "The underlying message is that there is something wrong with you because you have this problem with gluttony and sloth. But actually, it's a biochemical drive set up by high insulin. It's not that you're choosing to overeat. You must overeat because you are starving. Rather than being two distinct problems (overeating and inactivity), it is one problem: your biochemistry."

The biochemical cascade activated by the amygdala is the main driver for overeating and weight gain. One thing leads to another. When the amygdala is activated, the appetite ramps up and a drive for high-energy-density food – comfort food – kicks in. We do the natural thing and overeat, thereby "self-creating" hunger. Biochemically, our drive to overeat is on fire. The excess cortisol leads to insulin resistance, and the cells in our muscles, fat, and liver don't respond well to insulin and can't easily take up glucose from our blood. That can lead to the chronic oversecretion of insulin that blocks leptin signaling to the brain. Without leptin signaling the brain that we have plenty of stored fat to keep us from starving, we store excess blood sugar as adipose tissue. That is why stress makes us pack on pounds.

Let's talk about leptin. Leptin is a protein hormone regulating appetite and fat storage. It is predominantly made by fat cells, and its primary role is to control appetite and signal satiety to stop overeating when fat cells are large enough. The amount of leptin in the blood is directly proportional to body fat. Being overweight raises leptin levels and can result in a decreased sensitivity to leptin, or leptin resistance. When this happens, the brain doesn't get the message that fat cells have stored enough reserve and will continue to drive hunger. Combined with insulin resistance, leptin signaling is further impaired and our brain thinks we are starving.

The end result of the activation of a "hijacked amygdala" that is not contained by the emotional processing of the thinking brain, is the chronic elevation of cortisol, public health enemy #1. Cortisol in combination with ultra-processed foods torques the entire metabolic system and points fat deposition to the belly, right where it causes metabolic disease. Be aware of your cortisol level, which corresponds to your brain state, both to identify your stress level and to prevent metabolic disease. As food and weight are both highly cortisol-sensitive, use EBT to set limits with work and life so you do not activate your amygdala and force yourself to feel hungry, store body fat, or both.

The Reward Center

Brain Structure: Nucleus Accumbens

Primary Chemical: Dopamine

All three centers of the triangle interact in multilayered loops. Chances are, if you're stressed, your brain is under-rewarded. Your drive for pleasure will ramp up and eating is the most reliable, socially acceptable way to boost dopamine. Currently, more than half the calories Americans consume are from ultra-processed foods as they deliver higher than expected levels of dopamine.

I asked Jessica, "Are you reward-insufficient?"

She paused for a moment, then said, "Absolutely. I'm dying inside. I love my kids, but I feel like I'm about to crack up half the time. I hold it all in, get through dinner, put them to bed, and then attack the kitchen. I eat whatever I can get my hands on."

Jessica does not have a mental health problem, but a biochemical problem, and the interaction between the stress and reward centers of her brain causes it. Reward insufficiency is common if the amygdala is chronically activated or if stress-eating episodes are frequent. At low-stress levels, the thinking brain can consciously bring up a thought of a higher purpose that stimulates the septal region of the brain, causing intense pleasure to shuttle down to the reward center in the emotional brain. However, this reward system is hijacked by high stress and the high dopamine levels that come from artificial pleasures.

Thoughts of higher purpose are genetically imbued with the capacity to create dopamine surges that are internally sourced, endlessly accessible, and non-addictive. This ready supply of positive emotions is survival-based, as the stress response does not switch off until the positive emotions of the parasympathetic nervous system swamp the negative feelings associated with the activation of the sympathetic nervous system. To soundly switch off the stress response, a touch of joy always works.

The reward pathway of the brain involves the ventral tegmental area (VTA) and the nucleus accumbens. The VTA determines whether a stimulus is rewarding or aversive and sends that information to the nucleus accumbens, which releases dopamine. In a reward-insufficient, stressed-out state, the VTA is on the lookout for "sledgehammer" dopamine, sources of massive doses of the reward chemical. The subtle satisfaction from a dopamine release in response to eating healthy foods when hungry, going for a walk to relax, or gazing at the stars for inspiration is replaced by a dopamine surge from something else. Now, the drive for survival shows up and demands immediate access to unbridled pleasure. What delivers? Ultra-processed foods ("hedonic eating") are perfect, as are other drugs of addiction: nicotine, alcohol, and recreational drugs.

As the thinking brain's impulse control is not available in stress, and with compromised leptin signaling and insulin resistance both in play, eating for pleasure, albeit artificial, becomes a necessity, and the amplification of the reward value of food can skyrocket. This dynamic is particularly impactful after food deprivation, which makes it damaging to force rigid dieting and changes in eating without first clearing stress.

Rather than eating for hunger, strong bursts of dopamine amplify the drive to overeat highly palatable foods and to use them as a drug. Highly processed foods can be seen as substances manufactured by the food industry for their extreme palatability. The food industry capitalizes on our biochemical drives, delivering the customer to their "bliss point," which drives overconsumption and weight gain.

The lead chemical of the nucleus accumbens is dopamine. Sugar, salt, and fat produce an abrupt dopamine blast giving a temporary boost in mood, followed by cravings like other addictive substances. Pay attention to your dopamine surges. After thoroughly rewiring the four major circuits that cause overeating and weight gain, reassess how much of a dose of these substances you want to release into your body and brain. Literally, how free from stress do you want to be?

The Habit Center

Brain Structure: Hypothalamus

Primary Chemical: Insulin

The last of the three brain structures in the Stress Triangle is the hypothalamus, the master regulator of energy homeostasis. It helps to control body temperature, hunger and thirst, mood, sex drive, blood pressure, and sleep. But in stress with the amygdala activated, the nucleus accumbens seeking food as a drug, insulin levels high, and leptin signaling ineffective, the hypothalamus misreads the needs of the body and goes into starvation mode.

That makes people feel bad – lethargic and apathetic. Resting energy levels decrease, exercise seems odious, and the thinking brain's impulse control vanishes. Comfort foods beckon.

Given the compromised functioning of the brain due to the contributions of all three centers toxified by stress, it's a reasonable expectation that we feel out of control.

This is particularly important. The human brain is pain- and change-avoidant. It likes the status quo. If our stress and reward centers are making sure that we are consuming a processed food diet, not exercising, and sleeping poorly – all of which boost stress, overeating, and weight gain – we're in trouble. The biggest problem is we believe we are starving, but if the message is to starve ourselves more, that's stressful.

According to Igor Mitrovic, "Not only is eating the easiest and most reliable way to feel better, but hunger causes stress." The message we get from our brain in stress is that we have to stress ourselves more.

State-specific memory is the phenomenon that our brain will only remember an emotional experience when we are in a similar situation to when we acquired the memory. Due to this, any circuit in the brain that was encoded at the same level of stress is "hot" or online and more apt to activate spontaneously when we are stressed. This is not so bad if you have lived a charmed life, but about 70 percent of us have had trauma, so most people will activate other circuits when they are stressed.

This causes two problems. One is that the thought of restricting food will activate 5 Circuits. We call this a "scarcity panic." Also, if we restrict food and activate hypoglycemia, that can activate a trauma circuit. This can cause retraumatization, which can be even worse than the original trauma. Just by dieting, we are retraumatizing ourselves.

The lead chemical of the hypothalamus is insulin. Although all three structures of the triangle impact insulin, it is the blockage of leptin signaling by insulin that results in the starvation response. That feeling of being always hungry and lethargic, depositing all our calories into fat cells, blocks our joy. Who needs that? Although your physician may tell you to eat healthy to lower your insulin levels, an even more compelling reason is so you can feel vibrant, clear hunger and lethargy, and have a new zest for life.

A fresh new approach to eating and weight

The beauty of not forcing changes in our eating but rewiring the Stress Triangle instead is that we avoid suffering. Eating healthy and releasing extra weight can not only be easy, but a joy, because we are not going up against fight-or-flight circuits. We are getting the chemical benefits of purpose.

Start your EBT work by addressing your stress, not only momentary stress, but that backlog of trauma circuits that are still bullying you. That is part of the stress treatment in The EBT 1-2-3 JOY Program. That's also part of healing. When you are drawn to boosting reward, it will be so much easier. By the time you even think about changing habits – eating, exercise, and sleep, the three major factors that impact weight – you will be biochemically healthier.

The underlying message of countless weight-loss programs is that if you eat food, you must burn it or gain weight. With the Stress Triangle spiraling out of control, weight loss becomes self-neglect, self-abuse, or a little of both. You will eat foods that initially satisfy your craving, but then trigger starvation mode, hunger, more stress, and fat deposition. There is no way you will exercise because your metabolic rate has decreased, and you don't have the energy to burn off those calories.

What is really occurring is that you have been the victim of the weight-loss culture that does not honor the emotional brain. Weight-loss programs have bypassed the controller of food and weight, and instead have asked you to go against your amygdala and nucleus accumbens and change your hypothalamus. At the same time, these structures are still damaged by stress, and your body is still a fat storage machine through no fault of your own.

The functioning of three centers – stress, reward, and hunger – has become compromised by our current weight-loss thinking. The logical solution is to change your biochemistry so you aren't storing the food as fat before you have a chance to burn it, can exercise with joy because you feel great, and use food to fuel living a great life instead of just eating for reward or artificial pleasure.

How can we do that? We'll use the brain's power to change – neuroplasticity – to optimize the Stress Triangle.

Jessica seemed pensive about all this. She said, "I didn't hear anything after you said scarcity panic. I think I have that. I keep candy in my purse and stock my kitchen with chips and cookies. I must have ready access to comfort foods to feel safe. Any hint of food deprivation makes me incredibly anxious."

"That sounds miserable."

"It's miserable but safe. That's how I live my life."

"What if you could change your biochemistry by healing the hurts stored in your Stress Triangle, and you made no changes in your food or weight until your emotional brain tells you that it is both safe and rewarding to do so?"

"I can agree to that. My whole body just relaxed . . . "

4

Optimize the Stress Triangle: Fix the Glitches

Charlotte had enrolled in a 30-day intensive telegroup that Barbara Gabriel, psychotherapist and EBT Clinical Director, and I were facilitating. As always, a provider of the telegroup welcomes the new participant with a brief telephone call.

When Charlotte answered my call, she was very direct. "I have tried everything to lose weight. I can't have weight-loss surgery because the surgeon says my heart is too bad. I tried weight-loss drugs, lost 34 pounds, then gained all but five pounds back. I refuse to go on another diet."

I responded, "I completely understand."

Charlotte continued, "I've read hundreds of self-help books to the point I'm a self-help junkie. My bedroom has stacks of books, and I know I should give myself unconditional love, but I can't do it. I know I should think positive thoughts, but my mind makes a beeline for the negative."

I said, "When stress hormones are toxifying your brain, Charlotte, self-love and positive thoughts are biologically impossible. Anything that is good in life is natural. It's embedded in our genes. All you have to do is get to Brain State 1, the 'joy state,' and those optimal chemicals, emotions, and thoughts start flowing."

She replied, "Even when it comes to weight?"

I said, "Yes, even when it comes to weight. You just keep getting to Brain State 1, which is a physiological state. Everyone can learn how to do that by processing their emotions with symphonic precision, including you."

Charlotte had all of the typical health problems caused by chronic stress, which activates biochemical drives to consume ultra-processed foods. She had high blood pressure, high cholesterol, fatty liver, sleep apnea, high blood sugar, diabetes, and depression. The previous fall, she had started treatment for breast cancer and was planning a knee replacement surgery in the spring.

Although Charlotte had done her part medically, her eating was still out of control, and psychologically, she said she was "fried." Her self-help books mapped out sensible information, but their relevance was for a bygone era when stress was low. Now, with stress overload ubiquitous, our positive psychological state is routinely disrupted by fight-or-flight chemicals. None of those otherwise helpful strategies like thinking positive thoughts or giving yourself unconditional love is biochemically possible when the emotional brain is in stress. Stress drains serotonin, spews cortisol, activates extremes of dopamine, and spikes insulin all of which fuel negative thoughts, self-judgment, and self-created hunger.

Charlotte did not know that the root cause of both her physical and mental health problems was stress, or that she could not "think" her way out of the extreme stress levels we all experience today. Nobody put two and two together and said, "Charlotte, you need to update your approach to health. Treat your stress by learning a few exceedingly effective emotional skills and your health and weight will improve. You won't have to try to feel unconditional love for yourself or nudge yourself to think positive thoughts. Both will occur quite naturally."

The immense power of our emotional brain

Charlotte's problems were all largely preventable. If her parents, the school system, or the healthcare system had taught her how to engage her emotional brain and use its amazingly effective resiliency pathways, she might have avoided most or all of them.

Charlotte asked, "If I use EBT, what would I have to do?"

I said, "Focus on the power you have. Learn skills that shut off those harmful stress chemicals and activate healing joy chemicals. Scientifically, that is called deactivating 'allostasis,' or stress that careens us out of control, and activating 'homeostasis,' or self-balancing stress."

She said, "I like it that EBT is scientific."

I said, "It's based on capitalizing on the brain's capacity to change (neuroplasticity) and optimizing how the brain changes physiology (neurophysiology). The brain cannot concentrate on two opposing ways to control life. You can either choose to ignore the fight-or-flight chemicals that cause overeating and force yourself to eat healthy or clear those chemicals so that you eat healthy naturally."

Charlotte said, "I'll switch off the chemicals, but it's hard. I've been organizing my life around controlling my food for as long as I can remember."

I said, "I know. I used to do that, too. I put all of my attention on starving myself early in the day, stuffing myself by evening, and then devolving into blaming myself before the cycle started again. That left me no time to focus my attention on balancing my errant chemicals."

Charlotte sighed. For many, changing the habit of focusing on food is the hardest part of updating to the new paradigm.

I said, "You can stop tracking food, overthinking, and white-knuckling behavior change. Instead, you connect with your body and process your emotions in a brain-savvy way. If you do, before long, the spigot of those stress chemicals will shut off, the joy chemicals will take over, and healthy habits will magically appear. Many of your problems will fade away or go 'poof' and disappear on the spot. Any problems that remain, you can overcome with far more grace and ease."

Charlotte asked, "What do I have to do?"

I said, "You start spiraling up throughout the day, including before you eat, and you'll see it working. Watch videos on our website so you learn how to use the skills. However, for the best results think of EBT as going to the brain gym. You need to work out your brain, so it changes.

"There are daily drop-in 30-minute telephone sessions – Spiral Up Groups – and your brain changes just by sitting in on them. Start with them, and, in time, join a private premium group with a provider who knows you (and your brain), to complete the program together. These groups include Connection Buddies, people with whom to use the skills for a few minutes now and then between sessions, as research conducted at the University of Kentucky on EBT showed participants lose more weight with that extra support. You have an opportunity to share the amazing journey of EBT and raise your set point together."

Her face brightened and she stated, "I can do that."

"You stay on the daily prescription: 10 spiral ups a day, 10 minutes of watching the videos, and at least one Connection."

She wondered, "Why so many spiral ups?"

"Given the stresses of modern life, most human brains are in chronic stress. That's how neuroplasticity works: you change by doing. Each spiral up wires your brain out of stress and into joy."

She inquired, "What's a 'connection'?"

"When you listen to another person spiral up. That changes your brain. When they listen to you, your spiral up goes much deeper into your brain, to where those Food Circuits are stored. It only takes five minutes by phone."

She looked puzzled, "OK. What about the control part?"

What a heartbreak. I said, "Charlotte, you've been through so much suffering, and all of it is stored in your emotional brain. Sometimes it clears quickly, but some of those wires are stubborn and you must give it a good kick . . ."

She laughed, "A kick in the butt, you mean?"

"Absolutely. That makes it more fun! Those stubborn little buggers need a lot of kicks until they vamoose."

She asked, "How long does it take?"

"Getting through the whole 'build yourself a new brain' program takes a year, but go at your own pace. It's a matter of how much fun you want to have."

She wasn't sure, "Fun?"

"If you get in there and become a spiral-up wizard and start clearing circuits, who knows how quickly you can do it? Every spiral up counts. You focus on this moment, then the next, and spiral up each time, collecting a Joy Point. How many Joy Points do you think you need to collect to clear the stored stress in your brain and experience the joy of releasing extra weight?"

Charlotte paused, then sighed, "I don't know, maybe a thousand."

"Each one takes one to three minutes, so say two minutes each, so that is 33 hours of spiraling up. Plus, time watching videos and spiraling up with other people."

She agreed, "It doesn't sound that bad . . ."

"Part of it is switching to the new paradigm and stopping beating yourself up about your food. You eat precisely what your emotional brain finds safe and rewarding for you to eat, while your weight is the same."

She said, "Yes, my weight stays about the same."

"You are using new powers now. You are changing the circuits that control the chemicals and electricity in every cell of your body. As your circuits change, your eating and weight change easily and naturally."

Charlotte agreed, "OK, I'm up for it."

"Just keep dropping into those Spiral Up Groups and listening. Be sure to have fun, and your brain will change. Complete the intro course, then get down and dirty with rewiring the deeper circuits. That's even more fun!"

She was worried, "I can do it, but what about the glitches?"

"Glitches are what you rewire. When you lose your joy or have a craving, that's a glitch. I can take you on a tour of the three brain areas . . ."

Charlotte said, "Yes!"

Everyone has a few glitches

Most of our wires are pristine homeostatic circuits that hold us in a state of connection, even when the dog has an accident on the floor, our friend is mad at us, or we see injustice in the world and want to scream.

A few allostatic circuits, the glitches, sneak through and worm their way into the semi-locked memory box at the bottom of our brain. Most of this happens in childhood, as our limbic system is wide open to encoding adversities. Yet they can also be encoded later in life during traumatic experiences, scary situations, and anything that the highly sensitive amygdala perceives as threatening.

If you map out times of weight gain, within one year of that time, you will probably find that you had a loss, change, or upset. Consider that stored stress and blocked joy. Clearing those circuits takes releasing that packed-in stress and training the brain to see reasons for joy everywhere. I asked Charlotte to think about the onset of her weight gain and the times when she regained the weight.

Charlotte said, "I started being chubbier than the other children after my sister Maddie was born."

Losses during childhood, when we are completely dependent upon our parents for inner security and stability, can result in the encoding of trauma circuits that spew enough biochemical mayhem to cause weight gain. Vincent Felitti's research on adversity ("adverse childhood experiences or ACEs") include emotional, physical, or sexual abuse or household dysfunction.

In the US, only 32 percent of children have not experienced one or more ACEs. However, stress is perceptual, so even objectively small stressors, given genetic differences or a sensitized amygdala due to in-utero stress or preverbal adversity can encode strong and dominant enough circuits to cause obesity. The birth of a new baby, the death of a pet, if that pet was the child's only source of comfort, and the loss of emotional connection to a parent through a substance use disorder, divorce, health problems, or death are prime examples.

Charlotte explained, "My other big weight gain was in my 20s. I was engaged to Brian, and he ghosted me. He disappeared after I had moved to LA to be with him. Right after that, I was mugged at a gas station. In the year after that, I gained 40 pounds. I couldn't stop eating."

I replied, "All you have been through is so hard, and it is hard to rewire the neural residue – we call it emotional clutter – from it. The only thing harder is not to clear that clutter."

Charlotte asked, "What are you talking about?"

"Using traditional therapy takes so long to clear clutter that most people avoid the therapy or do it in a way that is not organized and fun."

"What do you mean fun?"

"You were a victim of trauma, but healing the brain glitches left behind is liberating. You don't have to house that clutter for the rest of your life. We live in the age of neuroscience, so we can clear it in an organized, joyful way."

Charlotte was catching on.

She said, "How dare those circuits live inside me?"

I responded, "And they don't even pay rent."

Then she laughed.

I said, "Emotional healthcare is changing rapidly because our nation is in crises caused by ignoring it. Just the way 20 years ago, people did not floss their teeth. Now flossing is considered basic self-care. Our goal is that within 10 years, "flossing the brain" will be integrated into normal self-care. Instead of just flossing their teeth before going to bed, people will use EBT to prevent the day's stress from accumulating in the brain."

Charlotte said, "I can do this, and I like the idea of making it fun."

The brain accommodates these glitches

One way of thinking about the cause of obesity is that we have a hunter-gatherer brain that is exceedingly adaptive. The good news is that that "hyper-adaptability" has enabled humans to avoid extinction.

Our motherboard of humanity, the brain, turns lemons into lemonade. For example, take blood pressure. At first, the brain resists a spike in blood pressure, but if it experiences it often enough, it relents and says, "OK, I'll keep your blood pressure up all the time," and then you have hypertension. This does cause less drama for the brain to deal with because the brain has reorganized our physiology to cope with it. Case closed. But the adaptation causes metabolic stress down the line.

The same is true for food. After one episode that could be characterized as gluttony, not much happens other than a food hangover and bloating. But if you keep it up, the brain recalibrates all your digestive chemicals, and voila, you overeat and all that food gets deposited in your fat cells. We have no inherent sense that we are overdoing our food intake, except the number we see on the scale.

We are often oblivious to many of the glitches in our brain because our body has done a chemical dance to make adjustments in our metabolism. Besides, repeated behavior is seen as safe in the brain, and the emotional brain likes sameness. However, the result is that we may be harboring glitches and not even see them as problems.

Separating physical from psychological stress

The most stunning error of our genetic code is that evolution missed being able to distinguish between physical and psychological pain. As our hunter-gatherer ancestors only had a couple of chances to run away from a hungry lion, the stress response had to let loose with crushing amounts of adrenaline and cortisol, being careful to guard against premature switching off of the latter, which is our chronic stress hormone, aka Public Health Enemy #1.

At a later time, psychological stress that is activated dozens of times daily can result in the same exaggerated response. When my brain encoded my Food Circuit, I was at Brain State 5, in stress overload. After that, my brain replayed the wire hundreds of times. And because these wires are tagged as life-saving, they are stored in the least plastic area of the brain and refuse to reveal their hidden message to our conscious mind. We are unable to rewire them unless we outsmart them.

The job of EBT is to help all of us outsmart our exceedingly adaptive brain. It's a snap to clear those faulty wires, and It's even clearly laid out on the app. Use Spiral Up #3 Deep Work option and memorize the information boxes. Drop into Spiral Up Groups so you can hear Certified EBT Providers coach participants in using Precision EBT.

It's not surprising, given that rates of stress overload are escalating, that every step of Precision EBT asks us to do something that our parents told us not to do. The process is the problem, and EBT is harder to learn because we have brains conditioned to process stress overload in highly ineffective ways.

I learned as a child not to complain. Actually, a brief complaint activates the faulty circuits, so the emotional processing can clear them.

First, complain. State briefly what that outrageous wire does to you – like make you nibble constantly on food, always have something in your mouth, or dive into a meal as if there is no tomorrow. That will activate the offending wire.

Next, do what your mother told you not to do: express anger. Unleash a quick burst of safe, effective, but intense fury (you will get good at this). This anger turns stuck emotions into flowing feelings, to avoid depression, panic, anxiety, and shame and lead you on a straight pathway to joy.

You are dismantling that wire in real-time, but the process is novel. Parents tell us to identify our sadness, fear, and guilt, but that gives too much power to the thinking brain. By using our thinking brain to identify one deep feeling for each of these three emotions and feeling the feelings until they fade, the process is faster and keeps the brain on track to focus on the offending circuit.

The rest is a lovely experience, as you quickly flow through your emotions, and discover the message encoded in that wire. This is the most magical part of using EBT. You make the unconscious, hidden message in your emotional brain conscious. The biggest joy in life is to "know thyself" and now you can plumb your unconscious mind on demand and meet yourself at a deeper level.

This "reveal" leads to many "aha" moments and a personal power. You don't have to run to a therapist each time you have an issue. You can take out your app and be your own therapist. You can peer into your own beautiful emotional brain and discover yourself. With self-knowledge, self-love grows.

Knowledge is power. You can use that inside information (literally) to juxtapose the opposite message. As the prefrontal cortex cannot hold onto two opposing messages at the same time, you can target and wipe out the wire! Once you have moved through your anger, sadness, fear, and guilt, the circuit is at your mercy. That hidden wire with its biochemical explosion that has threatened and harmed you for years is now completely vulnerable to being weakened, crushed, annihilated, and replaced.

The synaptic connections between its neurons (nerve cells) are unlocked and fluid. Now you feel victorious because, with enough repetitions and sufficient removal of emotional clutter, you can dismantle that wire so it can stop harming you. The big bonus is that you can rewrite the messages in your own brain. You can create a sparkling new wire with the healing and empowering message of your choosing.

The lopsided brain: It favors the negative

When at Brain State 1, everything goes right, and it is all so easy, but to fall in love with life takes accepting all your experiences, even those 5 moments. There is a devilish duo of two brain characteristics we all share: negativity and obsession.

The brain over-remembers what happens when we are exceedingly flipped out at a five-to-one ratio. It takes five good experiences to wipe out a bad memory. Who has time to manipulate the mind five times when we are stressed? Spiraling up gives us a pathway to do this. But what do we do without access to the pathway? We focus on the negative, think about it endlessly, and obsess about what happened, what we could have done differently, and how we can fix it. All this makes the amygdala smile because it has duped us into self-inflicted negative emotional plasticity. This is serious and a major reason why spiraling up 10 times per day is so powerful.

The consequence of this "double trouble" of the negativity bias of the brain and overthinking hit home for me after the loss of my mother. When my mother, Mackey, was being impossible, my father would throw his head back and laugh with loving affection. When my dad was being impossible, my mother would sharply say, "Oh Jack!" then collect herself and say, "I have a bone to pick with you, but not now." Then she would melt with compassion for him (he truly never did anything wrong in her eyes), and it was over.

After my mother passed away, my dad was grieving, and the stress went to his stomach. This seems to be genetic, as that's where my stress shows up, too. He was nauseated, not just a little, but to the point that he had his gallbladder taken out. He popped Zofran pills like lifesavers and even used medical marijuana. I still have vivid images of sitting on the tiny deck outside his room at the skilled nursing center, helping him light a joint.

The nausea kept him from eating, and he went from 180 to 128 pounds and was on hospice care. This is when his doctor diagnosed him with a condition of negative obsession. My father had always refused to use EBT before (our family is very stubborn), but he listened respectfully to the doctor and made the decision he wanted to live. After that, he used therapy, medications, and EBT (the Flow Tool), eventually regaining all the weight and his health. My dad lived another nine years, passing away peacefully of natural causes at age 95.

The new stress diagnosis: Chronic Physiologic Stress Overload (CPSO)

With the human brain so at odds with what we need in modern life, stress overload is ubiquitous, and that "elephant in the living room" is now in every health clinic in the US. We are treating the symptoms of stress but not the brain-based root cause. Stress is the underlying physiologic state that causes, prolongs, and intensifies all other pathologies. As much as we can measure allostatic load, identify set points, and track circuits, stress now needs its own clinical diagnosis.

At the EBT Annual Meeting on June 4, 2023, Drs. Mitrovic, Frassetto, and I proposed the diagnosis of Chronic Physiological Stress Overload (CPSO). With evidence of rising rates of toxic stress that is biologically based, we need to consider insulin and obesity as causes of CPSO. Insulin levels in individuals today are two to three times higher than 30 years ago based on glucose tolerance tests of comparable populations. Why is this? It has to do with the way we eat today – processed food – and our stress triggering wires in the brain that drive our eating behaviors.

During the past 30 years, obesity rates have nearly tripled. By adding CPSO as a diagnosis, patients can get to the root cause of the problem and use medications and treatments to alleviate the symptoms. Be sure to ask your physician whether they will add the diagnosis of CPSO to your problem list and support acceptance of going to the root cause of our epidemic of obesity. EBT offers certification courses for all health professionals, so check if your practitioner is EBT Certified.

The Stress Triangle

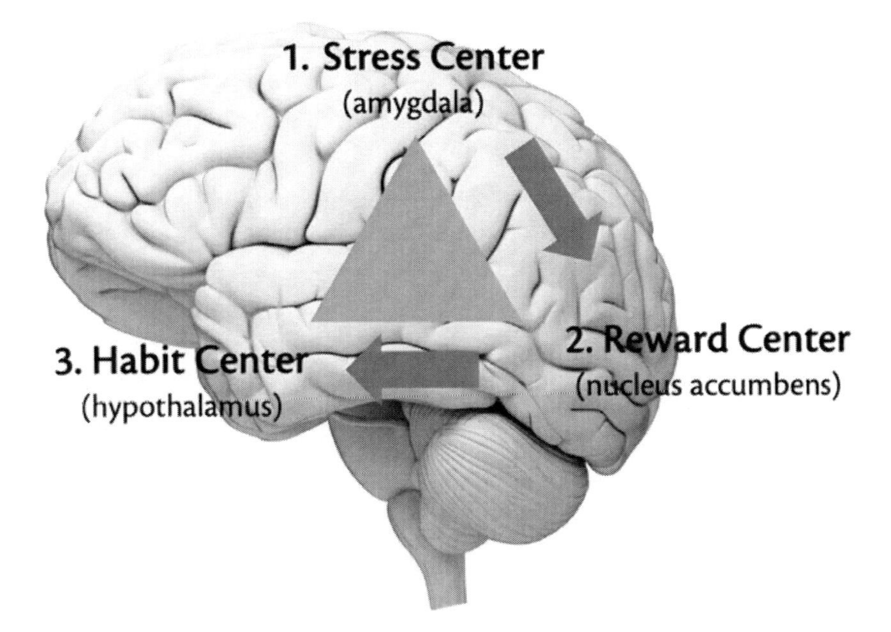

I asked my EBT participant, Charlotte, "Does this make sense to you?"

She said, "Everyone I know is stressed. People accept it, and they take medications, zone out streaming videos, and eat, drink, worry, and spend themselves silly. Something has to change."

I said, "You can change this with your own brain. Fix your glitches, and as you do, you will radiate joy and your health will improve in ways that were previously impossible."

"I'm ready for that!"

"Let's look closer at the Stress Triangle of the brain – the amygdala, nucleus accumbens, and hypothalamus. This triangle is the controller of our stress.

To understand glitches in each of the three structures of the Stress Triangle and how EBT is designed to fix them, let's take a quick look at the science, beginning with definitions.

The Emotional Brain

The emotional brain is the subcortical structure, the unconscious mind that reflexively controls everything that really matters in life, from survival, reward, and spirituality, to loving connection. It does not change by thoughts but by emotional experiences.

The Thinking Brain

The thinking brain is the cortical structure, principally the prefrontal cortex, that consciously controls our thinking, analysis, planning, and deciding. It is the brain area that learns and applies the EBT tools to change the neuronal stress circuitry stored in the emotional brain.

A Glitch

A glitch is any neuronal Stress Circuit (strings of neurons that coactivate) that causes the dysregulation of physiology and harmful extremes of thoughts, emotions, and behaviors.

Fixing Glitches

Fixing these maladaptive Stress Circuits is the process of optimizing the Stress Triangle to promote the prevention and treatment of stress-related health problems by identifying allostatic circuits, and then using positive emotional neuroplasticity to reconsolidate allostatic circuits into homeostatic circuits.

We'll start by focusing on the Stress Glitches, as it is by switching off these rogue circuits that the thinking brain comes back online to optimize executive functioning. The intervention to promote resilience can begin.

Stress Triangle 1. The Stress Glitch

The primary focus in medicine is to stop the damage of the stress response and clean up after failures to do so. The priority of the brain is survival, so it is always on the lookout for "threat detection errors" – circuits that grossly over or underestimate the threat. We rewire these in EBT.

The brain constantly evaluates risks and sends up warnings of possible threats: psychological, physiological, or environmental. These activations come from the sum of all our life experiences in the amygdala, which then activates a wire that replays past experiences and tries out each one to see if it is an appropriate response in the present. This is what starts the stress response, even though there is no real threat present. The dominance of wires stored in the brain, either homeostatic or allostatic, is significant as it is from this backlog of wires that the brain will activate warnings of threat.

I asked Charlotte, "What is your experience of these warnings?"

She said, "They are popping up all the time. When I wake up in the morning, my list of worries starts. If It's not my son and his depression or my granddaughter who is failing at math, it's all the emotional echoes of the way my neighbors treated me when all I did was park one foot into the red zone in front of their house . . ."

"Charlotte, you'll love spiraling up 10 times per day, the standard dose, because you'll switch off those little glitches. I don't mean just distract yourself. I mean do the wires in so they don't keep piling up."

"What a relief that would be, but what would I think about then?"

I said, "Only one thing: how you will make your dreams come true."

The problem is that the expectations embedded in these wires are stored during stress when the prefrontal cortex provides no wise filter. They are completely ridiculous, which is why we call them glitches. The more chronic stress and traumatic early life experiences we have, the greater the risk that constant warnings from our wires will cause us to suffer. Traumatic experiences later in life can also cause reflexive responses leading to suffering, and ultimately to harming our health and blocking our joy. Chronic stress and our life experiences, coupled with trauma, flood our amygdala and lead to these reflexive responses.

At the EBT Annual Meeting in June 2022, EBT Scientific Director Igor Mitrovic delivered a keynote address on this topic.

He asked the participants, "What is our brain for? Not just automatic functions, maintaining blood pressure, controlling the heart rate, or even the functions that are more or less automatic, like seeking food when we are hungry. What is the purpose of the prefrontal cortex, the cognitive part of the brain?" Several participants offered ideas, such as creativity, imagination, connection, and survival.

Dr. Mitrovic agreed that all were true but explained that he was asking for something more fundamental. He said, "It's actually to predict. From a biological standpoint, the brain is the most sophisticated future prediction device . . . All these things that have ever happened to us are constantly processed, constantly assessed, and compared with the present situation, and they are projected into the future, so we know what to expect. Whoever has the best predictive ability has the greatest chance of survival."

He continued, "If we don't detect any threat, then we relax. If we do detect a threat, we scrunch, and we start getting stressed. The more predictor circuits stored in the amygdala, the greater the chances of our survival with well-being, that is optimal health."

One of the most significant shifts you can make as you develop your EBT Practice is to reframe these glitches in the worst possible light because that is accurate. If you had a bomb going off in your brain five times a day, you would do something about it. These wires are chemical bombs. These glitches take three forms:

Survival Circuits: False Associations that Trigger Us

In his 2010 article, *Rethinking the Emotional Brain*, published in *Neuron*, a premier forum of the neuroscience community, Joseph LeDoux, director of the Emotional Brain Institute, formally documented the existence of Survival Circuits – false associations between a natural stress response (unconditioned response) and another response (conditioned response) that create fight-or-flight drives to do whatever the wire tells us to do.

Dr. LeDoux defined emotions, the so-called "basic emotions" that are universally expressed and recognized in people around the world. He believed that basic emotions are "conserved in our close animal ancestors, and supposedly hard-wired into brain circuits for another type of emotion." These are the emotions that are wired into our circuits. These basic feelings are not only psychological in purpose, but biological: to provide immediate information to alert us to our greatest need. (In Spiral Up 2, see the Brain State 2, Feelings Tool for access to processing these basic feelings.)

In stark contrast to the basic feelings, Survival Circuits have no direct role in emotions. Their function is to control behaviors and responses to support the organism's survival. They orchestrate vast swaths of internal and external stimuli and motivational systems to bring closure to the perceived risk. In contrast to basic feelings that involve the cognitive or reflective appraisal of emotions, Survival Circuits are prone to activating automatic, unconscious appraisal. They get the "survival job" done without consulting the conscious mind, as when these wires fire, we do not think or feel, we just do.

The message or expectation embedded in the Survival Circuit is based on the formula: I get my "X" from "Y." X is a universal survival need (unconditioned response), and Y is whatever other wire was consolidated with that circuit, that is, the conditioned response. Below is the basic structure and an example.

The Stress Glitch

I have a strong biochemical drive to meet my need for ___
(e.g., safety, love, existence, power, protection, or comfort),
and to disconnect from myself and connect to
something that does not meet my real need.

Example:
I get my safety from food.

At first, the memory trace changes the nervous system and synaptic consolidation occurs, but this is not serious because memories are encoded throughout the day. Some are competing, so storing the circuits only occurs after sleep. This is why spiraling up about the day's conflicts before sleeping is very wise. Only store the memories that you want to keep and clear the rest!

During sleep, the hippocampus shuttles the surviving wires into long-term memory that is relatively permanent unless emotionally activated and provided with a new contradictory message (Spiral Up #3 Deep Work). This involves reconsolidation, or the reactivation of previously consolidated memories, so most memories are updates. This makes them labile again and provides opportunities for continuing to update them. Every time a circuit is activated, it has the potential to change, which becomes the neuronal pathway to personal control over our lives in automatic, easy, and lasting ways.

If EBT were directed just at identifying Survival Circuits, it might sound like a more robust form of CBT because in cognitive methods it is core to identify unreasonable expectations. The difference with EBT is that by activating the circuit with strong emotions we do not reveal the contents of the conscious mind. The problematic circuit is not in the conscious mind but in the unconscious mind. We find the unconscious message by taking a nosedive into emotions (with joy, excitement, and vigor!).

As our fight-or-flight response fuels that message, we must confront it with its polar opposite message to rewire a Survival Circuit. Neuroplasticity will be compromised without discovering the message from the unconscious memory, which is often significantly at odds with what we "think" it is. The EBT method is designed so you can discover and verify the unconscious message as a key prelude to clearing it.

I wanted Charlotte to appreciate how important rewiring these circuits is, so I explained further:

"Charlotte, these Survival Circuits are exceedingly meticulous in ensuring that they are reactivated immediately and strongly so any sensation, emotion, thought, behavior, or state that occurred at its encoding is recorded. That means that a vast array of stimuli can reactivate it. They don't have to be logical triggers, as this is the nature of neuronal Stress Circuits. This is why we crush these circuits. Otherwise, who knows when they will be activated? We lose our freedom."

She said, "I know my most damaging Food Circuit, it's a monster circuit, it's binge eating. It is the ultimate collection of garbage because it crosses over to any environment. I get this buzz in my body that I gotta have something salty at parties or while watching television when my husband goes on a trip and I am alone – I can eat until I am sick then."

I explained, "The more you activate the circuit, the stronger it becomes, and then not only the original triggers are operative, but new ones form. They become super garbage collectors, and the brain starts generalizing activation of that circuit . . . and there you go, binge eating yet again."

Charlotte said, "For me, It's completely push-button. The circuit activates, my mind goes blank, and I eat until the food is gone."

What Charlotte observed is extremely important. Most traditional methods focus on complexity. The wire in her brain that activates a fight-or-flight drive is very primitive. It only rewires while it is unlocked, so we need a very simple process that we can repeat to change it, not abstract ideas and insights. Psychologist and minister Jim Billings, whom I met when I was a consultant for Dean Ornish's heart disease prevention program, taught me to focus on emotions rather than thoughts to facilitate meaningful change. He said, "Laurel, insight plus five cents only give us a nickel."

I said to Charlotte, "The good news is that your brain keeps this quite simple. You keep spiraling up until you notice that the drive to overeat is gone. Just spiral up by complaining that you are binge eating, and the EBT tools will do the work for you. Just keep spiraling up until the drive goes "poof" and stops. You know you have rewired that glitch when you have zero desire to overeat."

She responded, "OK, so I just spiral up, and spiral up, and spiral up."

"Correct."

As Charlotte learns how to use EBT and moves through the program, her spiral ups will draw her to identifying two other kinds of threat detection errors: Core Circuits and emotional clutter (trauma wires). This is the more profound work that is the most rewarding in EBT because it "cleans house" of the negative memories that lead to anxiety, depression, and overeating. Instead of living with the past that keeps us on edge, hungry, lethargic, enduring cravings, and gaining weight, we clear away those faulty wires.

Core Circuits: False Generalizations

Charlotte will begin to notice that sometimes when she is quite stressed, she does not feel triggered, the signature experience of Survival Circuits. That's because the other kind of circuit is often activated, a Core Circuit, a false generalization. Think of these Core Circuits as erroneous beliefs that are encoded in long-term memory. Their role as threat detection errors is indirect, as they create chronic stress that often sets off Survival Circuits. Fixing these core glitches is extremely important for achieving lasting weight loss, as when you are stressed enough to overeat, most typically the real reason is that a Core Circuit caused it by activating a Survival Circuit. This is why completing The EBT 1-2-3 JOY Program is so important.

How do Core Circuits work? The emotional brain extracts basic truths about ourselves, others, and life in general, especially those that are threatening or stressful. They are very forceful but simple statements that a two-to-four-year-old would make, such as "I am bad," "I don't matter," or "I have no power." Often, they are encoded early in life, so the brain treats them as sacrosanct. Use Spiral Up #3 Deep Work to rewire them.

Emotional Clutter: Fear Memories

Survival Circuits can be categorized by where they are stored in the brain, with the strongest wires encoded at Brain State 5. We call these 5 Circuits, and of all the experiences in EBT, rewiring these will be your most life-enhancing. Here's how it works. You discover a Survival Circuit, say "I get my existence from food." If it is a light circuit encoded at Brain State 3 or 4, it won't be that hard to rewire using the basic skills, but the real action happens with 5 Circuits. When you find one (See the How to Rewire Course), you can use two skills to clear away any wires that are tangled up with it. The two skills involved are the Travel Back and Clear the Clutter Tools. These fuel the threat detection error, and some clutter removal is essential for lasting relief from these circuits.

I asked Charlotte if she thought she had any 5 Circuits.

She said, "I do. A memory comes up of me in my bedroom, listening through the wall to my parents' bedroom. My mother was crying, and my dad was drinking heavily. Just thinking of it brings up a pain in my stomach. What did I need? Safety."

"That gives you a start. You'll discover the precise message as you learn how to dip into your unconscious mind and activate the circuit."

Charlotte continued, "I think that was when I started feeling so ashamed. That experience might have encoded some Core Circuits, perhaps I am bad, or I am not worthy. It was right after that when I started stealing food from the kitchen. What a relief to know they are circuits, something I can process, so I don't have to live with shame and feeling unworthy for the rest of my life."

"EBT gives us the power to be fully present as the tools can free us from replaying the past."

Charlotte said, "That's important to me, and it makes me value EBT even more."

Stress Triangle 2. The Reward Glitch

The glitches of the ventral tegmental area (VTA) and the nucleus accumbens are "reward detection errors." They are quite similar to the "threat detection errors" of the Stress Center, but given that food and stress are both involved, they are a lot more complex. Stress impacts the reward center and strengthens drives to overeat.

The reward glitch builds on the statement of the expectation and is constructed based on the formula: I get my "X" from "Y" to express the use of external artificial rewards of pleasure. Think of this element of the experience as taking the bonfire of the stress glitch and pouring kerosene on it.

The moment the thought of food enters the brain, even before the first taste on the tongue, the Stress Triangle goes berserk. Below is the basic structure of this glitch, and an example.

The Reward Glitch

I have a strong biochemical drive to meet my need for ____
(e.g., safety, love, existence, power, protection, or comfort)
and disconnect from myself and connect to
something that does not meet my real need but **gives me an abnormal dopamine high that is addictive.**

Example:
I get my safety from food and **escaping reality with a false high.**

One of the most disorienting aspects of eating to me is how one moment we are in control and at peace with food, and then a stimulus arrives in our brain and triggers the Stress Triangle. Nothing much matters other than getting that highly palatable ultra-processed food.

In low stress, eating healthy is easy because of our biochemistry. First, the Stress Triangle is not running wild, and the high-functioning prefrontal cortex can generate a thought of higher purpose, which activates the moral center ("septal region"). That sends input to the VTA and then to the nucleus accumbens, which releases dopamine. We feel good without overeating. Second, we receive accurate signals of when to stop eating. Our ability to sense, interpret, and integrate the inner body systems and determine hunger and satiety is strong. Due to state-specific memory, our Survival Circuits that trigger the chemical cascade that prompts cravings for luscious, yummy foods, are switched off. Our capacity to eat when hungry is very high.

In that low-stress state, sensations and feelings from the emotional brain bubble up to the thinking brain as basic feelings. We know whether or not we are hungry, and those signals are accurate. Eating practically any food tastes good because it relieves the discomfort associated with hunger.

Normally, dopamine is triggered intrinsically in small pulses to provide a brief reward in response to a perceived need. These small pulses are delivered immediately, and we associate them with our behavior. However, what if we eat ultra-processed food when we are in low stress? It will deliver a greater-than-predicted positive reward that is enticing to our brain, but we are protected. The food will activate a dopamine high, but afterwards, we are present to the aftermath: a blood sugar low, rebound hunger from the overshooting of insulin, nausea, or bloating. As we are in low stress, we learn from the experience as the brain associates both the positive and negative consequences of overeating. Quite naturally, we learn to eat when hungry and stop when satisfied.

In contrast, consider a person who is not hungry but is chronically stressed, and an image of a milkshake and cheeseburger on television activates a Survival Circuit. An activated survival drive forces a "sledgehammer" burst of dopamine from an external source, whatever we can find that is tasty in the fridge. This masks the awareness of the intrinsic dopamine surges. Our processing of daily fears also builds up and contributes to our epidemic of anxiety. We cannot numb out with food and properly process our reality simultaneously. With our thinking brain function compromised, our impulse control and the biochemical benefits of bringing to mind a higher purpose cannot help us, and interoceptive awareness deficits make being mindful of hunger and satiety biologically impossible.

Whereas intrinsically-triggered dopamine does not reduce dopamine receptor sensitivity, extrinsically-sourced high doses of dopamine do and render the next blast of ultra-processed food less effective in producing a dopamine surge. With more and more dopamine required, the potential for addiction is now in play.

However, the pulse of dopamine and its subsequent pulse of satisfaction are transient in the human brain. According to Peter Sterling, "We are never more than minutes or hours away from dissatisfaction, as satisfaction cannot be stored and must be continually renewed."

In low stress, small pulses of dopamine from small surprises, natural pleasures, and the subtle pleasures of purpose and things turning out better than expected deliver satisfaction. A positive prediction error is when a cue predicts a reward that is more valuable than we expect. But, when a positive prediction error happens, it is surprising. Eating artificial food is not a multi-layered, ever-changing emotional experience like stroking the cheek of a loved one, watching fall leaves shimmer in the sunshine and float down in waves, or bumping into a friend unexpectedly and both being in awe that you met. Food is just, well, food.

Consuming sugary, fatty foods shows the same decline in rewarding effect with length of access, just like drugs of addiction – nicotine, cocaine, alcohol, cannabis, and heroin. Increasing quantities are needed to deliver the same level of dopamine, and withdrawal causes dissatisfaction, anxiety, fatigue, and depression, all because of a dopamine low that makes people feel lousy.

What is the role of the reward detection error or "reward error" in the already toxic milieu of the Stress Triangle that is aching for overconsumption? In contrast to the basic emotions present in low stress, the Survival Circuits are knee-jerk reactions to ensure coordinated engagement in behaviors and responses for survival. In contrast to the more subtle positive and negative emotion motivations of low stress, any time there is a greater-than-predicted reward, a dopamine surge follows that locks in the propensity to repeat that response.

According to Peter Sterling, the neuroscientist who coined the term allostasis and author of *What is Health? Allostasis and the Evolution of Human Design*, the tricky challenge of the reward-detection errors caused by the consumption of ultra-processed foods results in "foods of despair." They are legal, cheap, and ubiquitous, and unlike shooting up with street drugs, eating in the absence of hunger and pouring substances into our body that cause metabolic mayhem is socially acceptable. Also, food has so many crosscurrents of emotional deprivation, body shaming, and scarcity panic that changing how we eat with EBT becomes . . . perfect. We develop the motivation to become wizards at processing stress and magicians at activating internal dopamine surges. If we can do that, we can do anything.

I checked with Charlotte about whether the Reward Glitch was relevant to her.

She said, "I sit there in my chair in my television room with my dog Raymond on my lap. Next to me is a bag of tootsie rolls. I watch television, play video games, and eat."

"What does that mean to you?"

"I am an extrinsic dopamine consumer. This definitely rings true for me."

"Super. After you clear the stress, your brain becomes more powerful because it is not chronically doused in cortisol. A bit of your EBT journey will be creating more natural joy in your life."

Then Charlotte laughed, "That scares me to death. What if I am not capable of joy?"

"Are you kidding me? You're already on your way. You've laughed more in the last 30 minutes than I have."

She smiled and said, "You're right."

Stress Triangle 3. The Habit Glitch

The last of the three glitches is the metabolic adaptation error or habit glitch. It is stored in the hypothalamus, which is the grand controller that manages hunger, thirst, fatigue, sleep, and basic bodily functions – our habits. It's the area of the brain with the errors we target in EBT.

The Habit Glitch is the simplest one of the three to rewire because it has widespread impact. It is the center of the starvation response, the culmination of the chemical dysregulation that the Stress Center and the Reward Center initiate. It activates a starvation response, which is why dieters feel so lousy. We have lethargy, lower resting energy levels, fewer spontaneous movements, chronic hunger, and weight gain. We're literally starving, even if we are gaining weight.

This error is rooted in the overall permissiveness of our genes, that the brain can adapt to anything. For example, the brain will adapt to our eating ultra-processed foods, resetting our biochemistry to expect it, but here is the bad news – we are then at risk of mental health problems, cancer, obesity, metabolic diseases, and more. When we decide to change habits, the hypothalamus laughs at us. Good luck! It likes the status quo, which makes habit change so difficult.

The habit glitch completes the story of the Stress Triangle. Not only is the message that I get my "X" from "Y" expressing the use of external artificial rewards of pleasure and then activating it as a survival imperative, but even when we find that there is a price to pay, we do not care. The habit center is that powerful. It will write off severe physical and mental health problems as not important, and make it very difficult to change our habits.

The Habit Glitch

I have a strong biochemical drive to meet my need for_____
(e.g., safety, love, existence, power, protection, or comfort)
and disconnect from myself and connect to
something that does not meet my real need but gives me an abnormal
dopamine high that is addictive,
even though it harms my health and blocks my joy.

Example:

I get my safety from food
and escaping my reality with a false high
even though it gives me a food hangover, adds belly fat,
increases my blood pressure, and decreases my joy.

Although these "metabolic adaptation errors," or habit errors, are daunting, the purpose of the 1-2-3 JOY approach is to use neuroscience to outsmart these errors and make habit change easier. The critical factor here is joy. The activation of the nucleus accumbens swamps stress, so we can overcome these wires and change our habits consistently enough to reset the hypothalamus to new habits that it then protects. That takes time and persistence, which is why lasting change, the goal of EBT, requires intervening for one year.

Adding the Habit Glitch to an expectation completes the story of why bypassing the emotional brain and not addressing the errors in the Stress Triangle has led to an obesity epidemic.

I told Charlotte that trying to stop overeating and release weight without the 1-2-3 JOY approach is called suffering, and we don't do suffering in EBT.

Charlotte said, "If I put it together, I would say I get my existence from stuffing myself with food to stop worrying, even though it doesn't work, and even if I get diabetes, depression, and zero out my joy."

"Can you now feel compassion for yourself?"

She said, "I have tears in my eyes. I understand why it has been so phenomenally impossible for me to lose weight."

"And do you feel compassion for yourself?"

Charlotte said, "Yes, I do feel compassion for myself, and I have hope."

How can we optimize the Triangle?

The above series of explanations of the three brain areas and their glitches puts into words the impact of all three errors caused by the clashing of modern life with our hunter-gatherer genes. As described by Michele Meitus-Snyder and Robert Lustig in their seminal article and summarized in Chapter 3, for scalable public health and clinical and self-care treatment of the biochemical consequences of the triangle's "conspiracy," we need the power of words.

Treating biochemistry alone would require a handful of pharmaceuticals, each with its own negative side effects and drug interactions, risks of dependency, and missed opportunities to address the root cause of obesity. The root cause is emotional bypass, as thoughts cannot overcome chronic stress at or near the fight-or-flight level most people face in daily life now.

Without engaging the emotional brain and harnessing its natural, universal powers to quickly and reliably switch off the stress response, threat protection errors (Stress Glitches), reward detection errors (Reward Glitches), and metabolic adaptation errors (Habit Glitches), wreak havoc on our physical and mental health. The most widespread impacts of these glitches are obesity and metabolic disease in the realm of physical health, and anxiety and depression in mental health.

We need words to treat the glitches in the triangle to target not just the array of biochemical perturbations caused by that triangle spinning out of control, but also to use self-directed, targeted positive neuroplasticity to reconsolidate the circuits that cause them.

Spiraling up rapidly performs the primary intervention needed, which is a way to clear stress and reset the prefrontal cortex to carry out executive functions effectively. With the thinking brain functional, spiraling up accomplishes the secondary intervention required – processing the circuit so that the unconscious errant expectation stored in the emotional brain becomes clear and can be verified by the conscious mind. Once verified, the now highly functional thinking brain can juxtapose the words of the glitch with orthogonal words ("adaptive opposites") to switch off the circuit for immediate benefits and repeatedly present that opposite expectation to the emotional brain to rewire it for lasting results.

As Stress Glitches are reconsolidated over time by this process, sustained improvements in prefrontal cortex functioning due to a rise in set point enable the fixing of both the Reward Glitch and Habit Glitch and the further rise in the set point from an allostatic state to a homeostatic state. Instead of the default state of the brain being allostatic (wired at Set Point 3, 4, or 5), the goal of treatment is a homeostatic set point of 1 or 2, and optimally, Set Point 1. Rather than being wired for stress, the goal is to be wired for joy.

The "fixing part" of the method is vigorous. Essentially, we only rewire one glitch at a time, and if you find one, you always choose if you want to "put it on the shelf" or crush it now. There is no in-between, as that does not work. These are nasty, primitive, determined wires, and they only succumb to dismantling by an equally determined, highly effective prefrontal cortex that won't stop hitting the circuit until it has been busted open, smashed, and broken. Only then will that wire stop terrorizing us. Then the new elegant and healing circuit takes us up and over to joy and freedom. Reconsolidating a circuit takes skill and passion, accurately seeing both ourselves and the circuit.

The above explanations of the three brain areas and their glitches put into words are a prelude to the actual techniques used to rewire the Triangle. The words you will use to break these faulty wires will be far simpler than the above. The unreasonable expectations that are up for rewiring are exceedingly diverse, yet the new words that will replace them are remarkably similar.

Mirroring the opening of Leo Tolstoy's novel, *Anna Karenina*, "All happy families are alike; each unhappy family is unhappy in its own way," the adaptive wires, the "glitch fixes," are expressions of what evolutionary biology has in mind for us, that is, optimal physiology. Interestingly, the emotional brain is our psychological organ, and the new words reflect secure attachment, the hallmark of psychosocial development. Last, as the emotional brain is the seat of the soul, the messages of these fixes are in harmony with the essence of spirituality, connecting to something accessible within us that is sacred and good. They convey that not only can we feel joy, but our true, natural essence IS joy.

Fix the Glitch

I have a strong biochemical drive to meet my need for (e.g., safety, love, existence, power, protection, or comfort) by connecting with myself to get a natural dopamine high that is non-addictive, to live in a way that improves my health, and to bring myself joy.

Example:
I get my safety from connecting to the deepest part of myself, eating healthy, and creating joy in my life.

The simplicity of the fix for these maladaptive Stress Circuits is that instead of seeking an external solution, we train our brain for an internal one. Connecting within is the solution. That phrase, "connect to the deepest part of myself," came from EBT Master Trainer Dr. David Ingebritsen, and conveys connecting to our spiritual core, so we can both transcend our bodies and have optimal physiology in our bodies, achieving unity from within.

I asked Charlotte, "Can you imagine that by activating an old food wire to unlock the connections between its neurons and stating repeatedly that you meet that need by connecting to the deepest part of yourself, not to food, you will experience such a chemical shift that you leave food on your plate effortlessly?"

She said, "Not really, but I'm willing to try it."

That was a success. If she used the tools, her drives would change, and she would prove to herself that she had the power to change her brain.

I asked, "What's the most important thing you learned today?"

Charlotte said, "That EBT is based on science, and I'm at the forefront of a new movement in which people change their own wiring. Also, I don't have to force myself to change, but focus on changing my wires and my habits will change automatically. I like that and I want to get going. I want to start fixing my glitches."

"You do?"

"Yes, I do, and I am getting the idea that this could be fun."

I said, "If it is not fun, it's not EBT."

Charlotte laughed, and so did I.

Once Charlotte rewired her first circuit, she would feel even more secure that she had a new approach to life. By her third or fourth rewire, she would trust the tools and start having fun rewiring her own brain.

EBT is not fun like blowing bubbles, but it is immediately rewarding, instantly riveting, and something that brings out the kid in us. When I encoded my Food Circuit I was 11 years old. I had to activate the circuit to rewire it, which took me back to my reality at that age. I could see the kitchen table of my youth. I could hear my mother vacuuming in the back bedroom and smell the thick white frosting on the cinnamon rolls. At that moment, I got to be 11 years old again! That is beyond science fiction: it is science – and that is fun.

Although not all memories are initially happy memories, they can all become positive and rewarding. This is partly because, as EBTers, we have the protective shield of the skills to spiral up so we are safe. No matter what comes our way, we can weather the storm and reliably guide ourselves out of Brain State 5 and into at least a sturdy, if not glorious, Brain State 1. Moreover, in several decades of coaching participants in their deep Cycles, I have never experienced anyone not being in awe when they activate a circuit and discover its previously hidden message. They bring the unconscious message into the conscious mind, delivering aha moments and the joy of self-knowledge.

Even more, once learned, EBT becomes an ongoing practice, and awareness of our choice to continually deepen self-knowledge can bring a sense of security. No matter our future circumstances, we will never be bored and can always self-generate dopamine pulses and endorphin blasts based on our inner journey.

This step-by-step pathway to transforming our glitches into new wires that raise our set point is The EBT 1-2-3 JOY Program. Let's look at the program and explore one special breakthrough moment in your EBT journey that changes everything . . .

5

Spiral Up: The EBT 1-2-3 JOY Program

As with any healing, gaining freedom from eating and weight issues is rooted in one emotion: love.

For some people, that love comes on gradually until one day they say to themselves, "Why am I making myself miserable about food?" or "I love myself, so why don't I love my body and take care of it?"

For others, that love awakening arrives in a burst, typically after a moment of despair. The emotional thrust of that moment can be indignation, which was the experience in my case. I was recovering after the birth of my youngest son, relieved that his arrival had gone so well, and adjusting to splitting my time between two children and work.

In many ways, it was one of the happiest times of my life. My daughter was magical, age two, with wisps of blonde hair and a drive to figure out the world and change it that she still has today. Joe was a happy baby, settling into life with an optimism and calmness that made the transition to being a family of four smoother. I was in a flow state with my work, developing the emotional tools, then called "the magic words," and my boss, Charlie Irwin, made it easy for me to take three months off for maternity leave.

One morning, I was curled up in bed, my daughter off to preschool, and my son sleeping peacefully in his bassinet. Yet, with numerous glitches firing from my amygdala, I found myself amid a rip-roaring body shaming session.

There was one new difference in this particular burst of self-denigration: I did not bypass my emotions. I was at Brain State 5, and the emotional blockade caused by that cortisol dump was raging, but like staying put on a bucking bronco, I somehow managed.

The toxic emotions, really vicious ones – self-hatred, body disgust, powerlessness, and shame – were front and center, but I stayed connected to them. Then, my mind went blank, and I felt empty. Normally, I would have gone to the kitchen to find something to eat. This time, I faced my emptiness. The word "spaciousness" came to mind, also love – and added to my surrender.

I knew at that moment that I was not willing to deprive myself of food anymore. I was more important than my food. What's more, my body shame was over. Instead, I would eat when I was hungry and find the right weight for me, whatever that was.

From then on, it was easy. I released the weight out of self-love, rewired a few more gnarly circuits, and was on my way to raising my set point. The only adjustments I would make in my experience, if I were to redo it today, would be giving myself a triple dose of the "clear the clutter" work of the method. That's not just discovering the glitch and changing the expectation but burrowing down to the tangle of fear memories and trauma circuits at the core.

Until the clutter is cleared, the brain easily reinstates old wires as a reminder that until we unpack the suppressed emotions from the past, they never really stop haunting us. Each spiral up is directed at trauma and clearing it creates wisdom not accessible any other way. It's best to dig a little deeper, do a few more Travel Backs to more fully grieve the losses, and know and love who you are – imperfections, quirks, and all.

That natural process of spiraling up until the drive to overeat fades and the joy of releasing weight ramps up is at the heart of the EBT Program. Just move through the courses, and throughout the many spiral ups of a daily EBT Practice, be in joyful anticipation. Watch for the moment when you have such a clearing of stress wires that you get excited about being a little hungry. You get upset because someone put too much food on your plate – you don't want it. Or you eat half your lunch and notice you are done. The joy of releasing extra weight has kicked in, and weight loss will be easy and even a joy from then on.

Now in its 4th iteration, The EBT 1-2-3 JOY Program has three components that are designed to be completed in order.

EBT Essentials: Learn How to Spiral Up

Like any project, our first need is to acquire a new mindset and essential tools. The first course in The EBT 1-2-3 JOY Program helps you shift to the new paradigm in which there are no problems in life, just circuits, and the circuits change by using emotions in a novel way: spiraling up. You learn how to use the three spiral-up options to clear chronic stress and make small but important circuit improvements. This course, EBT Essentials, takes about one month and gives you time to drop into a couple of Spiral Up Groups a week to hear the skills in action or, if you choose, to be coached through spiraling up by an EBT Provider. A gentle start is good, as we don't want to scare the amygdala. It likes comfortable changes, especially at first.

How to Rewire: Clear 4 Major Circuits

After about a month, the glitches start calling to you. Sure, we are spiraling up, but the Big 4 Circuits that control eating and weight don't move. They are deeper in the brain and coactivate with other wires, so they take more skill to rewire but yield far more benefits than the simple spiral up. You know you have rewiring success when the drive for that response stops. Changing the behavior is not the strategy. Rewiring the circuit that drives it is, and when that occurs, changes in your behavior are natural and more lasting.

It's essential to rewire all of the Big 4 Circuits until you see spontaneous, easy changes in your behavior for food, mood, relationships, and body. By clearing them now, the third component of the program becomes far more rewarding, and the changes come more rapidly. Most people take one to two months to finish this process, but it takes as long as it takes because by thoroughly "breaking" these circuits, you open up pathways to making profound changes in your life.

Advanced EBT: Raise Your Set Point

There are seven 30-day advanced courses in the program, one for each of the seven rewards and the seven Core Circuits. These courses focus on creating an acquired secure attachment, encoding every basic wire we hope we had encoded early in life. The courses give us a direct way to complete our own emotional evolution. The positive focus mirrors what the most comprehensive psychotherapy can bring, except you can do it with peers and do it for yourself.

The courses are completed in order because development requires that. First, you establish a safe place inside, a Sanctuary, and then add Authenticity. With both rewards strong, bring in more body pride and become healthy with a zest for life, Vibrancy. Then, enhance Integrity (healthy boundaries), and boost Intimacy, Spirituality, and Freedom.

Count on completing the program in one year. Keep your sense of humor. When you challenge those stubborn 5 Circuits that put the reptilian brain in charge, they will not be happy. They don't like you taking one year instead of 10 or even 20 to raise your set point. They particularly resent it when you clear a circuit and therefore threaten their preference to stay at your current set point. When you have rewired that circuit, are in a wave of rapture, and wonder if you aren't already at Set Point 1, the reptilian brain will throw a rage. It drops you into a pit of stress. That's when you laugh and say, "Oh, my inner reptile is ticked at me for transforming so much. I get that! It will pass."

Just pull back slightly but expect the reptile to try to convince you that you are back to square one. Wait it out, as after the 5 comes the 1. All you have to do is stay connected to the love inside you, even imperfectly, and magic happens. Within 24 hours of a real bruiser of a Brain State 5, having stayed present to your emotions rather than binge eating, numbing out with food, or departing your emotional reality in another way, doors will open. Out of nowhere, you will receive exactly what you need to move forward in your emotional evolution and make your dreams come true. I see it as the universe, the spiritual, or the planet rewarding us for our choice to connect deeply within.

Watch for some other strange dynamics, all in harmony with evolutionary biology, but still not logical. One is that the brain will only make you aware of circuits once it feels secure that your resiliency pathways are strong enough to overcome them. Our genes make healing feel safe. Next, after the rewiring is complete, notice that your Brain State 1 is enchanting but may be short-lived. Bliss can be far too boring according to your genetic code. Quite soon, notice that your mind travels to the excitement of the next circuit in the line-up that leads to being wired for joy. We lose interest in the old circuit.

Seeing the cleared wire is much like bumping into an old lover at a party. You say to yourself, "What did I see in them?" The love affair embedded in the survival drive is over, and the excitement is now about the new love – the next circuit.

This loss of interest in an erased wire was one of the most profound realizations of my years as an EBT Provider. I love helping participants dig down and discover a gnarly circuit blocking their joy, then having a "party" and clearing it. I didn't initially understand that they might not even mention it once it is cleared. Here I was so excited about their overcoming a circuit even though they typically cleared the wire between sessions, so it was old news by the next session. They were already falling in love with rewiring the next circuit.

I get so much energy from teaching Precision EBT to participants, the skills learned in How to Rewire, and seeing them discover their own power to transform their lives. Lily was ridiculed for her body and mocked for being fat by her mother, who favored Lily's slender and pretty younger sister. Lily came to EBT because she wanted to control her weight, but the real gift of EBT was something even more important. Lily was jubilant when she broke her wire but also amazed at the new life she was experiencing.

She said, "I came to EBT to have freedom from feeling as if I would die if I couldn't eat whatever I wanted to eat in whatever amounts I wanted. Now, I have that freedom, but the gift is much more amazing than that. I am experiencing life in a new way. I am a different person. I just picked my neighbor some flowers. I was on the phone with a very rude store clerk, and I felt compassion for them. Now I'm cleaning out my closets. I had no idea that my Food Circuit and Body Circuit were blocking me from being fully alive and in love with my own life."

Instead of trying to control overeating, we can focus on clearing the circuits that drive it. All that wasted energy stops, and not only can we break those faulty circuits but we raise our brain's set point. We start soaring, making magic in our life, and giving back to the world in just the way that makes our life complete.

You are raising your set point with 1-2-3 JOY

Move through the advanced courses rather quickly. Learn one skill each day as a personal practice. Day by day, you raise your set point, clear away the past, and discover who you are, what your life is about, and how you will fulfill your purpose.

This advanced training is essential based on what we know about neuroplasticity. Without raising our set point, traces of wires we have already rewired can remain in the brain and are more likely to be spontaneously reinstated. Also, the brain happily holds onto our set point in stress, giving us the illusion that we have changed by relinquishing one excess, only to transfer to using another. This can be a roadblock because solving problems seems to be a national pastime, as it is also addictive.

Given the negativity bias of the brain, it is so much fun to solve problems, but so time-consuming, expensive, and distracting that what really matters – our emotional and spiritual evolution – does not get the focused, intensive attention required for success. Instead, we delay or even miss the opportunity to do the work we came to Earth to do.

The goal of this program is for you to experience easy, natural, and lasting weight loss, and ultimately to have an abundance of all seven rewards of higher purpose. Right now, you may be flirting with EBT, or want to engage in it and work the program. It is not always easy to start EBT because it is a new paradigm, and it takes a while to get your head around the idea that the reality of life is the circuit that is activated at the moment – and that you have the power to control your circuits.

At first, your resiliency pathways may be narrow, or you might wonder if you can process emotions at all. That's normal, but even during the first month, you will become more resilient, and by rewiring the Big 4 Circuits, even more so. After you wire in all seven rewards, your brain will become spontaneously resilient most of the time. You will still go down to Brain State 5, and when you start doing a Cycle, you will need to complain and express a productive burst of anger to protest the hurt. However, almost immediately, you will feel gratitude and be at Brain State 1. You will have trained your brain for optimal resilience.

If you decide to move forward and start EBT, give yourself endless compassion. A sense of humor is essential (e.g., "Oh, my amygdala is throwing a fit today"). Then stay with it until you have completed the program and realize that you can say that you have an abundance of a purposeful life's seven rewards. Only then are you truly stress-protected with a lasting solution for life.

1 2 3 JOY!

Step 1: Clear Stress

6

Your Stress Center: Fall in Love with Your Amygdala

No one ever taught me I had an amygdala, much less to fall in love with it. However, to control the quality of your life, health, and longevity, centering your affection on that brain structure is a perfect start.

The amygdala warrants that affection because it stores our memories. Right now, I'm bringing to mind being on a beach in Hawaii, our whole family watching the blazing, yellow sunset in awe. That awe is the product of the activation of the amygdala.

This almond-shaped structure is so intimately connected to all other structures that we "feel" that memory throughout our entire body. It receives inputs from the thalamus, prefrontal cortex, hippocampus, olfactory bulb, and more. Its outputs go to the vagus nerve, hypothalamus, ventral striatum, prefrontal cortex, and other areas.

Falling in love . . . with limits

In calmer times (Brain States 1 and 2), the prefrontal cortex manages the amygdala and resolves the chaos, switching off negative memories quite easily. Yet, I could be on that beautiful beach, feeling completely in control of myself, when one of those little, brown geckos might climb onto my foot, and my amygdala would go crazy, instantly hijacking my thinking brain.

The role of EBT is to give us a way to recover control faster, and to get into the habit of switching off the amygdala at will and quickly. The payoff for this is huge because trauma circuits in the amygdala can sensitize it to stress, so overreactions are frequent and the set point declines.

More specifically, there is a tug of war between the thinking brain and amygdala. A goal of EBT is for the pathway from the thinking brain (PFC) to the amygdala to be dominant over the amygdala in the emotional brain. We are training the brain so that when a craving, overreaction, or fear memory crops up, the PFC's direct neural route to switch off the amygdala dominates, and based on both conscious control, and, in time unconscious control, deactivates negative memories and unwanted drives.

Dominance of the Thinking Brain Over the Amygdala

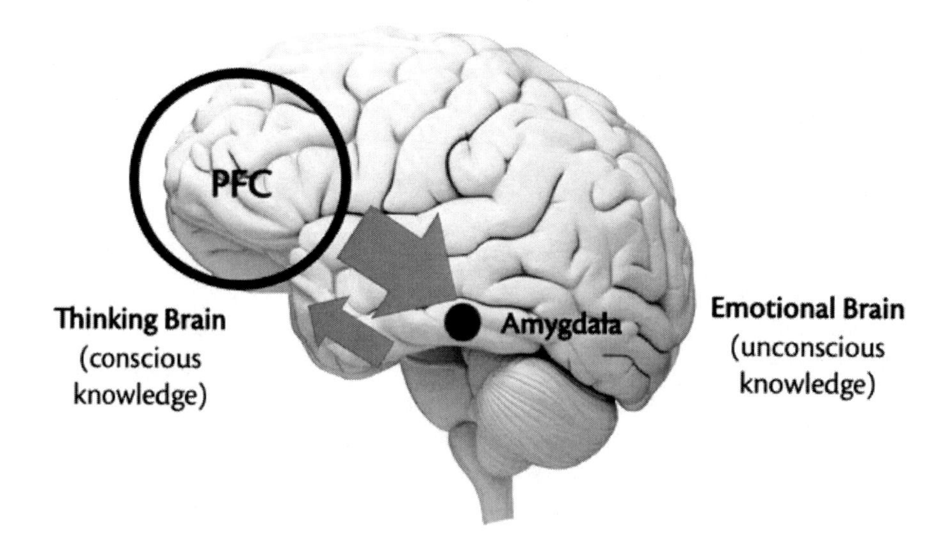

The average adult human brain can accumulate the equivalent of 2.5 million gigabytes of memory. However, the #1 job of the central nervous system is survival, as orchestrated by the stress response, the circuits in the amygdala fall into two categories. One is effective and promotes homeostasis, leading to joy, and the other is ineffective, engendering allostasis and leading to stress. Everybody has both. The health strategy in EBT is to notice when you are not in joy, recognizing that a Stress Circuit is the problem. What happens? Quite naturally, a Joy Circuit takes charge, and spirals you up to Brain State 1.

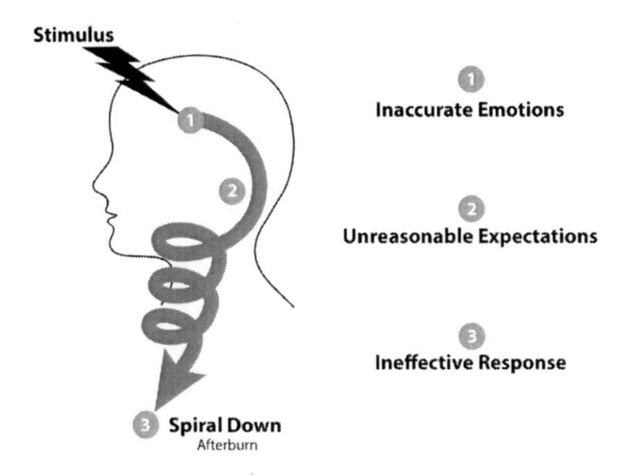

The anatomy of a circuit

All neuronal Stress Circuits have three phases, and you can track each one by the sensations in your body.

The first phase (#1) is a quick subcortical processing, which is a response of the Sympathetic-Adrenal-Medullary (SAM) Axis, with its immediate sympathetic activation to fight, flee, or freeze, releasing catecholamines such as epinephrine and norepinephrine. The Hypothalamic-Pituitary (HPA) Axis adds to this response with its rapid release of stress chemicals that tell the adrenal glands to produce cortisol. The associated sensations and emotions we experience range from calmness to terror.

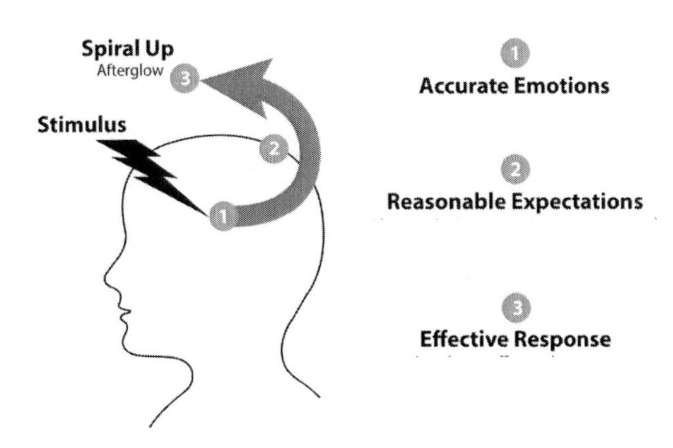

The next phase (#2) is the release of emotions from the messages embedded in the circuit, which are accompanied by biochemical drives to follow their directions. These emotional messages bubble up to the conscious mind as expectations that we believe are accurate. These feelings are generated by past experiences stored in the specific wire that the amygdala happens to activate.

The last phase (#3) is when the circuit generates thoughts and drives to take corrective action to meet a perceived need. The emotions and sensations are based on the wire generated, which varies considerably.

According to psychiatrist Bruce Perry, senior fellow of the Child Trauma Academy in Houston, Texas, and an adjunct professor at the Feinberg School of Medicine in Chicago, responses vary from either hyperarousal to dissociation. The hyperarousal continuum corresponding to Brain States 1 to 5 are rest, vigilance, resistance, defiance, and aggression. Dr. Perry points to headaches, stomachaches, light-headedness, and even fainting as signs of dissociation.

Spiral Up to Rewire Stress Circuits

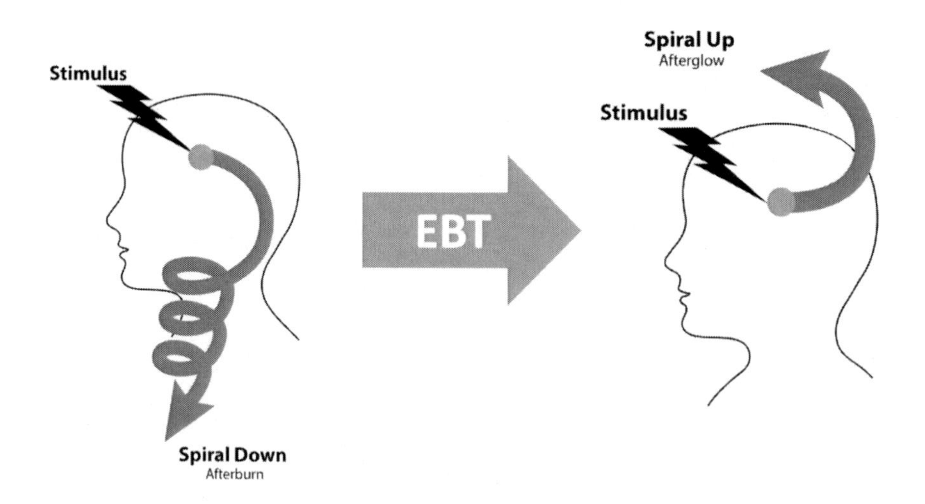

Afterglow or afterburn?

A Stress Circuit ("Glitch") spirals us down into allostasis. The ensuing emotional state includes an afterburn, bad feelings, and negative sensations in the body. As the wire has no shut-off valves, chronic stress is likely unless interrupted by distraction, external forces, or, best of all, spiraling up.

In contrast, when a homeostatic wire has been activated, it spirals us up, and the resulting emotional state is an afterglow of positive emotions and sensations. These wires have automatic shut-off valves, so they tend to flicker rather than become stuck, sustaining positive physiological states, emotions, thoughts, and behaviors.

Got the signal? Take immediate action

How do you manage your amygdala, even fall in love with it? Appreciate that it gives you immediate feedback. When you **feel good, savor it, prolong it, and extend it.**

Notice yourself spiraling down into stress? Do something about it, but first, just appreciate that you have received the signal. Your amygdala tells you to be vigilant that a fight, flight, or freeze response may be in the offing. Do not wait. Heed the call, reach for your app, and spiral up so you can identify and meet your needs.

Start your day by saying, "I am creating joy in my life." Then do it! Every time you notice that you are not in joy, say to yourself, "What's going on? Where did my joy go?"

You have natural resiliency pathways in your brain that evolutionary biology, the spiritual, or Planet Earth gave you. When there is a global stress pandemic that everyone is feeling, now is the time to use them,

Choose one of three pathways to spiral up and celebrate your beautiful emotional brain and the gift of life!

7

Spiral Up #1: Zap Cravings on the Spot

Kevin was a handsome, fun-loving restaurant owner with a big body and personality. He worked long hours, so his wife and three kids were used to him being away. Kevin loved good food and having a drink or two, sometimes three.

When the new weight-loss drugs came out, he decided to take a shot at using them, and they helped some. However, after four months, he was nauseated and only down 16 pounds. He decided to add on EBT to improve results and to counter the weight regain the physician told him to expect after going off the weight-loss drug.

Kevin was not happy when I told him to use the Instant Boost (also called the Cravings Zapper) skill to interrupt the stress response 10 times per day, the standard dose of EBT.

"I can do it during my off hours, but when I go to work, I leave my emotional brain at the door."

It's an adjustment for most people to be present to their brain state and connect with their emotions, so I wasn't surprised at his reaction.

Kevin responded, "It's an adjustment."

"I'm used to going flat out. That's the basis for my success."

"After you adjust, you'll probably say to me, 'I wished I'd learned EBT before. I would not have gained 50 pounds, wouldn't have needed the alcohol as much, and would have been far more successful at work.'"

"That could be, but I can't do it at work. What can I do? Tell people that I have to deal with my emotions, so please wait around? That I'll get back to them?"

"You do what physicians do between patients. They reach for their phone and tap through the app for one minute."

Spiral Up #1
Instant Boost
(Also called "Cravings Zapper")

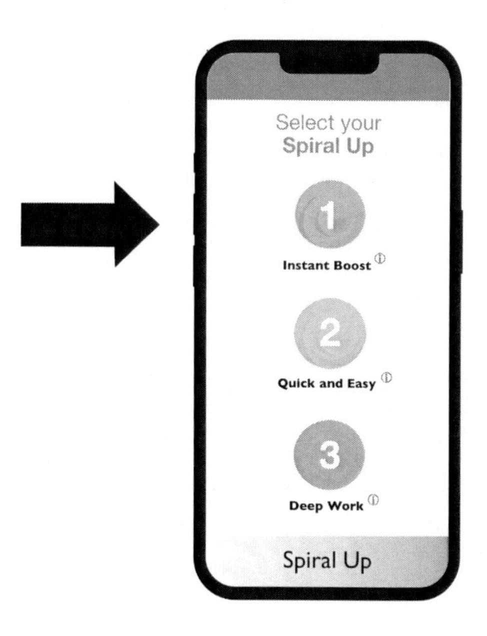

"I don't want to do that."

"You make it a habit to do it before you eat and whenever you are stressed."

Kevin said, "I do not want to do it."

"That's not a problem. Emotions are chemical. Your reluctance to do it is a circuit that spews stress chemicals. Those are allostatic or 'stress overload' emotions that hit us like a wall. Spiraling up tears down that wall."

He let out a big sigh.

"Kevin, getting started with EBT is the hardest thing. That's why, from the start, you need to identify your purpose for doing this. Everything is easy when you decide on a higher purpose. The brain starts spewing dopamine, which is the fun chemical."

"I told you. I want to lose weight. That is my purpose."

"How long have you wanted to lose weight?"

"Since I was 14."

"The brain demands a higher purpose."

"I want to lose weight because I'm tired of my physician telling me I am a candidate for a heart attack."

"You don't like listening to her say that, but weight loss is agony if you do it because you should. It's being aware of the deeper meaning of what you do that changes everything."

"What are my choices?"

"Sanctuary, which is to have peace and power from within. Also Authenticity, Vibrancy, Integrity, Intimacy, Spirituality, or Freedom."

Kevin chuckled, "I'll take them all."

"You will have them all when you complete the program, but which one motivates you the most now?"

"That would be Integrity. I have kids and a wife. I need to be there for them."

"Great, now I'll show you how to use this tool, and you can select a couple of Spiral Up Groups to drop into. Your brain will learn this best if you listen to others spiraling up. Later, you can teach your kids EBT for their stress. You and your wife can use it together. She can listen to you spiral up, and you can listen to her."

"Okay, I'm in."

Using Spiral Up #1: Instant Boost

The #1 pathway is your "go to" for EBT. Use it one to 10 minutes before you eat to calm your appetite. Feel completely satisfied on less food naturally. Use it between meals to ease stress and, most importantly, preventively. It takes only about a minute with practice and by creating a pattern of spiraling up throughout the day, you outsmart the reptilian brain's desire to keep the stress response stuck on. The trick is to pass through the pages quickly, not even feeling your feelings. Just make a blitz through the pages to feel far better in record time.

Move through the lead-ins on each page rapidly. Start by taking a deep breath. Put your shoulders back. Warmly observe yourself. Then, move through expressing eight feelings. Complete the sentence with whatever comes to your mind. It does not have to make any sense at all. Just blurt it out loud or say it silently in your mind. Your stress comes from suppressing your emotions, and your relief comes from expressing them. Use very few words, such as completing the lead-in "I feel sad that . . ." by saying something like, "I have so much to do." Brief is best.

There are four negative emotions (anger, sadness, fear, and guilt) and four positive emotions (gratitude, happiness, security, and pride).

The first four emotions clear the "emotional blockade." In stress, emotions stop doing their job of telling us what we need. Instead, they confuse us or tell us what we want (not what we need). No matter what the emotion (hostility, depression, anxiety, shame, numbness, or false highs), in EBT we use the same process to clear them. The blockade falls apart once we express anger, sadness, fear, and guilt. We're no longer stalled, but to soundly shut off the stress response, we must experience positive emotions.

There is only one lead-in that needs more of your attention. It is "I feel angry that . . ." Express it six to nine times. Expressing anger within this framework is very safe and highly productive. Anger releases stress faster than any other emotion and is the powerhouse of the spiral-up process.

After expressing anger and the other seven feelings, use the Take Action Tool. In just four taps, it clarifies how you will move forward with purpose and transcend the moment's challenges. That tool will keep you from backsliding into worrying about what you will do or over-analyzing your feelings. It is very powerful. You complete all spiral ups by planning how you will go forward.

Move forward with clarity and purpose

Often the plan to move forward is simple. For a spiral up about eating, it might be that I expect myself to eat healthy, or if eating healthy seems impossible to you, it might be that I expect to have compassion for myself. However, the lower the set point, the more likely you will miss learning procedures that make life easier, as having the prefrontal cortex available is essential for task learning. When you find yourself not overwhelmed but feeling a little lost about how to get something done, use this tool to lay out the process in an organized way. For example, I expect myself to spiral up to Brain State 1, and check if I am hungry or not. And if I am not hungry, I will not eat. If I am hungry, eat healthy foods, stopping short of feeling deprived. It's amazing how easy life becomes when you are at One and make an orderly plan responsive to who you are and what you need.

Always finish the Take Action Tool by facing the essential pain, the hard part, and being aware of the earned reward (higher purpose) in following through. This trains your brain to accept life's realities so you find everyday life much easier. The earned reward gives you a dopamine pulse to lock in your plan to move forward and reward you for doing it.

This tool is incredibly powerful. In giving a talk on EBT for the National Institute on Drug Abuse, one researcher who was familiar with EBT spoke up when I presented this skill, and said, "This is the most powerful anti-addiction tool I know of." How could that be? Using this tool requires that we see ourselves accurately, as the expectation must neither be permissive (too easy) nor abusive (too harsh). Then it gently guides us along with positive thoughts, helps us deal with life's realities, and finally rewards us in a way that furthers our emotional and spiritual evolution. Doesn't that sound like the perfect parent? We train our own brains to see, feel, hear, and love ourselves and be exceptionally effective in the world, to get stuff done. Life becomes so rewarding that we don't need food, drugs, alcohol, credit cards, gambling, or their substitutes as much. Our reward center, which had been hijacked by addictions, starts accessing pleasure again with small pulses of internally-sourced dopamine and health-promoting natural rewards rather than big blasts of externally-sourced dopamine that trapped us in addiction.

The emotional brain is the seat of the soul, and it has its own moral code. Give it a reward of just pleasure and comfort and it is not impressed. The dopamine surge is pathetic, not even worth registering. Prime this tool with an expectation that is challenging enough to nudge you to face a reality of life, thus boosting your resilience, and couple it with a reward of higher purpose. Robust but non-addictive surges of dopamine and endorphins guide you to follow through with your plans and experience an afterglow.

Once you have completed spiraling up, the app will prompt you to feel a robust surge of neurotransmitters. That fulfills multiple purposes. By checking for sensations in your body, like a tingle or a glow, your brain pairs spiraling up with immediate and meaningful rewards. This hastens the time when you reach for your app in joyful anticipation of your next reward surge and promotes automaticity – spiraling up effortlessly. Also, the prolongation of the dopamine surge supports locking in the wiring changes you made in your spiral up.

Last, honor what you just did. Say, "I spiraled up." Make that fun. You deserve it! Then you are done.

The easiest way to become proficient at EBT is to do it well right from the start. The first three times you use the app, from the Spiral Up page tap on the informational "i" button and read how to execute the lead-in on that page. These skills are stored in the unconscious mind, the "survival brain," and if you learn them without precision, it is challenging to unlearn the imprecise way and learn the ways that work.

For each of the three spiral-up pathways, when first learning one, use only that skill for three days. You'll learn EBT much faster! Start with Spiral Up #1. Give your brain a chance to create "tracks" of resilience so the pathways work more efficiently and faster. Then go on to Spiral Up #2, then Spiral Up #3. Your resiliency pathways will start becoming stronger. They may start out as paths that are bumpy, but they will soon become four-lane superhighways. Participants who have completed The EBT 1-2-3 JOY Program often say that the tools have become automatic, and situations that aggravated them before don't bother them a bit. That is the resiliency superhighways in action, which is just what we want. Keep it fun, spiral up often, and start making it automatic.

Spiral Up #1 is also called the Cravings Zapper because you use it before you eat, even if you are not experiencing a craving but instead preventing one. It is the best tool to use before

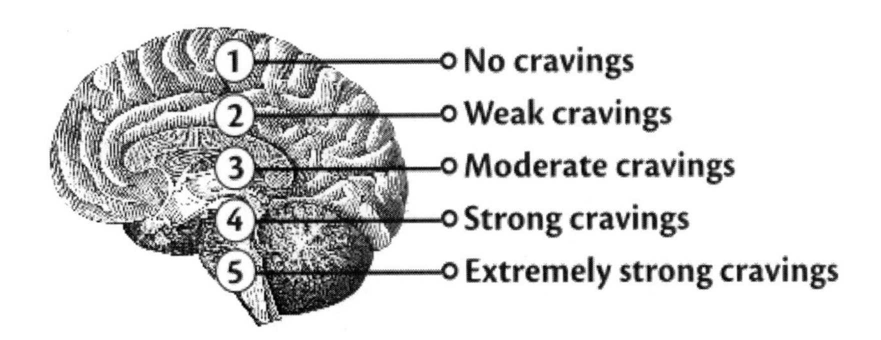

eating because it is so easy. Stress can increase in anticipation of eating, so making it a habit to use a quick, straightforward, and very reliable tool will decrease your drive to overeat earlier in the training. We also call it the Instant Boost. Use Spiral Up #1 throughout the day whenever you are not in joy and want a quick way to release your stress.

Making it easy

The emotional brain is stubborn and only changes when we deliver a very simple, consistent intervention. Do this 10 times per day and always before eating. After using it, do not hold yourself accountable for changing how you eat. Instead, be consistent with the practice of spiraling up. Over time, that changes your biochemistry, so you will spontaneously change how you eat.

Kevin had some concerns.

He said, "I don't want to use it before eating because it could make me stop overeating. I need a lot of food. I don't want my 'rations' cut!"

"Kevin, nobody is going to cut your rations. You need more food now because your Stress Triangle has been spinning out of control. Once those chemicals calm down, you'll feel completely satisfied eating less."

"The weight-loss drugs have decreased my hunger, but I'm still drinking, and I still eat a lot of chips, cookies, and candy."

"My job is to help you crush that food wire that has been living inside you since . . ."

"Age 14."

Kevin liked thinking of his eating in terms of biochemistry, so I told him, "When you get your cortisol and insulin down and your dopamine balanced, it will be easier to eat healthy naturally."

"But I tend to start something, then I drop the ball and quit."

"Are you going to quit this?"

Kevin said, "Hmmmm. I don't think so, that is if it works. But I don't see how expressing eight feelings is going to stop the appetites I have."

"Assess it for yourself. Cravings are driven by biochemistry. When you're excited about eating, say you are at your restaurant, and you're anticipating eating, what brain state are you in?"

Kevin said, "I'm at Brain State 1."

"So, you are in complete control. No cravings. No worry that you may start eating and not be able to stop."

"No . . . I'm more like Brain State 3."

I responded, "That would be moderate cravings. What if you could change your biochemistry so you went to Brain State 1 and didn't have cravings? You would savor and enjoy your food and be in complete control."

Kevin said, "I've never felt in control of my food. Never."

"You have been trying to control your behavior. Instead, control your biochemistry. Start earlier in the process. If you wait until the urge is strong, the thinking brain is offline, and it is virtually impossible to stop yourself from getting that food. It never worked for me. Instead, switch your brain state just before you eat. Even if you overeat anyway the first few times you use it, you're establishing a habit that will have a profound impact over time."

Kevin said, "Okay, I'll do it!"

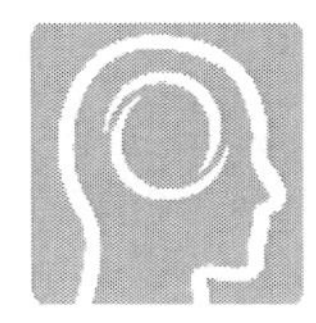

8

Spiral Up #2: Create Joy Anytime, Anywhere

I was worried about Jessica. Her situation with three children brought up the circuits I had of my years as a single mother of three. I felt her exhaustion and my own sadness that the days of cuddling up in bed reading my children *Noisy Nora, Good Night Moon*, and more had passed.

The fact that she was creating joy in her own life meant that she was encoding those spiral up Joy Circuits in her own brain that she would transmit to her children. For parents, EBT is the ultimate two-for-one: deal with your stress and transmit wires that create joy to your children.

At our next coaching session, Jessica had worked up to 10 spiral ups per day with Spiral Up #1 and was ready for more.

I started by asking her, "How can I help?"

"It was a little irritating because sometimes I forgot to spiral up, so I set notifications. All in all, I'm a happier person. It may have impacted my eating, because I left half my sandwich on my plate yesterday. I didn't want it anymore, which is strange for me. I *always* eat every last thing on my plate."

"The best news is that you have made the paradigm shift. You're not restricting your food, but instead powering in on those circuits so that clean-plate drive fades."

"I have three apps for tracking my food, and I don't use any of them."

"Excellent. You can't force behavior change and pound away at spiraling up at the same time. That switch is essential."

Jessica would have recurrences of that drive to control her behavior, but eating is the tail end of a fight-or-flight circuit, and trying to control food is like trying to control a dog by pulling on its tail. It takes a lot of energy and doesn't really get the job done.

"What we're looking for here is Freedom, and just think, if you forced yourself to change your food behavior, you could be successful, but you'd never know if you had rewired the circuit.

You need evidence of rewiring, and that only comes when you notice spontaneous changes that are easy and natural. You're on the right track."

Jessica had yet to learn to use the full set of EBT tools (Spiral Up #2) and had yet to take the How to Rewire course, so her brain was still storing the four big circuits that drive overeating and weight gain.

"Two things bother me. One is that Jeremy had a very bad day at school earlier in the week, and I used Spiral Up #1, but I was still a little stressed when I was done. Also, sometimes I don't quite get to Brain State 1."

"I think you're ready for Spiral Up #2."

Spiral Up #2
Quick & Easy

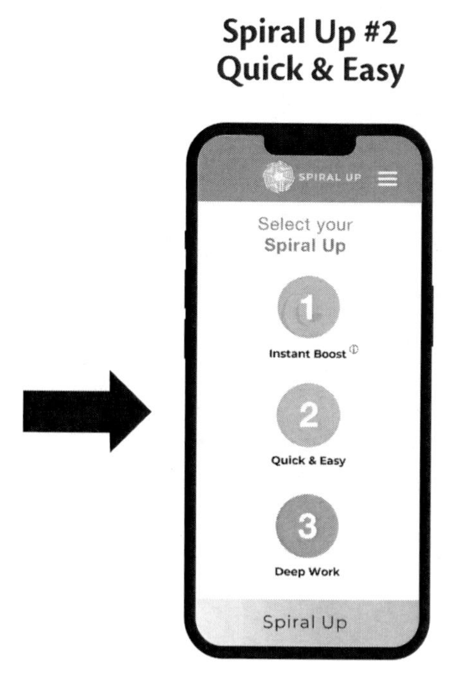

Using Spiral Up #2: Quick & Easy

What I love most about Spiral Up #1 is it is fast. You don't have to feel. You just tap through the pages. You switch off the stress response 10 times per day and all you do is read each lead-in that appears on each page of the app and say what comes to mind.

Spiral Up #2 takes more time, about two minutes, but delivers all five distinct resiliency pathways in the brain. The first few pages guide you through the standard check-in process, which is all physiologically impactful. They are: take a deep breath (diaphragmatic breathing), shoulders back, also called "Body at One" (proprioceptive posturing), and warmly observe yourself (decentering).

After that, you ask, "What's My Number?"

Five options give you enormous power to control the circuits in your amygdala that control your Stress Triangle and entire physiology.

The most immediate benefit of Spiral Up #2 is that you can tap on a number and be escorted through the state-specific resiliency pathway in the brain, ending up (most of the time) at Brain State 1. If you do not arrive at Brain State 1, that's not a problem because you can circle around and use another tool until you land in that state of supreme safety and reward.

You cannot go wrong by having access to all five skills, so you do not have to worry if you cannot identify your brain state. Just guess your brain state and follow along with the corresponding tool. Don't try too hard. Let the tools do the work for you. If it doesn't take you to Brain State 1, you try another tool until you get there.

As these resiliency pathways are evolutionarily based, the goal is always to stick with it, use as many tools as needed, and not quit. Do not stop until you feel the glow of Brain State 1. As a parent, you wouldn't see your stressed-out infant on the floor feeling awful, connect with them, start them along the emotional road to joy, but then drop them off when they are still cranky or sad. EBT is rewiring our earliest interactions with those who raised us. Even if they quit before we were in joy, we don't have to do that now. We can stay connected with ourselves until the job is done, which means we are at Brain State 1.

The reason for this persistence, other than the immediate gratification of selecting your brain state and using the state-specific resiliency pathway to get to One, is twofold. Both pertain to the impact of state-specific memory, the tendency for the stress level to activate other wires at the same level.

Spiral Up #2
The EBT 5-Point System

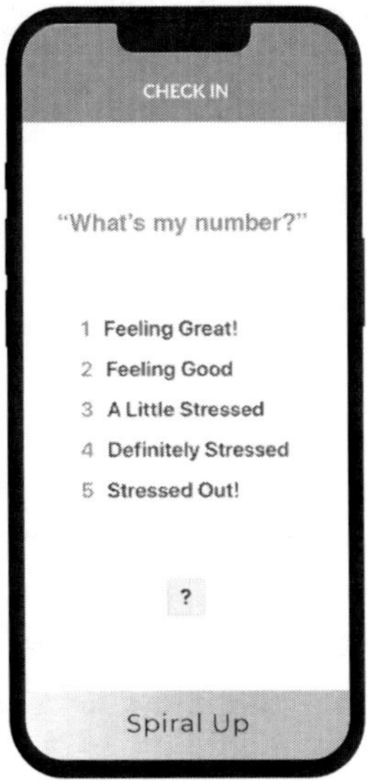

First, when you identify your starting number and, after spiraling up, the number at which you conclude, you have been under the control of two different wires. However, each wire has a forefield and a backfield. The forefield is the strong, direct emotion and whatever message it delivers, such as I get my safety from eating whatever I want, with a drive to find food. The backfield is the experience of the activation of legions of circuits encoded in the same brain state that are also prone to activation, creating a shimmering, multi-layered experience.

Having this backfield of the circuit to contend with is a definite plus-minus. The combination of the wire and its backfield impact on you has powerful impacts on your perception of life as it amplifies the reward of spiraling up many times a day when you are not in joy. The homeostatic Joy Circuit brings on happy, healthy, positive activations, while the allostatic Stress Circuit delivers sad, unhealthy, and negative activations. This is why we can ride the wave of the homeostatic circuit and "spiral up." We don't need to know where all those happy chemicals come from to enjoy them. But, that wave crashes when the circuit is allostatic and spirals us down into the wasteland of human misery. Which would you choose?

This is a neuroscience explanation of why to avoid what is referred to in the addiction community as addiction geographical, that is, changing your location and circumstances instead of changing your addiction wires and brain. We bring our circuits and our set point with us wherever we go.

For example, I live across the street from the grammar school that my three children attended. If I am at Brain State 1 and gaze across the street all these years later, I feel uplifted. All these unconscious wires are flashing images of my happy children enjoying the playground, and my dopamine and endorphins are flowing. If I am at Brain State 5, I don't see the school. I just see the sewer line and the busted wooden fence, and a wave of sadness – strike that – depression comes over me, how did my children have the audacity to grow up and not need me anymore? I cannot control my unconscious mind to clear those Brain State 5 backfields quickly unless I process my emotions.

Second, we all have a lot of clutter. It's the norm in modern life because of the speed of change, information overload, and an increasingly stressed, therefore polarized and extreme, world. Both eating and body size are controlled by our brain state. We eat and weigh precisely what our emotional brain tells us is safe and rewarding. It's not logical but physiological, and the way we control our physiologic brain state and the message of our wires is to spiral up.

The modern way to care for our emotional and physical health is to institute the practice of spiraling up as the foundation for how we live our lives. Hmmmmm, I'm not at One? Then spiral up, because it all adds up in the end. We each have a finite number of Stress Circuits that we need to activate and transform into Joy Circuits. We keep clearing clutter until the dominant circuits in the brain are Joy Circuits, and then something magical occurs. It all adds up, spiral up by spiral up, until the brain experiences the "emergent effect." The brain begins smashing the Stress Circuits more naturally, as if it shrugs and says, "Okay, I get it. The dominant state is going to be homeostatic. I can live with that."

Participants report this experience toward the end of the program when the brain has trained itself to rely on sustainable dopamine and endorphin surges from higher purpose and natural pleasures more consistently. They have far more energy to go out into the world and give back in just the way that makes their life complete and creates many new learning opportunities. What is the result? You will never be bored again, and you will be apt to live your life without judgment, with a warm heart and the abiding glow of purpose.

Learn to use Pathway #2 well from the start, as once your brain uses it ineffectively, it is hard to change. As with Pathway #1, the first three times you use the app, tap on the "i" button and read how to use each skill. You will learn more in The EBT 1-2-3 JOY Program, but this will get you off to a good start. You have a full set of skills. Spiral Up #1 is the simplest version of the 4 Tool. You just use it really quickly to stop cravings and for an instant boost. Spiral Up #3 is a deep dive into the two 4 Tools that rewire trauma, using them more effectively than in Spiral Up #2.

The 5 basic tools: Resiliency on demand

When you tap on Brain State 1, Feeling Great, the Compassion Tool will be at your fingertips. Feel compassion for yourself, others, and all living beings.

When you tap on Brain State 2, Feeling Good, the Feelings Tool will open up, and you can check how you feel, what you need, and whether you need support from others.

Spiral Up #2
Brain State 4
3 Variations of the Cycle Tool

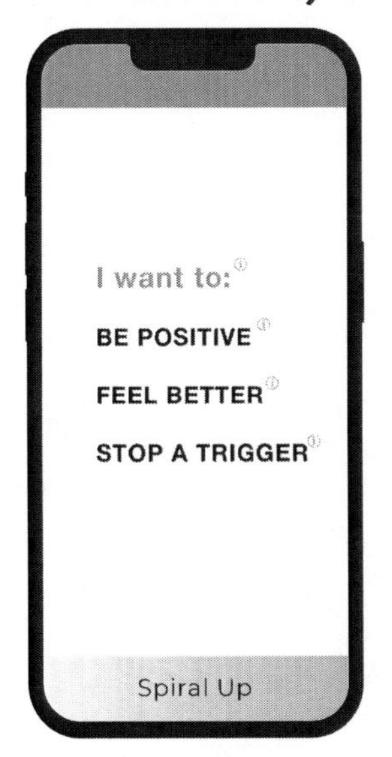

Brain State 3, A Little Stressed, leads you to the Flow Tool. The allostatic emotions are starting to create an emotional blockade. Don't let it continue. Instead, quickly tease apart the scattered feelings, where you are anxious and start overthinking. Use the Flow Tool to express anger, sadness, fear, and guilt, and then gratitude, happiness, security, and pride. Stop the glitch before it settles in!

Brain State 4, Definitely Stressed, brings you access to the Cycle Tool. It is the most powerful state and tool for self-directed, positive emotional neuroplasticity. The prefrontal cortex is online enough, given the boost of the EBT tools, to stay focused and rewire circuits, but the brain is in enough of a stressed state to activate trauma circuits.

There are three options for Brain State 4. One is the Be Positive Tool for situational stress (the same as in Spiral Up #1, except you feel and focus on your feelings). Another is the Feel Better Tool to switch off Core Circuits, and the last is the Stop A Trigger Tool to clear Survival Circuits. You'll spend a lot of time touching on the Brain State 4 tool as it gives a powerful burst of dopamine and the benefit of rewiring.

Brain State 5 is a full-blown stress response. The skill is the Damage Control Tool, which quiets the amygdala. Use it alone, or after making additional passes through it, use one or more additional tools until you find yourself at Brain State 1.

Becoming comfortable with all 5 tools

"Jessica, two things were bothering you when we started the session."

"That's right. One, what do I do when the Spiral Up #1 doesn't bring me to Brain State 1?"

I said, "Switch over to Spiral Up #2, so you have all the tools to choose from. Often, if the 4 Tool does not work, It's because we are at Brain State 5. Use the Brain State 5 Tool!"

This is a major wake-up call for most new EBTers. If we are in a full-blown stress response, our thinking brain cannot focus attention on emotions for long enough to spiral up. The best bet is to use the 5 Tool first, and then keep using the tools until you are at Brain State 1.

Jessica said, "I can do that!"

The brain changes with repetition, so I recommended that she use only Spiral Up #2 for three days. This is "Precision EBT," a natural form of brain surgery. It is best for her to learn it well, so I suggested she drop in for two Spiral Up Groups a week so she could learn this skill by experiencing it in action.

Jessica was using the tools before eating, and a total of 10 times per day, not judging herself when she forgot. I reminded her that the more consistent she is, the better her results will be.

Although persistence and consistency are essential, perfectionism and rushing cause suffering. The point is not for her brain to be "superglued" at Brain State 1, but to change her relationship with herself. For example, if she consistently sticks with 10 spiral ups per day, she'll be rewarded with a rise in her set point, but her amygdala will activate 5 Circuits because it doesn't like change, and they will put her reptilian brain in charge. She will probably hang out at Brain State 5 for a bit.

When that happens, her challenge is to give herself unconditional love and keep her sense of humor. Perhaps she might say to herself, "There goes my reptile again. That's a sign of my success. My reptile is threatened and grumpy because it wants me to stay in stress, overeating, holding onto extra weight, and blaming myself for it all. If I give myself even a touch of unconditional love now, Brain State 5 will soon transform into a beautiful Brain State 1. I will be aglow in dopamine and endorphin surges, and my set point will continue to rise. I will have won."

We now live in the age of the smartphone, and that has changed how we communicate our thoughts. However, we are in the age of emotional neuroplasticity now and are changing how we process our emotions. The new technology of EBT is giving us more power.

The best news is that Jessica does not have to take 10 to 20 years to raise her set point, or travel to a far-off land to facilitate it. She can do it after one of her son's meltdowns, when the twins are fighting over a toy, or when a particularly strong craving hits. These are all opportunities for rewiring when the circuit that is causing her to disconnect from herself is unlocked and vulnerable – she can spiral up and make small but important updates in that circuit.

It just takes falling in love with our amygdala and learning to spiral up in new and highly creative ways.

9

Spiral Up #3: Freedom from Old Wires

The basic strategy of EBT holds. Awaken in the morning and say, "I am creating joy in my life!" Then, whenever you are not in joy, reach for your app and spiral up.

The first two spiral-up options on the app deliver immediate results, optimal self-regulation. However, the real power of EBT is rewiring circuits.

The idea that we can target and rewire circuits is so daunting. As a health psychologist, I was taught to think in terms of constructs, issues, problems, and diagnoses. As an EBT Provider, now I think in terms of wires, what kind they are (Core Circuit or Survival Circuit), and where they are stored in the brain (A 5 Circuit, 4 Circuit or 3 Circuit). I think of which ones I want to put on the shelf, and which one I want to focus on and clear.

Using Spiral Up #3: Deep Work

It takes time and practice to understand how much power we have and how life-changing it is to have that functionality. We are used to updating our applications, but this is organic – we are updating the programming of our unconscious mind. Spiral Up #3, Deep Work is designed to give you the power to rewire circuits, much the way a programmer would identify a "bug," then fix it.

The deep work uses Precision EBT, the way of applying the method that rousts out 5 Circuits and gives us just the motivation we need to clear them. It boosts our prefrontal cortex's capacity to stay emotionally present to the contents of these wires, dismantling old circuits and constructing new ones, so that EBT works far more rapidly in crushing unwanted wires and raising the set point.

The Joy of Rewiring

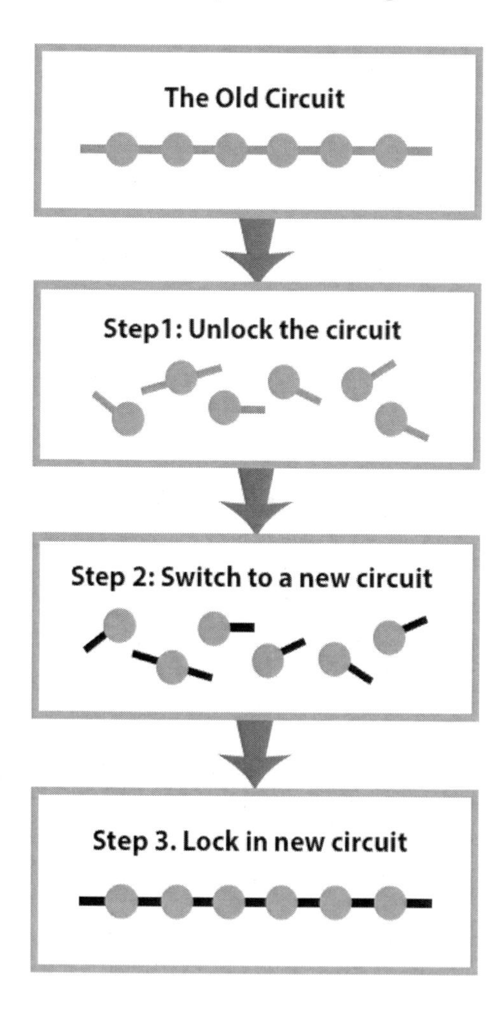

There are two skills, Stop A Trigger, which rewires Survival Circuits, and Feel Better, which rewires Core Circuits. Both tools also appear in Spiral Up #2, Quick & Easy, but the information buttons for them in that pathway provide a quicker way to use them that is designed for 4 Circuits.

In Spiral Up #3, the information buttons, prompts, and drop-downs are designed to activate and rewire trauma circuits. They help your prefrontal cortex weather the stronger emotions that arise after activating a 5 Circuit. They slow down the discovery of the circuit process to promote staying present to the contents of the unconscious mind and making it conscious then guide you to find a new reasonable expectation that is associated with optimal health.

Spiral Up #3
Deep Work

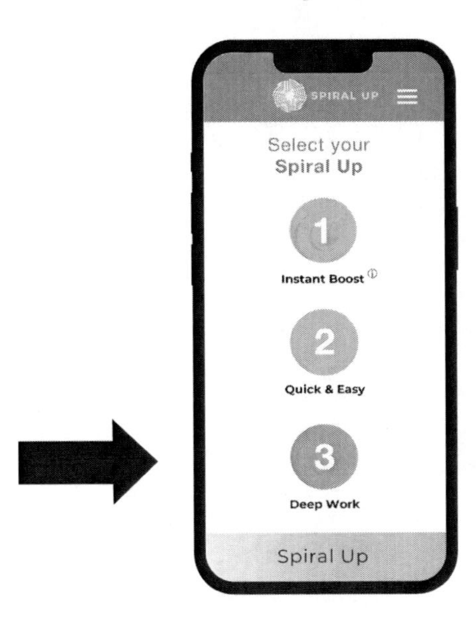

The various lead-ins and coaching prompts in Spiral Up #3 mirror what the best parent or best therapist would say to you to guide you in discovering your deepest feelings and motivating you to resolve conflicts and change behavior with greater ease.

Once you learn Precision EBT, you can choose a wire, dismantle it, and use your neurons to create a new wire of your choosing. You start by complaining about something that is bothering you and the circuit that is causing the problem is automatically activated. You unlock the circuit by following the lead-ins for this pathway, stay present to your emotions and change the message, then lock in the new circuit.

By using Spiral Up #3, we have a modern, neuroscience way to accomplish the goal of psychotherapy: activate 5 Circuits and rewire them. Rewiring requires staying present to the gnarly emotions that emanate from these trauma wires. Without staying present to the emotions, the brain switches off, goes "neocortical," and the reconsolidation process stops. The brain's preference to hold onto memories from trauma prevails. If the glitch wins, we run the risk of continuing to retraumatize ourselves with the activation of this wire for decades or, even, for a lifetime.

How does this "deep work" pathway mirror psychotherapy? Although EBT is skills training, not therapy, the processes are similar. The clinician co-regulates with the patient, sharing their emotional state so they "borrow" the therapist's functioning, making it easier to stay present to their feelings and process their emotions. The patient releases their stress and gains insights. Then, when the cognitive distortions caused by stress have been cleared, the

Spiral Up #3
Deep Work: 2 Options

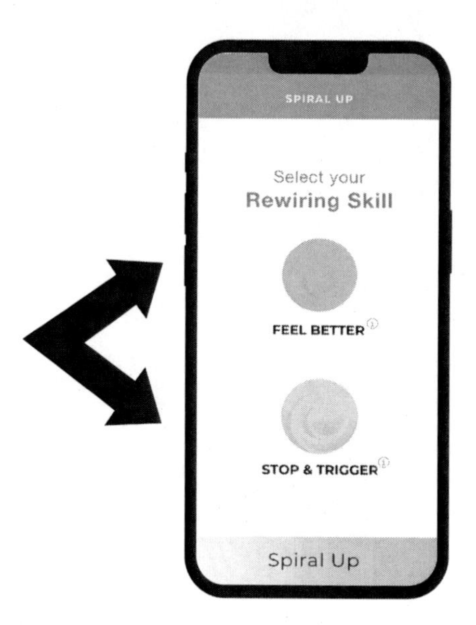

therapist gently identifies the unconscious, unreasonable expectation that has been made conscious by the interaction and replaces it with a reasonable expectation. The Stress Circuit transforms into a Joy Circuit.

Although this "dyadic attunement" and wise guidance in psychotherapy is deeply healing. what happens when we are on our own – say we wake up at 2 a.m. from a bad dream, we're triggered in a work meeting, or another night of binge eating awaits us? The precise use of emotional processing in Spiral Up #3 gives us a reliable and rapid process for staying present to our own stressed-out emotions, tearing down the emotional blockade of overthinking, depression, hostility, panic, shame, or numbness and turning it into flowing feelings that make it easy to self-attune. We can change our expectations ourselves and transform those Stress Circuits into Joy Circuits more effectively. Peer support and coaching definitely enhance our capacity to stay present to our emotions and rewire. Having the option to use it solo translates into changing the brain more rapidly.

These 5 Circuits are the primary neural causes of our healthcare crises. The more we use Spiral Up #3, the faster we can raise our set point, the more easily we can self-attune and use the brain's amazing capacity to heal itself. By using this pathway precisely and often, the brain heals itself and our physiology changes naturally. Our own brain becomes an organic pharmacy and we may need fewer medications and feel more vibrant with a zest for life.

As you did with Spiral Ups #1 and #2, read the information on each page the first three times you use Spiral Up #3. The instructions are precise for good reason. If you follow Precision EBT for Pathway #3, Deep Work, you can change your unconscious mind in ways of your choosing. What are the main differences between Pathway 2, Quick & Easy, and Pathway 3, Deep Work? Here they are:

- **Precision** – Each step is more precise. If one step is not done correctly, the rest of the spiral up will be less effective. You might rewire a 4 Circuit, but not a 5 Circuit. Follow the instruction buttons precisely.

- **Simplicity** – For the lead-in that identifies what you are most stressed about, keep it very simple, about five words. The 5 Circuits are very "pithy" and simple, so look for words a four-year-old would say. You seek to find the most extreme aspect of the problem, your "pain point," because if you state what *really* bothers you, you activate and rewire the circuit blocking your joy the most.

- **The Anger Procedure** – To activate a 5 Circuit rather than a 4 Circuit, the expression of anger must be slightly more robust, to the point that your mind goes blank for a moment. You have to release control in order to gain control. When the circuit was encoded, you were near or at a freeze response, and to rewire a circuit, we must re-experience the same level of stress we were in when it was encoded. It is only for a moment and not painful, but the sign that we have successfully activated a 5 Circuit is that moment of "blanking out." The perception is often that the mind is empty, and you have nothing to say. That passes, and you will be aware of the next emotion in this natural flow of feelings: sadness. The expression of anger in these highly effective ways has a monumental impact on the process, as it rapidly releases stress. You might even find yourself at Brain State 2. Also, your emotions are now homeostatic and flowing instead of allostatic and stuck or toxic. Without that expression of effective anger, it is not safe to feel sadness as it will likely turn into an unproductive and painful feeling of depression. Instead, expressing sadness feels tender, and the emotion fades when you feel it.

- **Tender Sadness** – After turning anger into sadness, the circuit has unlocked. The synaptic connections between the neurons are fluid, but more work remains. You slow the process down and pause until you feel emotionally connected to yourself, aware of the sensations in your body. Pause a little longer and refer to what you are most stressed about, staying on topic. The sadness is tender and sweet, and you reflect on how it is for you to experience that stressor. You are peering into the depths of your soul and grieving your loss. It is often very different from being sad about the situation. Instead, you are sad about the feelings you have, grieving what it has cost you. For example, if the topic is "I am out of control of my eating," you might otherwise (Spiral Up #2) say, "I feel sad I eat too much." However, in Spiral Up #3, you might say, "I feel sad that this is so painful for me." Once you have stated your sadness, you do not think or say any more words but focus on your body and feel your feelings until they fade. This is the therapeutic moment as you are staying present to the emotions that were suppressed long ago, but in a form that is not harmful but healing and often quite nurturing.

- **Fear that Motivates** – After expressing sadness, express fear, but when rewiring 5 Circuits, your statement is very pointed. Refer to the topic and state the consequences of not resolving it. The brain avoids resolution, instead holding onto pain because it is familiar, whereas resolving the inner conflict involved takes effortful control and the risk of facing the unknown. If it were easy to clear this circuit, you would have already done it. By stating the specific consequences of not resolving it that matter to you, motivation to change increases. For example, you might say, "I feel afraid that . . . my topic is I am out of control of my eating . . . my one deepest fear is that . . . the consequence to me that matters to me of not resolving this is . . . I may feel out of control for the rest of my life. I might get diabetes. I may harm my body." Once you have stated your fear of not resolving the stressor, feel your feelings until they fade. This is another healing moment. As you state this fear after releasing stress by expressing both anger and sadness, it is safe. You are not in an allostatic state in which you might experience anxiety or panic but in a flowing, homeostatic state. You are facing the actual fear of not changing rather than the amplified or muted fear that respectively is either hurtful or not healing. This expression of fear often feels sobering and cleansing. You are facing reality, and it is motivating, but it also includes an element of liberation.

- **Joyful, Empowering Guilt** – After expressing and feeling the fear until it fades, it is essential to produce a significant shift in your brain state. Again, this is a very precise procedure. Your goal is to shift your brain state to One, as you need to draw upon the memories stored in that state ("state-specific memory"). The guilt statement is not about what you have done wrong but clarifying what the wise child inside you wished you would have done. A touch of humor is helpful here, as the guilt statement is often something completely logical that eluded you because of the cortisol surges and dopamine extremes caused by the Stress Circuit. You use proprioception and put your shoulders back and chin up to boost your brain state. Use a joyful, powerful vocal tone, either aloud or in your mind (both work). For example, you might sit up tall and say, "I DO have some power here! I feel guilty. Why don't I do the logical thing and . . . let's see, my topic is that I feel out of control of my eating . . . Why don't I just

... eat healthy? This accomplishes two things: creating an image, which is a circuit of the adaptive response to get a head start on encoding the new adaptive circuit, and sharpening your accuracy in discovering the unreasonable expectation, the "all-important" articulation of the message from the unconscious mind. Rewiring a 5 Circuit more easily juxtaposes the precise message from the unconscious mind and the opposite expectation. This way of completing the guilt statement may be challenging as you may find it easier to state what you wished you would not do, such as saying, "I feel guilty... why don't I just ... stop eating?" Putting extra effort into creating an image and describing what you wished you would do is important. This becomes the perfect setup to discover the words of your 5 Circuit.

- **Discovering the Circuit: Double Dipping** – In Spiral Up #3, if you are using the Feel Better Tool to rewire a Core Circuit, discovering the circuit is similar to the process in Spiral Up #2, except that it has a more primitive feel and is much more exhilarating when you discover it. (Rewiring 5 Circuits is extremely exciting and fun.) If you are using the Stop A Trigger Tool, the formula for the statement remains the same, which is I get my X (need) from Y (something that does not meet that need, the "external solution"). To discover the circuit requires "double dipping," or having two experiences of listening to the message that bubbles up from the unconscious mind. First, check for the need, and once it bubbles up into your conscious mind, verify that it rings true. Be sure to err on the side of needs that are very primitive, such as existence, power, protection, or survival. These are survival drives! Then, restate the need and focus on discovering your external solution. Both must be articulated accurately for the easiest rewiring. Check to be sure that the statement elicits nausea in you. If it does not, it's unlikely that you will rewire it as these are addiction circuits, and the brain resists separating from them. We are "in love" with our wires, even if they cause us to harm ourselves, so we need motivation to end the love affair. This "ick factor" test not only gives us a needed nudge to "break up" with the circuit but is enormously fun. For example, if your first crack at discovering the unreasonable expectation embedded in a circuit, "I get my safety from food," does not produce nausea, try "I get my existence from food." That's stored a little bit deeper in the brain in the more primitive and extreme areas. If that does not produce the desired revulsion, then get serious about making it more "icky." Say something like "I get my existence from stuffing myself with food to the point that I hate myself, hate life, and fall into a state of misery, all of which I happily repeat night after night." Be sure to approach this with unconditional love for yourself and pride in using the wisdom of neuroscience to rid yourself of any gnarly old wires that are residing in your brain without paying rent. Have fun with it, then discover that you can actively dismantle that wire much more easily and feel the immense pride of "rewiring success" faster.

- **Deeper Healing** – Once you have discovered and verified the words of the circuit (the unreasonable expectation), the app will guide you in spiraling up. Just follow the lead-ins and use the drop-down menus. They give you options to get started and learn how to use the tool more easily. However, as your skills deepen, you will learn more powerful ways to rewire, including clearing away the other circuits that coactivate with 5 Circuits. The lasting results come when you both rewire the expectation and clear the related memories. Suppose you only change the expectation without doing a deeper dive into your emotional brain and clearing away the suppressed emotions from the trauma that occurred when it was encoded. In that case, results are less likely to be lasting. This is because the brain resists "giving up" the symptom, such as overeating, until you have cleared the related wires. It "uses" the symptom to get our attention so that we will do a more thorough job of rewiring. One way of thinking about Survival Circuits is that they motivate us to "go fishing." We have a symptom we don't like, so we cast the line and catch the "fish" of the unreasonable expectation. However, to catch the fish, we must "reel it in" with the extra effort to change the expectations and clear away the related emotional clutter. Learn more about how to do the more profound healing work in the How to Rewire course that is part of the EBT 1-2-3 JOY Program.

- **Pride and Joy** – As you conclude using Spiral Up #3, Deep Work, notice that you feel transformed. You are not the same person you were before, as you have much more knowledge of who you are and why you do what you do. Also, often the wire "pops" on the spot, and vanishes, instantly replacing an old circuit with a new one. That's the joy of rewiring. Yet pride factors in, too. The confusion and self-blame that come from not knowing why we feel the way we do and have those unsettling urges are replaced by self-love. The problem was one of those glitches that was encoded through no fault of our own. Everyone has them, but you are doing something about them. You may have a sense of pride as the unconscious mind used to "own" you. Now you own it! Your prefrontal cortex has prevailed over the amygdala, and this ultimate "mind over matter" has set you free. Bonnie Hoag, an EBT Provider whose wisdom always astounds me, once said, "Laurel, people come to EBT because they want to be present and stop replaying the past." Using our natural powers to free ourselves from the miscellaneous content that somehow wedged its way into our brain and be authentic in our life is enough to make anyone proud.

Throughout The EBT 1-2-3 JOY Program, you will learn how to use these tools with far more ease and depth. To get started, let's look at one example of each of the Big 4 Circuits for overeating and weight.

Crush Your Food Circuit

Charlotte already had an idea what her Food Circuit was and that it wasn't just a 4 Circuit, a strong craving or drive, but a 5 Circuit.

She was curious about her wire but wasn't excited about her power to crush, obliterate, and destroy it.

Of course she wasn't. How many years had she endured the struggle of starting fresh each morning, telling herself that she would be "good" today, then having all her plans fall apart by mid-afternoon, and tearing into food that evening? How many years of self-blame and shame could she stand?

Remember, if it's not fun, it's not EBT.

I told Charlotte, "I'm worried because you're not having fun."

"Of course, I'm not having fun. I have been blaming myself for my weight and torturing myself about my lack of control for decades."

"The problem is not you. It's a wire. A ridiculous wire that invaded your brain, like a virus invades your computer."

"I have an antivirus program on my computer for that."

"EBT is your antivirus program for weight."

Charlotte laughed.

Then she declared, "I hate that wire. I'm going to drill down into my emotional brain, find that sucker, and do it in. I'm going to crush it, obliterate it, and vaporize it . . . and then feel the glow of my victory – YES!!!"

"You sound ready to begin."

"I'm more than ready!"

In the next few minutes, I would guide her through her Cycle very carefully. If she learned from the start to do her deep work with precision ("Precision EBT"), she would need to do far fewer spiral ups to complete the program and raise her set point – and enjoy each one of them more.

First, target the circuit

"The first lead-in is: 'The situation is . . .' then pause. The power of the pause is that you turn your attention to your body, where you experience your emotional brain. We're not looking for your conscious knowledge, but the information in your unconscious mind that is controlled by the amygdala. I want five sentences – complain – sound irritated. Be four years old and state your complaint, just the facts, no feelings."

"The situation is . . . I start eating, and I can't stop. I'm ruining my health, but I keep eating anyway. I eat until I can't eat anymore, and then I have heartburn and feel like a failure. I am completely out of control of my eating."

Charlotte paused, a sign that she had told her story and activated the circuit.

"Well done. Take a deep breath and tell me when you are ready for more."

This pause gives her brain time to organize that information and find the most threatening aspect of it. This is done naturally, but a pause is needed.

"Now say, 'What I'm most stressed about is . . .' Pause and wait for about five words to appear in your mind. Tolerate not knowing. The words will appear."

"What I'm most stressed about is . . . I don't know what I am going to do if I do not stop stuffing and starving and worrying that the combination of my self-judgment and processed foods is going to kill me."

"I need five words. One topic. Be direct and state what is hurting you – the eating – not the consequences of it."

"Okay . . . What I'm most stressed about is . . . I stuff and starve."

"Pause. Does that ring true?"

Charlotte paused, "Yes."

"Great, write down those words. I stuff and starve. This is your topic."

"Okay."

"Stay on this topic – those precise words – for the rest of the Cycle. Words are extremely important in the brain. Do not change the words, or you will unleash more circuits and confuse your unconscious mind. You will not find your 5 Circuit."

"Okay."

Next, unlock the circuit

"You are doing a fantastic job. Now, use safe, productive anger to be sure you get to the bottom of your brain and unlock that obnoxious, hurtful, stupid 5 Circuit, then quickly release the stress it contains. This is the Anger Procedure. Do it the same every time. Don't mess with perfection. Say, 'I feel angry that . . .' then state your topic, the exact words you have written down. Then say, 'I can't stand it that . . .' then state your topic again. Then say, 'I HATE it that . . .' then state your topic yet again. Then let it rip. You must get slightly out of control to unlock the circuit, drain its stress, and gain control over it. Say, 'I HATE it, I HATE it, I REALLY, REALLY

HATE IT!!!' and continue to express red hot, but safe, productive anger until your mind shuts off or it turns into sadness. When it does, pause and wait for me to guide you to the next step. Go for it!"

Charlotte dove right in: "I feel angry that . . . I stuff and starve and don't do anything about it . . ."

I intervened right away: "You're almost there! Let's start again. Stay on topic. *No extra words*. You are trying to speak to your inner reptile, the most primitive part of the brain. If at all possible, stick carefully with the rules of clearing 5 Circuits. Let's discover that wicked wire!"

"I feel angry that . . . I stuff and starve. I can't stand it that I stuff and starve. I HATE it that I stuff and starve . . ."

At that point, Charlotte let loose: "I HATE it, I HATE it, I REALLY, REALLY HATE IT!!!! I really, really, really HATE that wire!!!"

"Continue with anger until it shifts, which it will."

Charlotte said, "It just did. My mind went blank. I feel a tender, sweet sadness now."

"Perfect. Be very, very loving to yourself now. If you had not cleared the anger, your sadness would be allostatic. You would feel depressed, but the red-hot anger cleared enough stress that your feelings are no longer allostatic and hurtful, but homeostatic and healing. Well done."

She said, "Good."

Turn stuck emotions into flowing feelings

"Tell me when you are ready for more."

"Okay, I'm ready."

"Use a tender, loving voice. Refer to your topic, which is that I stuff and starve, and say the loss of that for you. Just repeat . . . My one deepest sadness . . . about that I stuff and starve . . . say how it is hurting you, then feel that feeling until it fades. It's feeling that one feeling until it fades, without speaking, that is healing. Speaking activates the thinking brain and we don't want that because the healing is completely subcortical, in the emotional brain."

"I feel sad that . . . I have disappointed so many people by gaining the weight back."

"Charlotte, I know you care how other people feel, but the foundation of your health is your relationship with yourself. It is essential that you see yourself accurately and honor that you have been hurt by this stupid wire. It invaded your brain through no fault of your own and hurts you. To release this wire, you must feel your sadness and grieve the loss – the loss to YOU."

Charlotte spoke in a loving tone, "I feel sad that . . . let's see, I stuff and starve . . . my one deepest sadness is . . . the loss to me is . . . this wire has tortured me."

Her voice was tender and loving. The success of her Anger Procedure turned what would have been stuck, dry, and damaging depression into warm, healing sadness that was flowing.

"Beautiful. Now feel the feelings until they fade."

I waited. She was staying present to her feelings. This was very safe, very loving, and quite tender. This was a healing moment for her as she was acknowledging her pain and then releasing it.

She said, "It faded. It's gone."

"Well done. Next, say, 'I feel afraid that . . . about the topic, which is I stuff and starve . . . If I don't resolve this, the consequences in my life that matter to me are . . . I feel afraid that . . .'"

Without keeping her focus on the topic and the consequences that matter to her if she does not resolve it, she could wander off into expressing many fears. That would be fine if she used Spiral Up #2 and expressed old, suppressed emotions. However, she was using Spiral Up #3, which is self-directed, loving, effective brain surgery. The precise rotten wire that had caused her suffering for decades was now unlocked. By discovering and expressing the consequences that mattered to her of not resolving it, she would tap into a new level of passion for frying that wire. However, in that moment she was at war – between her prefrontal cortex and her amygdala. Winning that war is the ultimate mind over matter.

Charlotte said, "I feel afraid that . . . about the topic, which is I stuff and starve . . . If I don't resolve this, the consequences in my life that matter to me are . . . I feel afraid that . . . I will die . . . I will not have joy in my life . . . and I will leave my daughter without a mother to love her and make her feel special . . . that's it."

The emotional brain's strong drive to maintain the familiar is hard to shut off, but holding two opposites – the drive to stay the same and the most extreme yet plausible negative consequences of not disrupting the familiar – has a powerful impact in promoting high-charged drives to change.

"Beautifully done. Do those consequences matter to you?"

Charlotte answered, "Absolutely."

"Perfect. Now, take a deep breath and feel your feelings until they fade. Please do not rush this. You are doing a magnificent job."

She was quiet for almost a minute, then said, "It's starting to fade."

"Keep feeling it until you have used up all the healing benefits, and it has faded completely."

"Okay, I'm there. It has faded completely."

This technique of finding the one deepest feeling that is on the topic and feeling it until it fades is at the heart of positive emotional neuroplasticity. Being present to our emotional experience changes the brain.

Charlotte would learn through experience that when she surrenders to feeling the feeling, it will at first be effervescent, then release slowly. She will feel connected to the deepest part of herself and be at peace. However, as emotional and spiritual growth is impatient, she will feel slightly charged up and ready for the next lead-in. The emotions that otherwise would become stuck and toxic flow beautifully, taking her to states of rapture, and pragmatically switching off the HPA Axis and the stress response. It is just a matter of making the healing technique automatic, which is just what Charlotte was learning.

Boost your power to change

The next step calls for a dramatic shift in posture and energy, all carefully calculated to keep the prefrontal cortex at Brain State 1 for optimal effectiveness in boosting pride and preventing the damage caused when guilt is mixed with stress, causing shame.

"Now, change your energy. Put your shoulders back, chest out, and your chin up. Be in your power posture, and use a strong, joyful voice, and say, 'I DO have some power here. I feel guilty, why don't I just . . .' and state what the wise four-year-old inside you would do. Use humor. What logical thing would that four-year-old inside you say?"

"I don't feel joyful."

"This is a brain procedure. For this step, we are using emotions as medicine, not as a psychological expression."

"Okay."

She adjusted her posture then she belted out, "I DO have some power here. I feel guilty, why don't I just do the logical thing the four-year-old inside me would know to do and . . . stop overeating?"

Charlotte gasped, "Yes, that's a good question, why don't I do that?"

"Because you have a glitch and we're just about to find out what it is, but do not think. Pause and listen to your body where you receive the messages from your emotional brain."

"Okay."

Discover the message hidden in your unconscious mind

I said, "This is the aha moment. To find the unconscious memory that drives you, state the following, and again use humor. Have fun. Say, 'Of course I will not do the logical thing that the four-year-old inside me would say to do and stop overeating, because I have a wire in my brain that is telling me that I cannot get my . . .'

"Pause here and wait for a need to come up that rings true, like safety, existence, power, protection, survival, or love . . ."

"Of course I will not do the logical thing that the four-year-old inside me would say to do and stop overeating, because I get my . . . I don't know . . . It's not safety . . . I get my . . . power . . . no that doesn't ring true . . . because I get my . . . oh, this is it . . . I get my EXISTENCE . . . from . . ."

"Now pause. That rings true? If it rings true, that means the words in your unconscious memory match the words in your conscious mind. Those precise words give you the power to dismantle, smash, and transform that circuit. Does it ring true?"

"YES!"

"Pause again as you are doing deep work, to get separate readings on the need and the external solution you are using to seek to meet that need. Say, I get my existence from . . ."

"Of course I will not do the logical thing and stop overeating, because I get my existence from . . . stuffing myself with food."

"Does that ring true?"

"Yes."

"Charlotte, we can stay with that, but if this is a 5 Circuit, your amygdala is doing everything it can to hold onto it because it is familiar, so if you want, we can add the 'ick factor.'"

"What's that?"

"If saying I get my existence from stuffing myself does not make you feel sick, chances are you will try to rewire it, but covertly your brain will want to keep it. So, with 5 Circuits you have the option of adding some words that reflect the extreme nature of the expectation. The point is to separate from the wire and crush it, rather than to cozy up to it and allow it to stay firmly planted in your brain."

"Oh, I want the ick factor."

"Try it several times until something rings true but brings up nausea."

Now Charlotte was laughing. It was fun.

"I get my existence from stuffing myself to the point that I ruin my health and block my joy."

"Does that work?"

"Yes, I feel completely revolted. I want to get rid of that circuit. Every cell of my body tells me this statement rings true."

"Perfect, now just sit with that circuit. That means to feel your feelings and be aware that this circuit has been living inside you for a long time."

"Since I was . . . eight years old."

Want to rewire it or put it on the shelf?

"You have a choice now. There are two distinct options. One is to 'put it on the shelf' and rewire it later, and the other is to crush that circuit now. If you want to crush it, do not stop doing the Spiral Up Grind In on your app and clear whatever emotional clutter is attached to that wire. You don't stop until the wire has been obliterated, as evidenced by its drive being gone. For a food wire, that means the love affair with food is over because the wire is gone, and you are getting that deep need met in ways that work. You are not depriving yourself of food, but you eat less and leave food on your plate. What is your choice?"

Charlotte exclaimed, "Are you kidding? I'm going to crush that circuit. I'm obliterating it. I don't care if I have to spiral up and do the grind in 50, 100, or 1000 times. I want that circuit GONE!"

Now we were both laughing.

"What's the most important thing you learned today?"

"That I have a 5 Circuit. All that blaming myself is history. The problem was always a random circuit that my brain encoded. Hah! All that suffering. All that confusion. It's gone!"

I asked, "How is that for you?"

"It is fantastic!"

Rewire Your Mood Circuit

Kevin had a slow start with EBT. He didn't drop into any of the Spiral Up Groups and averaged only five spiral ups per day, not enough to change his physiology. He said he was too busy to watch the videos and learn how to use the tools.

He said he was using weight-loss drugs and had become used to the nausea and diarrhea, but he was still trying out EBT for two reasons. One was that he knew he would regain 95 percent of the weight he lost within one year, and the other was he had several stress-induced problems.

Physiologically, all of us do. If the set point of the brain is in stress, cracks in the functioning of all domains of life start appearing.

I asked him how I could help.

He said, "My stress is getting to my wife. She confronted me last night, saying that I didn't care about the family, only about work, and then I blew it. I started yelling, saying I was working my behind off and doing the best I could. It was a bad scene."

"How was that for you?"

His voice was gravelly, "Bad. I realized afterward how much she loved me and that I was mean to her. My worst problem is not food or alcohol. It's rage. Sometimes I lay into people at work, too."

"Kevin, the goal of EBT is to raise your set point. I'll support you on tackling any circuit you like."

"My family's the most important thing to me. I want to crush that Mood Circuit and never do that to my wife again."

A Mood Circuit is the unbalanced emotion that is the brain's "go-to" in stress. These emotional states are not problematic when they are brief. Who doesn't feel anxious, depressed, ashamed, panicked, or hostile at times? However, over time and with repeated prolonged states, that mood becomes like an addiction, as it is a way to escape feeling our feelings.

I first began to understand these Mood Circuits when treating bulimic patients in the Division of Behavioral and Developmental Pediatrics at the University. Rhonda, a 14-year-old, had stopped binge eating temporarily but started again, explaining to me that she didn't miss the food, but the shame afterward was so familiar to her that it was comforting. Soon after that, a 16-year-old who had been diagnosed with bulimia nervosa said she vomited into empty mayonnaise jars and lined them up on the windowsills in her room. Her Mood Circuit was a seething chronic rage.

Mood Circuits can take many forms. They can trigger Food Circuits, prolong or intensify the overeating once the Food Circuit has been activated, or provide a special comfort or reward after the Food Circuit has run its course. The most common triggers of overeating are anxiety and depression. Numbness and false highs are also common while eating, and shame, depression, or numbness often crop up after overeating.

As everyone has a Mood Circuit, and most people have several, how do you choose one to rewire as part of rewiring the Big 4 Circuits? Choose the one that harms you the most, which is often the one that triggers the Food Circuit.

Rewiring any circuit has two aspects. One is to directly change the expectation, such as "I get my safety from being anxious." You can do this with the "Spiral Up Grind In" integrated into the Spiral Up #2 (a lighter version) and Spiral Up #3 (a deeper version). More advanced techniques for rewiring and "power techniques" are covered in the How to Rewire course that is part of The EBT 1-2-3 JOY Program.

The second aspect of rewiring is to clear the emotional clutter. That is any wires that coactivate with the circuit, causing it to be stronger, more dominant, and more challenging to rewire. Stress Glitches are usually encoded during a traumatic experience and clearing the related memories "loosens up" the circuit. Clearing the clutter makes it easier to "pluck" that circuit from the brain and discard it.

The Spiral Up Grind In involves three stages:

The first is slowly stating the opposite of the unreasonable expectation embedded in the circuit to weaken it. Even though with repeated statements that expectation may stop being emotional, it takes staying emotional to rewire the circuits.

The second stage is to restate the opposite expectation, but again to ensure the process stays emotional you must ridicule it. Make fun of the wire.

Once that no longer feels fun, the third stage begins. It is to state the new reasonable expectation. The entire process takes less than a minute.

I asked Kevin if he wanted to use the app with my coaching him as he moved through it. He agreed and began.

What's bothering you? State the facts, no feelings

"The situation is . . . I have a problem with anger. I am the guy everyone likes, and I stay positive, but then some wire goes off in my head, and I start raging."

His voice trailed off, a sign he had told his story.

"What I'm most stressed about is . . . I am a jerk."

Setting up the Cycle is extremely important. If the topic is off, the Cycle will not hit the mark of clearing the circuit that is causing the unwanted response. His topic was off the mark as it was not a statement about what he did that harmed his health or happiness. If he proceeded based on his original topic, he would feel better but not get better. Getting better means rewiring circuits, as changing circuits promotes lasting, natural improvements in how we respond in daily life. The provider's role is to help participants counter the natural tendency of the brain to protect 5 Circuits and guide them in "outsmarting" their reptilian brain and supporting the most powerful rewiring experience.

"That's a good start, but if you choose that for your topic, you will rewire the circuit that perceives you as a jerk. You will not stop raging. Instead of cycling on how you feel about your raging or how you feel about yourself or the consequences of raging, choose your pain point. That is what you do, that you wish you would not do."

Kevin said, "Okay, here we go again . . . What I'm most stressed about is . . . I rage at my wife . . ."

"Very effective! Great."

I suggested that he write down the topic to ensure the rest of his spiral up pertains to that topic. Changing the words even slightly can activate additional circuits and make it harder to discover the precise words conveyed by the offending wire, the Stress Glitch. It would be fine if Kevin used Spiral Up #2 and only wanted to switch off his anger in the moment. However, he was using Spiral Up #3 Deep Work, which is designed to reconsolidate the circuit. That pathway is the "brain surgery" option and requires precision.

Unlocking the circuit in a highly effective way

Kevin started using the Anger Procedure, but rather than following the lead-ins on the app, he flew into a rage.

"I hate it that I rage at my wife. I HATE that I am such a jerk. I HATE . . ."

Although raging felt good to him, it would not help him rewire.

I intervened right away, "Kevin, that's correct. Protest that wire, but the safe and effective way to use the Anger Procedure is to start with a very balanced expression of anger and say, 'I feel angry that . . . I rage at my wife.' Your thinking brain can stay present to that emotion. Then go in small steps, expressing more extreme feelings, but staying present to your emotions. Say, 'I can't stand it that I rage at my wife,' and finally, 'I HATE it that I rage at my wife.' At that point, the topic is clear, and then your job is to switch gears and rage until your mind shuts off and you feel tender sadness."

"You mean a controlled and safe rage?"

"Exactly. Taking that process in stair-steps and restating the topic lets you stay present to your feelings and target the circuit. When you switch to rage about the topic, you both soundly activate the most extreme circuit your brain can access at that time, then immediately calm down so your emotions are no longer allostatic (out of control), but rather, homeostatic and healing. Using this procedure is a major aspect of establishing an EBT Practice."

Kevin followed my instructions, did a very effective Anger Procedure, and then moved through sadness, fear, and guilt correctly. Then he discovered the unreasonable expectation embedded in the wire: "I get my power from raging at people."

As Kevin verified that it rang true, he said, "I see an image of myself with my father, and he was raging, his face beet red."

He had activated a 5 Circuit and some emotional clutter. Although acting on that experience immediately and doing a Travel Back Tool would be immensely gratifying for Kevin, using this more advanced skill early might feel unsafe. There is no rush in rewiring circuits, as whatever we choose not to rewire deactivates, remains in the amygdala, and can be reactivated later.

"Kevin, fantastic work! However, the priority of EBT is keeping it safe. There is no rush to travel back and clear that trauma. You can discover a circuit that is pretty deep in the brain but choose to 'put it on the shelf' and rewire it later. The method is designed so we can decide when and if we want to rewire a circuit."

Choosing to slow down and take it one step at a time

The Take Action Tool completes the spiral up, and not only quiets emotions that may be still flowing, but also enables us to decide the next steps.

I suggested Kevin continue tapping through the app and completing the Take Action Tool.

He said, "I expect myself to do the best I can to be proud of myself that I got started and to take it slowly."

"Well done. What are the positive, powerful words you need to hear to encourage you to go forward?"

Kevin said, "I need to do that."

"Now face the essential pain, the hard part of following through with that expectation. When you identify it and feel your feelings, you become unstoppable. You can follow through more easily."

"The essential pain is . . . I am not perfect."

"Feel your feelings until they fade, so your brain encodes that reality and accepting it becomes more automatic."

"I get it. If I can accept that, my earned reward will be Authenticity, feeling whole and being genuine."

"Now, notice what is happening in your body because you have changed your physiology. You might notice tingles, lightness, relaxation, or a glow. That's the evidence that you have had a biochemical effect."

"Yeah, I feel tingles in my feet and hands, and I am smiling. I can feel the muscles in my cheeks."

The peace of knowing yourself at a deeper level

"You did it! You discovered a 5 Circuit and have a plan for going forward."

Kevin said, "I learned a lot today . . . especially that I don't have to live with this circuit. I can change it."

"That's an intergenerational wire, Kevin, and by rewiring it, you stand the best chance of not passing it along to the next generation."

"So, my reward for rewiring this is the same as my Food Circuit: Integrity."

"How is that for you?"

"Very good. I have a plan."

Kevin's response supported the importance of rewiring the Big 4 Circuits. They often coactivate or trigger each other. Kevin's Mood Circuit was rage, which amplified his Love Circuit, which was to distance, and his Body Circuit, which was to use his large body size for power. These three circuits alone were enough to keep his set point in the allostatic range, in which behaviors are unhealthy.

Having discovered his first 5 Circuit, Kevin was on his way to having control over his unconscious mind. He could rewire any circuit that mattered to him and ignore the ones that didn't.

Even after discovering his first circuit when he asks himself, "Why do I do what I do when I know I shouldn't do it?" he will have an answer: "It's just a wire and I can rewire it."

Transform Your Love Circuit

Jessica had rapidly picked up enthusiasm for EBT, first dropping in for Spiral Up Groups and then joining a weekly premium group I facilitated that included access to five-minute Connections between sessions with other group members.

One morning, I received a notification that Jessica had scheduled a coaching session with me.

Soon I would learn that she had been triggered by a sensitive issue, and she wanted to clear the circuit quickly. It was her Love Circuit.

Jessica said, "Thanks for seeing me right away, as something happened with my son, Jeremy, yesterday that stunned me."

"What was it?"

"I realize that I am merged with him. I am blocking his development as I get a huge stomach ache at the thought of him having any pain at all."

The Love Circuit is one of the Big 4 Circuits because everyone under stress either merges with another person (being hyper-aware of the other's feelings and needs and not taking care of themselves), or distances (being only aware of themselves and not the other person). This is normal. It's what stress does to us.

The problem is that merging and distancing cause much of the stress we experience in life, and that stress can trigger overeating. In addition, by rewiring the Love Circuit we find that "sweet spot" of intimacy where we can be separate but close. That activates the hormone oxytocin, which is an appetite suppressant.

"The situation is . . . I am really sad about . . ."

"Great start, but just the facts, no feelings: five sentences, then what you're most stressed about, around five words. This makes it much easier to find the circuit."

"I get it. The situation is . . . I spoil my son rotten. I can't bear it if he has any pain, and he already has special needs, and I am making him into a baby. What I'm most stressed about is . . . I am a bad mother."

"You can choose that topic, Jessica, but it will take you 10 Cycles to clear it, and you will still not find why you do what you do with Jeremy. I'm worried that you won't find the circuit that will knock out what you are doing that bothers you and blocks your joy."

Jessica said, "So . . . what I'm most stressed about is . . . I spoil him."

She had nailed her topic. Excellent. Then Jessica went right into using the Anger Procedure to unlock the wire and move to expressing tender sadness.

Sadness is tender and loving, fear is our wake-up call

She said, "My one deepest sadness is, the loss to me is, that it is so hard to raise Jeremy . . . every day is so hard . . . "

I said, "See if you can feel your feelings until they fade, which they will."

She was quiet, just feeling her feelings and allowing herself to heal. She was learning EBT quickly.

Jessica continued, "I'm ready for more. My one deepest fear is . . . the topic is that I am spoiling him, and if I don't resolve that, the consequence to me is that I will . . . be a bad mother . . . he will not grow up . . . I will not have done right by him . . ."

Again, Jessica paused. She felt her feelings until they faded. Just six weeks into her EBT Journey, she had learned to trust herself and the tools.

At this point, she launched into a robust, "Hey everybody, I DO have some power here. I feel guilty, why don't I just . . . STOP spoiling him?"

I realized that she didn't need me. She had the process down.

She said with a laugh, "Of course I don't stop spoiling him, because my unreasonable expectation is - I get my security from Jeremy having no pain."

She identified the unreasonable expectation of the circuit, but something was still missing: her joy.

Healing is intrinsically fun because our genes reward us for evolving and contributing to the gene pool of people who can be of service to others.

I asked, "What just happened? Where did your joy go?"

She needed to have a fire-in-the-belly drive to crush that circuit, as passion is essential for a crisp rewiring.

Faster results and so much fun: The ick factor

To get to joy, Jessica had to have some fun and use a technique that brings better results faster by making the expectation more extreme.

I said, "What about adding the ick factor?"

She said, "I'll try that. Let's see . . . my unreasonable expectation is that I get my security from Jeremy having no pain . . . even if it keeps him a baby and ruins his life."

Then she started clapping and laughing!

Jessica said, "I love that. It's precisely what I am doing. Precisely."

"Go for it then, and finish with a Take Action Tool."

Still excited, she said, "I expect myself to do my best to fry this wire. Positive, powerful thought? It won't be that hard. It's a disgusting wire. The essential pain? I am alone. The buck stops with me. Nobody can rewire this merge circuit but me. The earned reward is Sanctuary, peace and power from within."

"How was that for you?"

"It was beautiful. I have compassion for myself as raising Jeremy is hard, but what he has given me is so much. In those moments when it is most difficult, he forces me to figure out who I am and who I want to be in this world. I have learned far more from raising Jeremy than from my work or mothering the twins."

When adversity comes our way, it delivers life-defining moments. Brain State 5 unlocks the circuits that are out of date or harmful, and by engaging our emotional brain, they turn into Brain State 1 and raise our set point.

Jessica said, "I will start crushing it right away. I'll get support from some of my Connection Buddies in my group."

"What's the most important thing you got from the session today?"

"That I love EBT. I had a glitch, and now I'm clearing it."

"How do you feel?"

"I'm at One."

Why the Big 4 Circuits are so important

Jessica was at One, and grateful that EBT could help her with Jeremy. She had identified food as her problem, but in the tangled-up brain circuitry of any person living life well, there are always a few errant wires to clear.

Our circuits play their own music, whether it is a symphony or a garage band. All of them are encoded through no fault of our own, so the EBTer is on their own journey. Any of the circuits they want to rewire will help with the diagnosis at hand (Chronic Physiologic Stress Overload – CPSO), so Jessica can rewire the four circuits in the order that works for her.

All that matters is that Jessica only rewires one at a time, and keeps crushing whatever wire she has selected until the drive it activates stops and she has more freedom in her life. After rewiring four of them, she will be close to playing Beethoven's 5th and can start raising her set point for lasting results.

Heal Your Body Circuit

Of the Big 4 Circuits, the most important to rewire to achieve easy, natural weight loss is the Body Circuit.

Most participants rewire the Food Circuit first and that shifts their relationship with eating, but it is not until they have soundly trounced their Body Circuit that the joy of releasing extra weight kicks in.

Once a participant rewires their Body Circuit, the weight feels "extra." They have so much self-love and body pride that being a little hungry now and then feels nurturing. The impact is often quite dramatic.

For example, my husband Walt was rather chunky when I met him, and he had a lineup of drugs he was taking. His weight was a significant medical risk, but he was casual about his eating and loved packing small candy bars into his backpack. He had joined Master Trainer Judy Zehr's weekly group and was spiraling up, making Connections, and using the tools with me. However, his body was not releasing extra weight.

Then one evening we were chatting about how the other three boys in his family of origin were athletic while he was a 150-pound weakling of sorts. Walt did a quick Cycle to discover his Body Circuit. Soon after that, the joy of weight loss set in. Instead of wanting more food, particularly those chocolate candies, he admonished me to "put less food on my plate." I hadn't said a word. Rewiring his body circuit spoke in volumes.

There are two types of Body Circuits. One is a self-judgment wire, that we do not love our body. That's a massive insult to our ego and perhaps even to the spiritual, as we are so fortunate to have a body. As self-image and body image are intertwined, if we do not love our body regardless of how it looks, then that transfers to not loving ourselves, and all healthy, lasting change comes from self-love.

The other type of Body Circuit is a self-protection wire that keeps us at a particular weight because it gives us safety. That weight speaks volumes to us and others, and if we dare lose weight without clearing that circuit, there is a telltale sign: we start eating even though we have no interest in the food. We pack on weight either with the munchies or outright binging. Our emotional brain is screaming at us through our behavior and telling us that we have to regain the weight or die.

The Body Circuit: Body judgment or self-protection?

Most people have both kinds of Body Circuits, and that was true for me. At age 33, when I started releasing weight with joy after my son Joe was born, I had broken my body judgment wire. I was sick of controlling my food intake and hating my body. I was going to love my body no matter what my weight, and eat when I was hungry, but not when I wasn't, to heal my relationship with food. Somehow, my body judgment wire was swept away with the Food Circuit.

Yet years later, a Body Circuit encoded itself in my brain, this time a self-protection wire. About 10 years ago, I met Walt, who later became my husband. As I mentioned, Walt was a little on the chunky side, and in our first six months together, that "in-love" phase, there was a fair amount of chocolate going down after dinner, and the last thing I was thinking about was my weight. I was in love, and after years of being happily single, I was exploring this new relationship with its layers of meaning and new joys. Then, one day, I realized that the evidence of those early chocolate fests on my body was still hanging on. I wasn't releasing that weight. My brain had encoded a Body Circuit.

I did a quick Cycle and discovered that wire: I get my safety from being a little chunky, like Walt. That was hysterical! My unconscious mind had encoded it so quickly that I dispensed with that wire, grinding in a new circuit: I get my safety from connecting to the deepest part of myself and being at the weight that is right for my body, not Walt's body. The extra weight came off rather effortlessly.

Charlotte first rewired her Body Judgment wire. I told her that she had to love her body as it was, as every single pound was evidence of her unconditional love for herself. I asked her to touch her body all over and give love to every square inch. If she found any judgments, she should spiral them up and clear them. At first, she was resistant.

Charlotte said, "I can't love my body. It's ugly, and there are veins all over and bunches of fat on my belly and thighs. How can I love that?"

I said, "Charlotte, that fat is there because you had more stress in your life than you had the skills to process, so your Stress Triangle unleashed biochemical drives to overeat that took your thinking brain offline and made it virtually impossible for you not to overeat. That weight is historical. Each pound is a testament to having more stress than you could process. Also, nobody told you the problem was a few wires or how to rewire them, so what else could you do but eat?"

It took Charlotte many spiral ups, but within a month, she stopped judging her body, and her love for her body and herself flowed. However, the joy of weight loss did not kick in. She was not releasing the extra weight.

I told her, "Charlotte, you may have a self-protection Body Circuit."

She agreed, and I coached her through a Cycle to discover it. Like many self-protection wires, Charlotte's Body Circuit was encoded about a year after a traumatic event. The teenage boy who lived next door had touched her inappropriately. She never told anyone until she was in psychotherapy in her mid-forties when going through a divorce. The therapy helped her stop blaming herself, but it did not rewire either her Food Circuit or Body Circuit.

As her nutritionist had focused on what Charlotte ate and bypassed the emotional brain, she had no support for connecting and rewiring either circuit. However, it was a classic circuit and she could see what happened not as a psychological trauma that led to an issue, but as a wire that she had the skill to discover and dismantle when the time was right for her to do so.

At the time of the abuse, Charlotte had been developing rapidly, and boys started ogling her, which made her feel extremely unsafe. She endured developing earlier than some of her friends but was uncomfortable talking with her parents about it. Then, the sexual abuse incident occurred and food became her way to escape emotionally. Her brain encoded a Food Circuit, and she gained 15 pounds immediately. Charlotte noticed that the boys noticed her less and that she felt safer. Her self-protection Body Circuit was encoded.

Charlotte started her Cycle to discover her wire, as usual, with a complaint: "The situation is . . . no matter what I do to lose weight, I gain it back. I always gain the weight back, even after working my tail off to lose weight. I keep gaining the weight back. What I'm most stressed about is . . . I gain weight back."

Melting the wire: Becoming skilled at EBT

Charlotte launched into the Anger Procedure, melted her sadness and fear, used her power to embrace what she wished she would do, and then found her circuit. It took her three minutes flat, and she said: "I get my protection from being big."

I said, "Beautifully done, Charlotte. Fantastic. You did it!"

It's easy to verify that the words are correct because when the words in the thinking brain match the message in the emotional brain, we get a "body feel" that it rings true. In addition, if we have activated a 5 Circuit the glow will fade, and we may feel slightly nauseated. If both do not occur, we try other expectations until one rings true.

I asked, "Does that ring true?"

She said, "Yes."

"Now, do you feel slightly nauseous?"

"Not really."

"Charlotte, you never have to rewire that circuit. You can put it on the shelf and rewire it later."

"I want to clear it."

"If you want to rewire it now, you'll need to embellish that expectation and add the 'ick factor.'"

Charlotte said, "Being big is a major part of my identity. I'm not sure who I would be without it."

"As long as that drive to stay big remains in your emotional brain, you will self-sabotage. You will not experience joy releasing that weight. To feel that joy may take a lot of spiral ups."

"How many?"

"It takes as many as it takes, but you never know when the next spiral up will change everything."

"I want to start working on it now."

The sought-after rewiring target of 5 Circuits takes two forms. If it is very low in the brain, very primitive, it is to the point and brief, usually five words or less. These are the rusty wires that are so gnarly that they activate legions of 4 Circuits. However, there is another kind of 5 Circuit that is slightly higher in the brain, bordering on a 4 Circuit. These need a "crowbar" to loosen, as although our perception is that we want to clear them, the brain covertly will do everything to make us believe we are clearing them, but instead hold onto them tightly. The solution for that is the ick factor.

"Then, let's add the ick factor. Add on to your expectation a few words that accurately describe the message in your emotional brain."

Charlotte said, "Okay . . . I get my protection from . . . being as big as I need to be to keep anyone from ever hurting me again . . ."

"Keep adding to it until it rings true."

". . . even if it ruins my health and blocks my joy."

I said, "How was that for you?"

Charlotte laughed, "I am very nauseated."

"Great work!"

A soft glow in her body and the reward of freedom

Charlotte had discovered her Body Circuit, but now she needed to plan what she would do about it.

I said, "Let's boost your safety by using the Take Action Tool."

She said, "I expect myself to do the best I can to . . . be gentle with myself and slowly rewire this Body Circuit at the pace that is right for me."

"What's your positive, powerful thought?"

"I have the power to do that."

"The essential pain?"

"I am not perfect."

"The earned reward?"

"Authenticity: feeling whole and being genuine. I have had trauma in my life, and I am not going to dodge healing it anymore. And there is another reward."

I asked, "What is it?"

"Freedom."

"Feel a surge of joy! Do you feel the biochemical effects of using spiraling up as medicine?"

Smiling, she said, "Yes, I do. It's a soft glow in my body. A feeling of peace inside and a slight tingle."

"Do you want to finish your spiral up by acknowledging what you just did?"

Charlotte was now in joy.

She said, "Absolutely, I spiraled up!"

Charlotte's joy was catching, and she had reason for hope. By rewiring her Big 4 Circuits – soundly trouncing each one of them – early in her EBT Journey, healthy eating and weight loss would arrive sooner.

She would be a "different person" biochemically, and functioning at a higher level, one that nourished her spirit the way that food never had. All it took was a few hundred spiral ups and a commitment to herself.

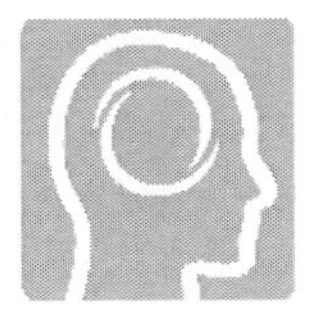

10

The Turning Point: Do You Want Freedom?

EBT is fun, and it works. Everyone likes to spiral up! However, about two months into using the tools, participants either find that they have enjoyed learning how to de-stress, or they sense that there are deeper rewards for them from EBT if they stay the course and complete the program.

By two months into using the program, the amygdala realizes that it is being threatened. You are on your way to living a new and better life. The brain responds to this disruption by activating wires you didn't even know you had!

Yet It's a very enlightening time because each person must decide if they just want to lose some weight or they want freedom. I first learned about this from Cathy, a lawyer who drove every week to the University from the East Bay and arrived precisely on time for the 5:30 p.m. group session.

However, when Cathy hit the two-month mark, her brain had changed enough that her amygdala was getting the message that the dominance of Stress Circuits stored there was being threatened. She was happier than she had ever been and could see some spontaneous improvements in her eating. Chicken tasted good to her and so did eggs, and sandwich rolls and candy bars were losing their appeal.

That week she showed up at the meeting 45 minutes late. She said she had made a wrong turn and had ended up at the San Francisco Airport. This was a brilliant woman whose thinking brain knew exactly how to drive to the university, yet her unconscious mind was at work, foiling her conscious mind's intention to come to the session.

Then, the next week, she did not come at all. The following week, she appeared on time but was clearly upset. At the start of each session, I led a brief check-in during which everyone relaxed into connecting with themselves and identifying their brain state. Then, each person had a chance to share their brain state and any "amazing learnings" or breakthroughs they had from using the skills in the past week.

When it was Cathy's turn, she said, "I'm at Brain State 5. I'm afraid I'm going to finesse EBT."

I wasn't sure what she meant.

Cathy continued. "I am going to put in an effort, but I will just skim the surface. I am not going to connect with the deepest part of myself. Instead, I will find a million excuses why I don't have time to do this work. Also, I'm afraid you won't call me on it and will let me get away with it."

I listened, sensing that she had a lot more to say.

She said, "I can talk my way out of anything."

I asked, "What do you need?"

She said, "I need to feel my feelings and be quiet during the rest of the session."

"Don't rush yourself, Cathy."

"I won't."

Cathy came to the next session.

She said, "I realize that I am not the same person I was two months ago. I'm scared of where spiraling up will take me, but even more scared that if I don't seize this opportunity, I may never know Freedom. And if I don't know Freedom, I may never know joy. I am in."

Cathy stayed with the program for an entire year, releasing her extra weight and accessing all seven rewards of a purposeful life, including Freedom. Taking all the time she needed early on and waiting until her unconscious mind had worked it through was essential to her success.

Now, 20 years later, that two-month mark is recognized as the time when participants reach that decision point. Jessica experienced the two-month mark in a very different way. Her brain started using "finding wires everywhere" as a distraction from doing the deeper work.

She said, "I find lots of 4 Circuits that tell me I eat because I'm happy, crave carbs because I'm depressed, or eat mindlessly because I'm bored. But I'm still binge eating."

The brain is organized in a hierarchy, with the most primitive and powerful circuits stored at Brain State 5. If we reach these wires and clear them, the circuits that are less primitive and strong fade. As reaching these wires takes emotional precision, they are generally not rewired outside of many years of deep psychotherapy. Without rewiring them, the default treatment is medications and surgery.

I said, "That makes sense. Your binge-eating wire is a 5 Circuit, and it fuels your 4 Circuits. Once you rewire your 5 Circuit, the other circuits will be easier to rewire, or your brain may even clear them spontaneously."

She said, "Everybody I know is either using medications or still eating, drinking, or spending too much. Some are zoning out on technology or staying constantly busy. I can see myself doing that, too."

"There is nothing wrong with doing any of those things. The basis of EBT is non-judgment, but because of the method, you have choices."

Suddenly, she had clarity, "I want to hedge my bets. I want to learn how to rewire my 5 Circuits, but if it doesn't work, I want to keep my backup plan and use other ways."

"Why do you want to rewire your 5 Circuits?"

"Because I want the rewards, I want all seven of them, or at least to know that I tried to get them."

"Is there one that particularly calls to you?"

"That would be Freedom. I don't want to stop overeating and then start drinking or spending, and I'm tired of losing weight and then regaining it. I want Freedom, definitely."

"Okay, then let me show you how to rewire those 5 Circuits right now."

She said, "I can't wait because I just had a rip-roaring binge last night, and I'd love to find the 5 Circuit that triggered it."

How to find the 5 Circuit

"First, let's sharpen your Anger Procedure. Think of the Anger Procedure as how you dig down to those 5 Circuits. Be bold. In fact, be really angry. How much trouble has that circuit caused you? Express that anger. Protest the hurt that wire has caused you!"

Jessica responded, "I do that. I do a primal scream every once in a while. It's not on purpose, but when I can't take it anymore, I let loose with a scream."

I said, "Excellent, just apply that intensity to anger."

"Why can't I just scream?"

"You can, but where does that take you? You've let off steam but haven't crushed the wire itself. A scream leaves us powerless. What do we do next? Scream again? Instead, state your grievance, say the essence of that complaint, and step past the power of a scream to protest that this has happened to you. Express your anger."

To find the 5 Circuit, use the Anger Procedure more lovingly. This circuit has harmed us. Loving ourselves means that we stop pretending that we are not hurting. What that wire is doing to us is repeating a traumatic experience with each activation of the wire, then, before we can process and clear it, engaging in the same harmful response that we used on the day it was encoded. Do not minimize the pain caused by that stupid wire. Activating that circuit takes a spark of the same level of distress we were in when it was encoded, nurturing ourselves by expressing the emotions we denied ourselves because of the circuit in the past.

"How do I do that?"

I said, "Learn by doing. I'll show you in a moment."

Treating Your 5 Circuit

Second, once you've activated and discovered the circuit, you have two to four hours to deliver a new experience to that wire, which updates it. This is the reconsolidation window, when the synaptic connections between the neurons are fluid and you have the most impact on the wire. The new experience you offer updates the old wire, replacing it with a new wire, increasing the chances of fixing the glitch and experiencing lasting and profound changes in your responses in daily life.

When you activate a 4 Circuit, the treatment is a Spiral Up Grind In, the one that appears on the app. However, when a 5 Circuit is activated, you give yourself two more options and use whichever feels most rewarding. Evolutionary biology is so skewed toward healing that you will naturally be drawn to: 1) sitting with your feelings, just feeling them until they fade, as a way to see the circuit and yourself in a new way, or 2) traveling back to the time that the circuit was encoded and replaying that experience in a way that is healing, whichever one will deliver the most potent rewiring experience.

I said, "Jessica, start wherever you are and complain about last night's binge."

She began, "The situation is . . . I ate a box of strawberries, then a bag of chips, then chocolate cookies, half a box, then I had ice cream."

"Find the deepest hurt. What bothers you the most? Keep it simple: about five words."

"What I'm most stressed about is . . . I am out of control of my eating."

"Is that what distresses you the most?"

"Yes."

"Write it down and use those words as your topic."

"Okay."

"Jessica, that wire is butchering you. It's hurting you. Protest!"

"I feel angry that . . . I am out of control of my eating. I can't STAND it that I am out of control of my eating. I HATE it that I am out of control of my eating. I HATE it! I HATE it! I HATE IT!"

She was still in over-control. She would need to temporarily release control to gain control, before discovering her 5 Circuit.

"Jessica, stay in anger until it turns to sadness, which it will, but to unlock that 5 Circuit, you must release control – just for a moment. You are a lioness. Let yourself roar! Expletives work well, too!"

She let loose with: "I HATE it, I HATE it, I HATE it, I #$%& HATE IT! I @&#$ HATE IT. I HATE IT, I HAAAAAATE IT!!!!!"

"Jessica . . . keep going until your mind shuts off, and after a moment, your emotions turn into tender, sweet, loving sadness."

"Ohhh . . . that's what just happened . . ."

She slowed down, connected with the deepest part of herself, and then stated her most profound sadness about the loss her eating had caused her and her fears if she did not resolve it. Both times, she felt her feelings without speaking, until they faded. Then she put her shoulders back and her chin up, and used the most positive, joyful voice she could muster.

She said, "I DO have power here. I feel guilty. Why don't I do the logical thing that the wise four-year-old inside me would do and . . . be kind to myself?"

As often happens with a 5 Circuit, the stress of the process was impacting her ability to stay on topic. If she cannot do that, she will not discover her 5 Circuit.

"Jessica, the topic is: 'I am out of control of my eating.' Put your shoulders back, chin up, and use a powerful, joyful voice! Use humor here!"

She said, "I DO have POWER here. I feel guilty. Why don't I do the LOGICAL THING that the wise four-year-old inside me would do and control my eating? In fact, not eat at all as my body is not hungry after eating dinner!"

In discovering 5 Circuits, sometimes it takes using a long sentence in the guilt statement, before the brain can generate the words to describe what you wish you would do in the best of all worlds.

"Pause for a moment until you feel connected, then state it briefly."

"I DO have POWER here. Why don't I enjoy my evening rather than overeat?"

"Great, now discover your 5 Circuit!"

"OF COURSE I wouldn't just enjoy my evening rather than overeat, because my unreasonable expectation is . . . I get my . . . safety . . ."

"Does that ring true?"

"YES!"

"I get my safety from . . . food."

"Does that ring true?"

"Absolutely!"

The 5 Circuits are often very pithy, as they are stored in the brain area that is associated with a freeze response and functioning like an infant or toddler. A simple statement often rings the most true.

"Would it be more rewarding for you to travel back, sit with your feelings, or spiral up?"

She said, "I'm already traveling back . . ."

The Travel Back Tool

Jessica would ask herself four questions. If she answered yes to each of them, I would guide her in a "reattachment experience." If she answered no to any of them, that would indicate that her brain was not ready to reattach. Instead, it would be more efficient for her to clear some emotional clutter. The brain does not permit the healing process without first grieving losses, as so much wisdom is gained from emotional clutter removal.

This processing of stored emotions is fundamental to success in achieving lasting results with EBT. The stress symptom of overeating was disturbing enough to motivate Jessica to discover her circuit and rewire it. However, the clean, light, pure feeling of rewiring a circuit will elude her until she has cleared her clutter, and it is by clearing it that she reconnects to the part of her she left behind when the circuit was encoded.

I began, "Question #1. Can you settle on one image?"

Jessica said, "Yes. I was six years old, and my younger sister was an infant. We were at the dinner table, my dad was drunk, and he and my mother were arguing. The baby was crying."

"Question #2. Can you see yourself in the image?"

"Yes."

"Question #3. Can you feel love or compassion for yourself?"

"Ummm . . . yes."

"Question #4. Are you drawn to traveling back and stepping in as the older you, giving the younger you exactly what you needed at the time: safety, love, and wisdom?"

"Absolutely."

The Reattachment Experience

If Jessica had not answered yes to all the questions, I would have guided her to either "put it on the shelf" and grieve her losses later or, if she chose to clear the clutter now, to plan on doing clusters of five spiral ups about this experience until she was at peace with the past.

However, she had answered yes to all the questions, so her reattachment experience could be very healing. I guided her through it.

I said, "Now, step into the image. Be authoritative. You are the only protection the younger Jessica has. You are not a peer to her. You are a strong, loving parent to her. Do whatever you need to do to give her safety."

Jessica said, "Okay, I'm telling my parents: back off. Stop ignoring her. She is scared. Grow up and stop yelling at each other. Stop drinking. Give her the safety that she needs and deserves."

"Are they responding to you?"

"No."

"Your job is to be the secure base she needed. Do not abandon her. Instead, try another way to give her the safety she needs."

"Jessica, we are getting out of here. Come with me right now. You deserve to feel safe. Come with me."

"What is she doing?"

"She's coming with me. She feels safe."

Jessica had completed the first of the three parts of the reattachment experience.

"Well done. Next, give her love in just the way she needs."

"Okay, I'm taking her outside and we are sitting on the grass, and I am saying to her, 'I love you. I am here for you, and I will always be here for you.'"

"Is she taking in your love? Does she feel loved by you?"

Jessica said, "Yes."

"Then give her wisdom. Correct the unreasonable expectation in the Stress Glitch. Mirror the Spiral Up Grind In."

"Okay, I am saying to her: Jessica, we do not get our safety from food."

"Be loving but authoritative."

"Sweetheart, we . . . do . . . not . . . get our safety . . . from food. We . . . do not . . . get our safety . . . from food."

"Excellent, be very loving and gentle but firm. She needs to know you are not telling her how to eat. You are telling her how to be safe."

"Sweetie, we . . . do . . . not get our safety . . . from food . . . that's ridiculous. Safety does not come from food. That's completely ridiculous. We get our safety from connecting to the love inside us. We get our safety from inside us and not from food. Do you hear me? We get our love from inside us."

"Is she listening to you?"

Jessica said, now with tears, "Yes, It's wonderful. She is listening to me, and I am giving her just what she needs."

Then she was quiet.

"How was that for you?"

Still with tears, she said, "I feel more peace right now than I ever imagined possible."

I smiled and said, "I'm so happy for you."

This was Jessica's first Travel Back Tool. She would complete many more during her EBT journey. Some would lead directly to a reattachment experience, and others to clearing more clutter first, then traveling back.

Either way, she now had a way to discover and rewire 5 Circuits. Any unwanted behaviors would change more rapidly, and most of all, she had a brain-based simple process for reconnecting with herself and knowing and loving herself more deeply.

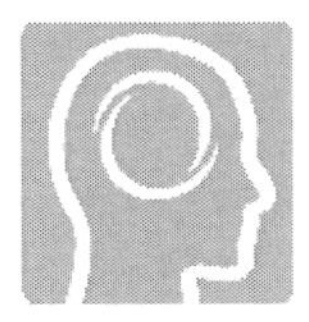

11

Honor Your Nature: Be in Joy

After rewiring the Big 4 Circuits, the set point typically rises. With stress quieting down, the brain turns its interest to creating joy.

Prior to that rise in set point, natural pleasures like eating when hungry or going for a walk on a spring day do not deliver dopamine quickly enough and in a high enough dose to counteract the stress chemicals and activate joy. We not only want, but need, that slug of dopamine from a donut, candy bar, or chips.

As spiraling up 10 times per day on most days changes our biochemistry, the prefrontal cortex now becomes nimble. It can give and receive love more easily, and prayer, meditation, and kind acts start becoming even more pleasurable. And rewards of purpose – they outshine donuts.

Making two additional shifts in our EBT Practice is the perfect preparation for moving to Step 2 and Boosting Reward. These are asking three questions, and then beginning to rewire Core Circuits.

Ask the three questions

Addressing each of the Big 4 Circuits results in transforming the wire from a reactive circuit promoting an insecure attachment style, to a resilient circuit promoting a secure attachment style.

This is profound healing and brings on an awareness of safety from within. Love begins to abound.

That's when it happened for Kevin.

He said, "I'm feeling so much better. I'm starting to like myself, not because I'm Kevin the character, the fun guy, but more than that."

"You might be ready to add more depth to your EBT Practice. The basis for EBT is the relationship with yourself. As your set point rises, you realize that there are questions you want to ask yourself."

Kevin responded, "Tell me more . . ."

You want to know who you are, the challenges you are facing, and your aspirations – who you want to be in facing those challenges. The answers to these questions are stored in the neural circuits in the emotional brain. To a great extent, emotional health is rooted in what these unconscious memories tell us, so in EBT we change them. All the negative self-concept wires are 3, 4, and 5 Circuits, but mainly 4 and 5. The ideal way to rewire them is to confront the negative ones after they have been unlocked. After doing a rip-roaring Cycle, the 4 and 5 Circuits are more apt to be "hot" or "online," with their synaptic connections fluid and open to change.

Presenting contradictory information first, then positive information just before using the Take Action Tool, accomplishes several things: 1) the Stress Circuits are unlocked; 2) you are at Brain State 1 so it is easy to generate positive and wise thoughts; and 3) a positive self-concept and clarity about the challenge you are facing and your aspirations produce the ideal mental state for making plans and going forward.

I said, "Kevin, ask yourself these questions when you are doing deep work. Slip them in just before using the Take Action Tool. I'll show you how to do it when you do your Cycle in a few moments."

"Sounds good."

The 3 Questions

- **Who am I?**
- **What challenge am I facing?**
- **Who do I want to be?**

What is my essence?

The loving nature of the emotional brain always astounds me. At a past three-day conference on EBT, Lori Karan, an addiction medicine physician, showed some advertisements for addiction medications that claimed, "You can have it all." The participants laughed.

Actually, that is truer about the natural properties of the emotional brain than it is about pharmaceuticals.

I asked Kevin, "Do you recall the first time you spiraled up and felt that glow?"

He said, "Vaguely . . . no, really . . . I do remember that. The experience surprised me."

"That moment at Brain State 1 was created by you. Your brain can do that."

Kevin said, "I get that."

"You had that ability right from the start. You are a person who can create joy."

"It's natural."

"Exactly. That tingle, glow, or lightness is the experience of joy chemicals. It's the Joy response. You use EBT to sustain that experience and wire your brain to activate it spontaneously most of the time."

Kevin said, "So my nature is joy right from the start."

As his set point rises, Kevin will be more aware of times when he is not at Brain State 1 and become curious about some of the beliefs encoded in his brain that seem foreign to who he is and who he wants to be.

Once Kevin becomes aware that he has core beliefs that are at odds with his essence, to be in joy, he will be drawn to using the Feel Better Tool to update faulty Core Circuits. As the unconscious mind has no walls, experiences are encoded in the brain that automatically extract "truths" that are pure fiction. This is a normal awakening and ideal for motivating us to change core beliefs that have found their way into our long-term memory through no fault of our own. In stress, the brain accepts whatever experiences arrive without filtering them, and then extracts truths from those experiences. It most strongly remembers experiences early in life when we are entirely at the mercy of our environment.

In EBT, we operationalize these early wires as the 7 Core Circuits. To raise the set point, we must build a scaffolding of core beliefs that promotes resiliency. That means fixing these glitches by driving them out, pulling apart their neurons, and refashioning them as joy wires that give us an acquired secure attachment and a set point in joy ("Set Point 1").

The 7 Core Circuits

Stress Circuits	Joy Circuits
I do not exist.	I do exist.
I am bad.	I am not bad.
I have no power.	I have power.
I cannot do good.	I can do good.
I cannot love.	I can love.
I am not worthy.	I am worthy.
I cannot have joy.	I can have joy.

The last circuit is the Joy Circuit, and the program builds up to encoding that wire. Stress tells us that joy is for others, that it was all used up by the time we reached the front of the line. Now, by raising our set point our unconscious mind informs us that we cannot only have joy but that joy is our very essence.

We become aware that evolutionary biology begs us to clear glitches so we begin to understand the deeper truths of life: that our essence is joy if we engage the emotional brain and surrender to trusting its resiliency pathways – and using them.

Use Spiral Up #3

Although most participants use the Feel Better Tool periodically when they start the program, they often become more fascinated with updating their core beliefs after their Survival Circuits are triggered less and less often.

The process is exactly the same as in Spiral Up #3 Deep Work for Stop A Trigger, except when you connect with your body, do not look for a drive that is urging you to move forward. Instead, watch for a "thud." It is a sense of sinking, a bad feeling in your neck, your chest, or your stomach.

The core expectation is a false belief. It seems true for a nanosecond when you are in a full-blown stress response, but it was encoded inaccurately. It is a false generalization, but the Cycle Tool transforms it into an accurate generalization, giving you a more secure base in daily life.

Appreciating your essence is joy

Kevin was ready to do a Cycle and learn how to ask the three questions, finding his first Core Circuit glitch.

"Kevin, start right where you are. Could you give me five sentences and five words?"

"Okay, the situation is . . . I had been really good at not raging, but I had been triggered by an employee who didn't do his job and then lied about it, and I have to go to the dentist and I go to Brain State 5 at the thought of anyone going into my mouth, and then my wife called and criticized me again and . . ."

"That's good, Kevin, but if you keep explaining it, you will drain all the emotion out of it, and there won't be any stress left to use to discover the circuit. Try this: pause and collect yourself until you have a complaint in mind. Be an irritable four-year-old and sound aggravated. Just complain for five sentences or so."

"Alright . . . the situation is . . . I had a bad day, then my wife called and told me what was wrong with me, and I started raging and lost control."

"Have you said what you needed to say to map out the story, the complaint?"

"Yup. What I'm most stressed about is . . . I lost control."

"Excellent, that's your topic. Go for it, the Anger Procedure."

"I feel angry that I lost control. I can't stand it that I lost control. I HATE it that I lost control. I HATE it, I hate it, I HATE it. I HATE myself for losing control. I HATE myself!"

"That's off-topic. Return to your topic."

"I hate it that I lost control with my wonderful wife . . . It's turning to sadness. I feel sad that . . . my topic is that I lost control . . . I feel sad that . . . I was so stressed that I was out of my mind, which was hard."

"Well done. Feel your feelings until they fade."

Kevin paused for quite a while, extracting every bit of power from that emotional experience.

"I'm ready for more. My one deepest fear is . . . my topic is I lost control . . . that if I do not resolve this . . . the consequence to me that matters to me will be . . . I will judge myself . . . my wife will leave me . . . and my wires will be downloaded into the brains of my children."

Kevin was deep into feeling his feelings until they faded.

"Kevin, now this is a change. You can state the Survival Circuit glitch but then go under it to the Core Circuit that is blocking you from rewiring that survival drive. Put your shoulders back. Use your powerful, joyful voice to keep your prefrontal cortex functioning at its best."

"Okay . . . HEY, I do have some power here. I feel guilty . . . why don't I just . . . stop raging? Of course I don't stop raging, because my basic expectation under that is . . . I am not worthy. That's it. I am not worthy, that's right."

"Do you want to spiral up?"

"Sure, first slowly . . . I . . . AM . . . WORTHY . . . I . . . AM . . . WORTHY . . . I AM . . . WORTHY . . . That's ridiculous. OF COURSE I am worthy. That's completely ridiculous. I AM WORTHY. How ridiculous. I am definitely worthy. I am DEFINITELY worthy. I am DEFINITELY WORTHY!!!! YES!!!!"

"Now, three more times with joy to lock it in with a dopamine surge."

"I am WORTHY!!! I AM DEFINITELY WORTHY!!! YES, I AM. I AM DEFINITELY WORTHY!!!! YES!!!!"

"Well done. Are you up for the three questions?"

"Kevin said, "I need some guidance."

"Ask yourself, 'Who am I?'"

"I'm a father . . . a business owner . . ."

"Use one simple statement to convey your essential goodness, like 'I am a good person' or 'I am loving and kind.'"

"I'm not always loving and kind."

"This is about you without Stress Circuits, the essence of you."

"Okay, I am a very . . . sensitive, kind, person who wants to do good."

"Great. Now ask, 'What challenge am I facing now?' The point of this is that you are bringing your best self to this, but it is a challenge!"

"The challenge I am facing now is to honor that I am worthy and have a sense of my goodness wiping out my rage circuit."

"Who do you want to be? People all over the globe are facing the same challenge, but what is your aspiration? Who do you aspire to be in facing this challenge?"

"I want to be a man who does not repeat his father's raging. I want to be someone who overcomes his personal history. I want to be someone who copes without raging or stuffing his feelings into overeating and drinking."

"Great. Now, the Take Action Tool. I expect myself . . ."

Kevin said, "I expect myself to do the best I can to fry this Core Circuit, and when that's blasted apart, to erase my rage circuit."

"Positive, powerful thought?"

"I am perfectly capable of doing that!"

"The essential pain? The hard part for you?"

"That's odd. What's coming up in my mind is, I must receive."

"That's the essential pain for Spirituality, as once it is clear how much you matter in this world, there is a need to surrender to the goodness of life and its deeper meanings, taking really good care of yourself so you have more to give back."

"Hmm, so I must stop pushing myself so hard and begin to receive the goodness of life, and my reward is Spirituality."

"Sit with that and feel it, as feeling it changes your brain."

"I'm doing that. I have warmth in my chest and a glow in my hands and feet. A surge of joy. I spiraled up!"

"What was the most important thing you learned from your work today?"

"That this work is deeper than I thought and that I feel touched. I have tears in my eyes, and that never happens."

"You did that, Kevin. You connected with the deepest part of yourself. That's why we engage the emotional brain. It's magical!"

Kevin was on his way to raising his set point and accessing the seven natural pleasures of a purposeful life.

1 2 3 JOY!

Step 2: Boost Rewards

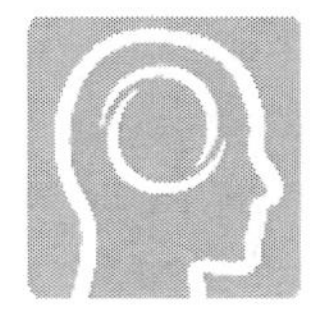

12

Your Reward Center: Balance Your Nucleus Accumbens

With the set point rising and stress cleared, the emotional brain calls us to shift our priorities to pleasure. The cortisol surges that block our joy have faded, and much like a child released from the classroom for recess, we want – and need – to play.

Marna Cohen, a social worker in pediatrics at the university, was the first person who taught me to see play as medicine.

I was learning how to evaluate the contribution of parents to a child's obesity, and she coached me, "The most important question to ask yourself is, 'does this parent know how to make themselves happy?'"

In today's world of brain science, she would probably say instead, "Ask yourself, 'Does this parent have a dominance of Joy Circuits so they are naturally happy?'"

Ultimately, it comes down to circuits. When running a Joy Circuit and at Brain State 1 or 2, we're happy and angelic, loving and kind in everything we do, all fueled by higher-purpose chemicals. We feel like going for a walk and enjoying the sight of puffy white clouds in the brilliant sapphire sky. Biting into an apple when hungry is divine.

Activate a Stress Circuit, taking us to Brain State 3, 4, or 5, and the stress chemical cascade makes thoughts of kindness absurd and stops any access to higher purpose. We are still the same loving person at our core, but the thinking brain's connection to the emotional brain breaks down. The prefrontal cortex cannot shuttle thoughts of higher purpose down to the reward centers in the emotional brain. It's not that we won't be altruistic, spiritual, or emotionally evolved, but that our brain can't let us bring out the best in ourselves.

Resetting for natural pleasure and higher purpose

Once Stress Circuits are running the show, appetites for artificial pleasures drive us. The quickest, easiest, cheapest way to reward ourselves is with ultra-processed food. The drive to reward ourselves is biologically driven and strong. If anything blocks us from getting our fix of food, we'll find a way to rationalize it, as survival drives for reward are operating.

For example, I asked Kevin whether he ate mainly ultra-processed, artificial foods or real foods. He answered flippantly, "You can't avoid sugar. It's in everything. I eat cookies and candy every day. Who doesn't?"

Kevin will defend his use of a mid-morning donut because he is "hungry," or order a salad at lunch to make up for the indulgence but then pour 1000 calories of ranch dressing on it so it is tasty.

In EBT, once past the first phase of clearing stress, we run up against our Reward Glitches that block us from enjoying natural pleasures and tapping into the power of purpose to make eating healthy effortless. Our job is to fix those glitches and train our brain to experience healthy pleasures as far more rewarding than unhealthy ones.

I said, "Kevin, you've beaten back the Stress Circuits, weakening them so you feel safer, but It's time to rewire those Reward Glitches so you start swooning about how great it feels to eat healthy food when you are hungry."

Kevin laughed, "It's not that easy. I always have two voices calling to me, one over each shoulder. On one shoulder, the voice says, 'Eat everything in sight,' and on the other, the voice says, 'Who needs food? Go get some joy.'"

"Of course you have two voices, because you have two different circuits, and they are dueling! As you keep spiraling up, the Joy Circuits will become dominant, and you will only hear one voice. Eating healthy will come naturally."

What did Kevin need? Someone in his court, a cheerleader of sorts to inspire him to use EBT with so much intensity and precision that the adaptive wires would become dominant.

Kevin said, "So, I need to become a master of rewiring – a ninja warrior – crushing any other circuit that gets in the way of my joy."

My job as Kevin's provider was to inspire him to use EBT with such intensity and precision that he created a monumental circuit of higher purpose for eating healthy.

I said, "And to have that passion, you need purpose. Would you like to spiral up and find your purpose?"

He said, "Yes, and began.

Spiraling up to break free of resistance to change

Kevin said, "The situation is . . . that I don't want to change. I like overeating. I like doing whatever I want to do: eating, drinking, and doing whatever I please. What I'm most stressed about is . . . I do not want to change."

"Excellent."

"I feel angry that I don't want to change. I can't stand it that I don't want to change. I HATE it that I don't want to change. I HATE it. I HATE it. I really HATE HATE HATE it! It shifted. I feel sad that . . . I have a war going on inside me . . . I feel afraid that . . . I will always have a war going on inside me . . . I do have some power here. I feel guilty . . . why don't I just . . . change? OF COURSE I won't just change, because my unreasonable expectation is . . . I get my . . . power . . . from staying stuck."

Then he stopped speaking entirely.

"What just happened, Kevin?"

"I feel stunned. I can't believe I get my safety from staying stuck, but that is spot-on accurate. That's the story of my life. I get my power from staying stubbornly stuck. That feels better. No, It's not about everything. It's about food and weight."

"Change the expectation until it accurately reflects the message in the circuit in your emotional brain and, thus, rings true. See yourself and this circuit accurately."

"I get my power from staying stubbornly stuck when it comes to food and weight. That rings true."

Kevin went on and spiraled up, then completed the Take Action Tool.

"I expect myself to do the best I can to have freedom from eating and weight wires. Positive, powerful thought? It is time. The essential pain? I am alone. Nobody can do this for me. The buck stops with me. The earned reward? Sanctuary. I will have peace and power from within."

"Is that your reward?"

"Yes, that's it. My body is tingling. I will do whatever it takes to clear these circuits and have that peace inside."

Kevin used the Cycle Tool to help him discover his higher purpose for raising his set point, but Charlotte didn't need to spiral up. All she needed was to relax and experience an Imagine, a guided imagery process that is used in the EBT Program.

"Now I'll guide you as you imagine yourself at Set Point 1, with all seven rewards, and typically, one reward will be the most alluring to you."

Charlotte agreed, so I guided her through this Imagine.

▪ ▪ ▪

Imagine: Me at Set Point 1

Relax: Begin by relaxing. Turn your attention to your body and your breathing and breathe in through your nose and out through your mouth, or in any way that feels comfortable and comforting to you. Then, when you are ready, begin to imagine.

Imagine: See yourself awakening in the morning and realizing that you have an abundance of all seven rewards of a purposeful life. You have:

The 7 Rewards

1.	Sanctuary	Peace and power from within
2.	Authenticity	Feeling whole and being genuine
3.	Vibrancy	Healthy with a zest for life
4.	Integrity	Doing the right thing
5.	Intimacy	Giving and receiving love
6.	Spirituality	Grace, beauty, and mystery of life
7.	Freedom	A life of joy and purpose

"See yourself moving through your day, having all seven of these rewards. You are at peace with food, and the joy of releasing extra weight makes it easy and natural to reclaim a body size that is healthy and right for you.

"You had the passion to rewire the circuits blocking that peace and joy because one of those rewards called to you. Bring to mind that reward. Was it Sanctuary, Authenticity, Vibrancy, Integrity, Intimacy, Spirituality, or Freedom?

"Bring to mind the reward you wanted most, which inspired you to rewire with passion. Take all the time you need, and when you are ready, please share what you learned about yourself from this experience."

■ ■ ■

"Charlotte, what was the most important thing you learned from that Imagine?"

She said, "That I wanted all of them."

"And the one that you wanted most and that inspired you to marshal the passion needed to gain freedom from stress eating and activate the joy of releasing weight with ease?"

"That would be Vibrancy, healthy with a zest for life. I love to walk on the beach with the waves splashing at my feet, or paint paintings that lift people up and give them hope. I wanted that zest for life."

"That's the reward you knew you must have, so you saw yourself crushing every wire in your way to get it."

"Yes, that's the one."

The reward that calls to you is undeniable. Once you identify it, you become unstoppable, because it is not a thought. It is a passion that comes straight from the deepest part of yourself, that which is sacred within you.

Although raising your set point until you have all seven rewards is the overall plan, use one or both techniques to find the reward that will light your fire within.

Identify the one reward so important to you that you become a rewiring ninja and happily clear any rusty old wire that dares to get in the way of your dream coming true.

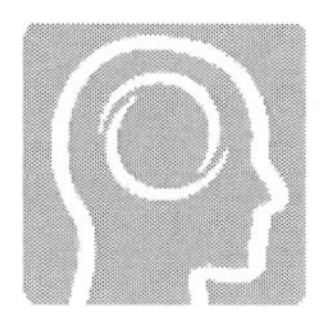

13

Clear those Glitches: Become a Master of Rewiring

It's our job to be sure we feel rewarded day by day. That's an essential pain of life, nobody can rescue us from our misery and no person, place, thing, or food can satisfy our deepest needs.

If someone whispered in my ear, on those Friday evenings when I baked meringue cookies and devoured them, that I could use a mental construct – a thought of higher purpose – and turn off my desire for sugar, I would have said, "You are crazy."

At the time, I was way too stressed.

However, fast-forward to that same girl with her stress cleared and I might have listened. In the world of the emotional brain, timing is everything. Once our stress has been largely cleared and the set point starts rising, the "why" of what we do becomes more interesting.

Then, It is just a matter of becoming a ninja warrior and getting excited about rewiring Reward Glitches. It's just a project, a pivotal one, and who doesn't like a good project?

Lynda Frassetto, one of the four scientists who conceptualized EBT as rewiring the stress response, once said, "There is a complex relationship between obesity, stress, and reward." To do a good job of rewiring Reward Glitches that prevent us from loving eating protein foods because they block cravings, for a reward such as Freedom, Vibrancy, or Spirituality takes rewiring how we reward ourselves, but also soundly clearing our stress. Let's further explore both types of glitches.

What are Stress Glitches?

These wires misinform us of how scared we need to be. Stress Glitches either overestimate or underestimate the real threat we face. They turn us passive, so we do not protect ourselves or have us so on edge that we wear ourselves out for no reason.

Both are allostatic circuits that have no shut-off valves ("positive feedback loops"), so if the wire gets it wrong and tells us we're in peril when we are not, the Stress Triangle goes bonkers, and our thoughts, emotions, and behaviors become completely out of line with our reality.

Initially, epinephrine and cortisol ramp up, then comes an extended secretion of cortisol, which is public health enemy #1. We may go into a social situation where there are no lions, but we still see lions everywhere, and with the buffet presenting all sorts of stimuli that trigger our Food Circuits, we overeat. This is an overestimating False Danger Glitch. They are such a bother!

The other Stress Glitch underestimates the danger we face, causing us to lose all perspective on life's dangers – a False Safety Glitch. Call it denial, delusion, distortion, or blind spots, but these wires make us overly accepting of situations, so we do not take precautions to save ourselves before bad things happen. We are fear-deficient, and the healthy bursts of stress chemicals that can spark us into action fail to appear. Cortisol remains low when we could really use a higher dose of it. We overeat because of False Danger Glitches, but that wouldn't be much of a problem if we didn't have the False Safety Glitches operating. Instead, we put the overeating out of our minds or shame ourselves, even asking ourselves silly questions like, "Why did I do that?" when It's obvious why we did it. A wire made us do it! The ways we cope distract us from rewiring the circuit, which is the only brain-based way to stop doing the same unfortunate thing repeatedly, and sometimes for the rest of our lives. False Safety Glitches cause this.

How Reward Glitches fit in

Neither of these two stress glitches alone would be all that harmful, except that there are two Reward Glitches that amplify their extremes. They dump kerosene onto the fire. The first is the Extreme High Glitch. Few of us binge on broccoli, but enough normal daily stress causing Stress Triangle activation can put us on edge. The first bite of a chocolate bar can activate a circuit that causes such an extreme elevation of dopamine that we gobble up the rest of the candy bar without even thinking. We don't think, because we are under the spell of an Extreme High Glitch.

Wires that cause damaging extremes of dopamine were encoded because we happened to experience a "more-rewarding-than-expected" moment. Perhaps we were anticipating pleasure from eating an apple when hungry, but instead found ourselves biting into apple pie a la mode, and a dopamine reward extravaganza ensued. This gets our attention (we "like" it), and the dopamine itself causes the circuit to strongly remember that we liked it. After that, even the slightest stimulus activates the overshooting of dopamine and the "I gotta get it" drive to repeat that self-sabotaging behavior.

Rewire the Stress Circuits

Type of Wire	Chemical Consequences
Stress Glitches	
1. False Danger	**Over-secretion of Cortisol**
2. False Safety	**Under-secretion of Cortisol**
Reward Glitches	
3. Extreme High	**Damaging Dopamine Highs**
4. Extreme Low	**Damaging Dopamine Lows**

This would not be all that bad, except for the last of the four glitches, the Extreme Low Glitch, which comes about because of the brain's overlapping pain and pleasure pathways. Evolutionarily, we need both, so these pathways work together to reward us for healthy practices and punish us for unhealthy ones. This teeter-totter of ups and downs biochemically stays in the self-correcting range when in homeostasis. Every time you spiral up, you experience a slight pain ("essential pain") that strengthens your resiliency pathways, and bingo, as you bring up the higher purpose reward for following through ("earned reward"), the teeter-totter moves back to positive emotions that enhance health.

Yet, if the set point is low (chronic stress) or a cavalcade of glitches transpires (e.g., false dangers, false safety, and extreme highs), two problems occur. One is that we are in allostasis, which wipes out the forgiving nature of homeostasis, and the other is that there is a price to pay in the pain-pleasure pathway of the brain. It's payback time, and that means a necessary extreme low happens. We cannot get ourselves out of the chemical ditch because the reason we got there – nobody taught us how to spiral up – is also the pathway to balancing the teeter-totter and returning to homeostasis.

So, we do what any brilliant, talented, and kind person does. We take care of ourselves the best we can, which means repeating the same cavalcade of circuits. Except each time, our set point is lower, and the glitches are stronger.

The brain's pain-pleasure pathway

Psychologist Richard Solomon proposed this pain-pleasure pathway, which is an opponent-process mechanism. In this application, when we experience pain, pleasure is temporarily inhibited. The greater the pleasure, the more the after-effects are painful. Pop a few blueberries into your mouth, and the pleasure is lovely but modest, then it fades. You notice that the pleasure is gone, but that's okay, you can handle that. Dish yourself up some hot blueberry pie with vanilla bean ice cream, and you are in rapture until it fades into an afterburn of "Why did I eat that much?" and a food hangover, followed by a craving for more pie or anything with the same rapid delivery and extreme dopamine surge.

Stopping that teeter-totter of extreme pleasure followed by extreme pain takes staying present to the negative emotions and riding them out. The craving disappears. Positive emotional neuroplasticity is self-directed, as it is only by staying present to the intense emotions and letting them fizzle out that we can counteract that teeter-totter effect.

Negative plasticity occurs if we do not call a halt to the extremes of the pain-pleasure pathway. The number of dopamine receptors on cells decreases, and the ones we have become less effective. More of the dopamine-activating substance is required for the same impact, and in time dopamine receptors poop out. Even binge eating to improve the rush or consumption of large amounts of ultra-processed foods habitually fails to deliver. It may blunt the pain with numbness or truncate depression, causing a level of unhappiness that is tolerable, but joy is no longer in sight.

Brain States and Addiction

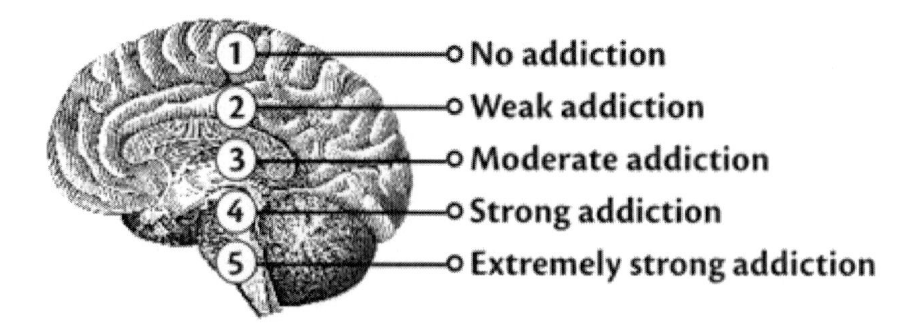

How do we classify addiction based on physiologic brain state? All allostatic circuits (Brain State 3, 4, and 5) promote the disengagement of the thinking brain and the reflexive activation of glitches and have at least a moderate addiction potential. All of them matter in EBT, but the rewiring of 5 Circuits improves health and quality of life the most.

These 5 Circuits cobble together multiple unconditioned, natural survival drives ("the fight-or-flight response") with any emotion, thought, behavior, sensation, or state, so we can categorize them based on the type of external solution we think we need: such as mood, behavior (e.g., food), relationship, and body image.

Survival Circuits vs. Core Circuits and Set Point

Another way to categorize addiction is based on the rapid-fire drive for excess versus chronic, habitual use. The EBT Program applies that approach. Survival Circuits activate a "phasic" delivery of dopamine, a short-term, high-amplitude dose. The other dopamine signaling is "tonic," which is long-acting with a lower amplitude. Core Circuits cause the latter resulting in wear and tear and adaptation of the brain ("allostatic load"), which is reflected in our set point. In the short term, stopping the triggered behavior is essential, but maintenance depends upon rewiring Core Circuits and raising the set point.

The EBT Program addresses both kinds of dopamine release. EBT can be integrated into any obesity or addiction program with relative ease. Providers are certified in the method, use it in their own lives, and teach from their personal experiences and scientific and clinical training in completing the EBT Program. EBT can be "bolted on" to any other program, procedure, or therapy.

The glitches are the problem!

Given that so many of us are trapped in the painful pattern of weight cycling or stuffing ourselves, the first step toward freedom is appreciating how hard it can be to change if we do not rewire our glitches. I was a card-carrying dieter for 22 years. I wish I had known back then that my food issues were not issues at all but a few random brain glitches that were tormenting me. I would have healed far sooner!

Let's take Jessica, for example. One evening, while putting her twins to bed, she is at her typical "baseline" pleasure level. Then, a "buttered popcorn circuit" is triggered in her brain. Immediately, she feels a glow as her nucleus accumbens has activated a slight dopamine surge. She enjoys that pleasurable feeling, but then her dopamine drops to sub-baseline levels. She feels worse than before she thought of food. This puts her in a reward deficit and motivates her "I gotta get it" response.

Jessica will quickly tuck the twins in for the night and turn her attention to getting to the kitchen, slipping the popcorn bag into the microwave, adding some extra butter, and pouring it into the large, white bowl she loves. All this is met with only a very slight increase in her dopamine level, as she works to get her "fix."

Finally, Jessica sinks into the soft sofa with her bowl of hot popcorn on her lap and places the first kernels in her mouth. Her dopamine level skyrockets, delivering just the extreme dopamine that keeps her trapped in dependency. Later, her dopamine will sink below baseline levels, increase her stress, and strengthen her glitches, but that is only half the story. The other half is what she is going to do about it.

The next evening, still with her Extreme Dopamine High Glitch alive and well in her brain and no awareness that the problem is perfectly rewirable, she proceeds with one of the three typical torture routines that millions of people go through daily across the globe. Her wire is a 5 Circuit, and her set point is 4.

Option 1.

"Let's do it again!"

The most common option is to do it again. Jessica's brain activates the Extreme Dopamine High Glitch. She is charged up, flooded with dopamine extremes, and overeats. Her better-than-expected-reward wire has her repeating the same drama as the evening before. She strengthens her glitch so the drive will be stronger the next time the wire is activated. Jessica distracts herself – the children's needs are constant, and work is incredibly demanding – and "reawakens" from staying busy the following evening, starts on the "glitch train," repeating the same process.

Option 2.

"I'll try to be good."

Most of us try to compromise, but any deal with the devil is fraught with pain. Jessica heeds the call of the Extreme Dopamine High Glitch but decides that she will override it. She tells herself that she will eat celery sticks and baby carrots instead. That's so sensible. They are so delightfully "crunchy!" Yet this is a biochemically-driven response, and although she dutifully downs the veggies, her nucleus accumbens is not impressed. Her worse-than-expected-reward wire, Extreme Dopamine Low Glitch, fires. She feels unrewarded and returns to Option #1. At least then she can count on meeting her "needs," even if that makes her feel ill, ultimately unrewarded, and lowers her set point.

Option 3.

"I'll cope in another way."

We are enormously resourceful, so finding a "good substitute" makes perfect sense. Jessica continues with the emotional bypass of her Food Circuit and engages in "healthier" ways to cope. However, biochemistry does not lie, and until she has balanced her nucleus accumbens, she will be at risk of an addiction substitution. A little casual internet shopping turns into serious credit card debt, and playing fun video games may become obsessive. She neglects the children because she can't wrench herself away from the computer. One glass of wine quickly leads to draining the bottle, and even staying active does not clear her Extreme Dopamine High wire. She finds herself addicted to being busy-busy-busy, or obsessed about her work – hooked on the position's power, money, or prestige. Access to joy and purpose escapes her as she trades one Extreme Dopamine High Glitch for another.

Option 4.

"I failed again. What's the use?"

If the first three options are not effective, Jessica may decide to force herself to stop overeating and make herself get on the scale daily, becoming the weight police. According to Peter Sterling, what might ensue may reflect the interaction of dopamine and serotonin. Jessica sticks with her program of dieting and weighing herself, riddled with self-judgment and amplified by perfectionism, and finds she is not losing enough weight. She has failed. Success in a formidable challenge delivers dopamine, but failure to achieve that goal produces serotonin, the endogenous offering of evolution to ease our disappointment. She quits the program, but then starts second-guessing herself and feeling like a failure, activating a worse-than-expected-reward wire, a Dopamine Low Glitch. That pain is so devastating to her psyche and soul that she vows never to try again. She is done with all of it, and naturally returns to Option #1.

Option #5

"I'll fix that glitch."

This is the EBT "crush the circuit" option. It's to see the problem as the wire, and "externalize" that Stress Circuit. That unwanted response? It's not us. It's just a wire. The process begins with discovering the circuit. Jessica and Charlotte had identified their Stress Glitches, so they set out to find the Reward Glitch that bothered them the most.

The Reward Glitch that triggers the drive

Jessica was confused about how she would find her Reward Glitch, the one that over-delivered dopamine and caused her to feel out of control.

I said, "Whenever you don't know why you do what you do, just complain about it as you start your Cycle. Be specific. That's why the topic is so important. The Cycle will take you right to the unconscious expectation driving it. Complain! Sound irritated!"

Jessica charged forward, "The situation is . . . I binge on salty, crunchy, sugary, fatty, fake food. I have to have it. Nothing else satisfies me. What I'm most stressed about is . . . I am addicted to fake food."

Then, like a ninja warrior, she let loose with a rip-roaring burst of safe, effective anger, and three minutes later, she revealed her glitch.

With her shoulders back and chin up, she said loudly and joyfully: "I DO have some power here. I feel guilty. Why don't I just . . . the topic is . . . stop eating fake food?"

I jumped in, "Jessica, see if you can state that again, this time with the image of what you would do. See yourself doing what, in the best of all worlds, you would do. That will pinpoint the glitch."

Jessica said, "I do have some power here. Why don't I just . . ."

"Stay on topic. What do you wish you would do instead of being addicted to fake food?"

"Why don't I just enjoy real food?"

"Keep going! You're almost there! Dig deeper. What is the expectation under that one?"

"OF COURSE I don't enjoy real food, because my unreasonable expectation is I get my . . . security . . . from . . ."

"Keep it simple. Then, repeat it as the circuit is very clear and simple."

"OF COURSE I don't enjoy real food, because my unreasonable expectation is I get my . . . security . . . from . . . getting high on food."

"Does that ring true?"

"Yes. I drain myself all day, taking care of everyone else's needs but my own, then I get my inner security from getting high . . . on food."

Then she paused, somewhat surprised.

"Oh, and it accomplishes the ick factor. I feel nauseated. I don't want that circuit in my brain. I hate that circuit."

"Jessica, that circuit was encoded when you had no better choices. It was what you needed in the past, but you have more skills now and you don't need it anymore."

"I know. Compassion, right?"

"Always, then, after compassion comes ripping the eyes out of that circuit!"

"Okay, I have compassion. That's enough for now. I want to spiral up."

"There are three parts: first slow, then ramp up, then state the new expectation with joy."

"I . . . can . . . NOT . . . get . . . my . . . security . . . from getting high on . . . FAKE Food . . . I . . . can . . . NOT . . . get my security . . . from getting . . . high . . . on FAKE Food. Even if I got high on fake food all day and all night, it would not give me the self-worth I need . . ."

"Now, ridicule it!"

"That's ridiculous! I can NOT get my security from getting high on fake food. No, I can't. How ridiculous. I can NOT get security from getting HIGH on fake food. Absolutely ridiculous! I can NOT get my security from being high on #$%& fake food. That's absolutely ridiculous!"

"Well done! Now create a new wire of your choosing: I CAN get my . . . "

"I CAN get my security from connecting to the deepest part of myself all day long, every day, for the rest of my life!"

"More joy. Dance if you like. Be bold!"

"I CAN get my security from connecting to the deepest part of myself all day long and creating joy in my life. I REALLY CAN get my security from connecting to the deepest part of myself and making each moment a moment of JOY. Yes, I CAN!!!"

I said, "You did it!"

"Yes, I feel the tingle all over my body, and that's what I am going to do."

I asked, "What is your reward for doing that?"

Jessica paused momentarily, then said, "I will like myself better because I will be genuine, not running around taking care of everyone else. So my reward is Authenticity."

I said, "Beautiful work, Jessica!"

Jessica had discovered the glitch that made the reward of fake food binges seem reasonable. Now, she would stop judging herself, point her finger at the problem, that glitch, and then rewire it.

The Reward Glitch that sabotages success

Of the two Reward Glitches, the one that bothered Charlotte the most was the Extreme Dopamine Low wire. For the last eight years, she had lost all interest in changing her eating and weight, and, watching her health deteriorate, her family had badgered her to change.

Charlotte said, "My Stress Glitch has been entrenched for so long that food is my everything. I eat for pleasure, power, love, comfort, safety – all of the above, but my glitch doesn't let me do anything about it."

Charlotte is dealing with natural biological forces, the pain-pleasure pathway, and the brain's need to follow the extreme dopamine highs of her binges with extreme lows. As she had gradually let go of any serious attempt to change, a serotonin surge may have helped her expect less of herself, but her disappointment in giving up may well have led to an Extreme Dopamine Low Glitch. By finding the offending circuit, she could get off the teeter-totter of highs and lows and find the sustainable, natural dopamine surges that would fuel her healing.

The Extreme Dopamine Low Glitch often keeps us avoiding change when it is really not that hard. Eating healthier and zapping a few of these wires is also not that hard. Avoiding change is what causes suffering.

Charlotte began, "The situation is . . . the moment I think about not eating exactly what I want to eat – and that is at least one candy binge per day with late night eating, too – my amygdala goes berserk. I eat double what I would otherwise. What I'm most stressed about is . . . changing my food feels abusive."

Her topic statement was critical. She ate and weighed exactly what her emotional brain found safe and rewarding. She needed to discover and rewire that glitch.

Charlotte launched into the Anger Procedure to unlock the circuit.

"I feel angry that . . . changing food feels abusive. I can't stand it that . . . changing food feels abusive."

Charlotte felt so beaten down by years of dieting that she was going numb as she expressed anger.

I checked with her, "Charlotte, let's pause. It may not be safe for you to do this Cycle."

She said, "I know. My emotions are drying up."

"Whenever that happens, It's not a problem. Let's circle around and begin again."

Charlotte complied, "The situation is I never want to diet again because dieting has ruined my life. The minute I think about changing my food, I go numb."

"That might be your complaint."

"What I'm most stressed about is . . . I go numb."

"Does that ring true?"

"Yes."

This time, Charlotte became a ninja warrior. She performed her most passionate burst of anger, which rapidly turned into one deep sadness, one fear, and then her brain was ready to identify her power.

She put her shoulders back, her chin up, and enthusiastically said, "Hey everybody, I DO have some power here. I feel guilty. Why don't I just . . ."

We both took a deep breath. She turned her attention to her body and waited for words to appear in her conscious mind.

"Why don't I just do the sensible thing that the bright, full-of-life four-year-old in me would do and . . ."

No words came out.

Again, she said, "Why don't I just do the sensible thing like the bright, full-of-life little girl in me would do . . . and face my fears and change my food?"

She wasn't at Brain State 1 yet, and the ick factor was not apparent.

"Dig deeper, Charlotte . . . the expectation that is under that is . . ."

Charlotte paused, then launched into discovering her wire, "OF COURSE I don't just do the sensible thing and face my fears and change what I eat, because my unreasonable expectation is . . . I get my existence from staying stuck."

She was stunned. Then she started laughing.

Her glitch was a Core Circuit, a fundamental belief buried in the least plastic area of her brain. Now that she had discovered it, she had the power to change it.

I said, "Does that ring true?"

"Yes, it makes so much sense now that I would do anything to avoid changing my food. It was a survival need to stay stuck. That's totally ridiculous! I want to clear it up. I want to do a Spiral Up Grind In."

I sensed that she would have some emotional clutter to clear later, but I always support the gut feeling of the person if they are at Brain State 1. Charlotte was in joy, and as our enteric nervous system from the brain to the gut is bi-directional, it was telling her what she needed to do."

I responded, "Let's do it!"

Charlotte stated it six times slowly: "I . . . can . . . NOT . . . get . . . my . . . existence from . . . staying stuck." Then she ramped it up, ridiculing the circuit: "That's ridiculous! I can NOT get my existence from being stuck, slowly killing myself by eating until I am stuffed. That is ridiculous! I can NOT get my existence from staying stuck." Finally, she was ready to transform it.

"How will you fix your glitch? What is your reasonable expectation, Charlotte?"

"I can get my existence from trusting myself enough to change at the pace that is right for me."

This was a deep 5 Circuit, so I suggested that she use the three Questions.

Charlotte said "Who am I? A loving person. A deeply good human. What challenge am I facing? I have had a lot of pain and my brain is telling me to stay stuck."

I said, "There are people worldwide facing the same wire right now, but all that matters is you. Who do you want to be in facing this challenge?"

She responded, "I want to be someone who knows and loves herself and gently begins changing step-by-step."

I could feel her loving connection to herself. At this point, she was giving me more than I had given her. This is the path of the EBT Provider. In contrast to many traditional therapies, we openly experience the joy of connection and cherish it, continually raising our own set point for our benefit and as a foundation for our effectiveness as clinicians.

I said, "Oh, I'm feeling the glow of what you said, Charlotte . . ."

Smiling, she completed her spiral up: "I expect myself to do the best I can . . . to clear the clutter about this . . . I think I have some Travel Backs to do and then crush that circuit. . . Positive, powerful thought? Now is the right time. The essential pain? I must give. I can't let myself off the hook. I cannot remain less than fully alive. My reward? Freedom."

I asked, "What did you learn from your work today, Charlotte?"

"I learned that I love myself more than I know and that change is not really that hard."

Then, she laughed.

Jessica and Charlotte had both established a reward that mattered most to them in their EBT journey by identifying their Reward Glitch. They were on their way to rewiring it, but each of them needed to strengthen their brain's capacity to enjoy the natural pleasures of life so that these extreme glitches would further lose their appeal.

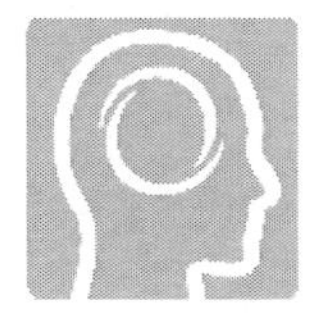

14

Customize Your Joy: What Pleases You?

It's not unusual to choose what you want to eat, but how about choosing the way you create joy in your life? That's a new endeavor born out of understanding that joy dismantles stress and that we have the mental tools to produce bursts of high-intensity pleasure at will. Joy is medicinal, and you cannot overdose on it.

Starting the day off right

An EBT morning does not begin with taking a hot shower, running around the block, or drinking a great cup of coffee, although you may do all of those things. It starts with intention.

Get into the habit of saying to yourself in the morning, "What am I doing with my day? I am creating joy in my life."

These words hold a great deal of meaning. "I" clarifies that nobody is responsible for your joy but you. "Creating" suggests that you must do something that requires effort and ingenuity. "Joy" conveys that having a mediocre mood doesn't make it. Finally, "in my life" conveys the value of each person's life and that your life and your day matter. Don't stop repeating these words until you "pop," which means that the amygdala switches off the nucleus accumbens and activates a dopamine surge.

Once you have made your "create my day" statement, keep it in the back of your mind, and whenever you are not at Brain State 1, reach for your app and collect a Joy Point.

Be generous with yourself – Collect a lot of Joy Points

During this second step of The EBT 1-2-3 JOY Program, focus more on counting Joy Points. You are rewiring Reward Glitches and the brain changes through experience. Right now, you need a lot of joy. Every spiral up includes scoring a Joy Point but be sure to add on self-created moments of chemical surges of neurotransmitters.

The app will help you with this. Touch on the Joy Point button, and you will see six options for generating that neurotransmitter surge. Choose from feeling that glow from relishing the higher reward for what you are doing, savoring a happy memory, enjoying sensory pleasures, bringing up a nurturing inner voice, taking a moment for spiritual connection, or engaging in an act of loving-kindness. Most participants try out all of them, then settle into using a few of them that light up their brain's reward center in the way that pleases them.

When Jessica started experimenting with Joy Points, she had some surprises.

I asked, "How did experimenting with the six ways to collect Joy Points go?"

She said, "Pretty well. The easiest for me was to bring up a happy memory. I thought of when my son was born, the moment I realized I was in love with my husband, and a special moment with my father when he told me he was proud of me."

"Most Joy Points come from moments of connection, and when you bring up the memory you not only activate the circuit, but you feel the benefits of a neurotransmitter surge."

"I could feel it, and bringing up these memories stopped me from eating mindlessly. I have been collecting a Joy Point whenever I start thinking about food."

"Was there another standout?"

"Sensory pleasures. I am eating slowly now and savoring each bite, but I am also learning how sensory-deprived I've been. I am so busy I don't take responsibility for giving myself sensory pleasure, and it's not that hard. When I put lotion on my legs, I focus on the sensation of stroking my legs and feeling their softness. My senses are coming alive."

Collect Joy Points

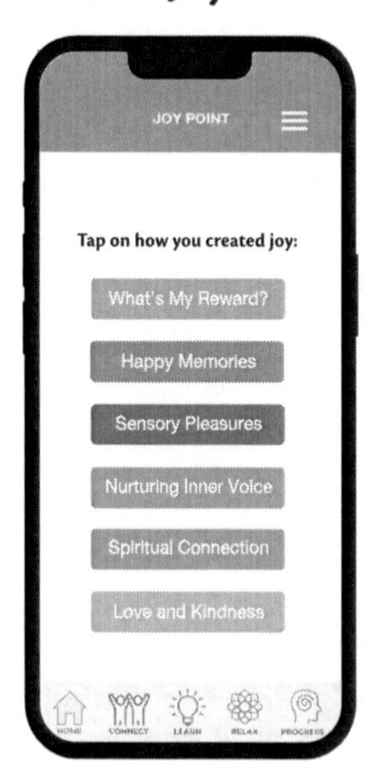

Could I be "joy insufficient"?

Obesity is associated with deficits in dopamine that increase our vulnerability to using food to self-medicate, boosting our reward chemicals by consuming ultra-processed foods. If we are dopamine deficient, it makes no sense to force ourselves to stop eating ultra-processed foods. We "need" the food because we are low in dopamine. The EBT approach is to honor our need to feel rewarded and meet it not by ingesting cupcakes, chips, and candy but by collecting Joy Points. They are calorie-free and when they deliver a sufficiency of dopamine, those ultra-processed foods begin to look incredibly unappealing. We have a certain personal pride that we choose to be selective in how we get our dopamine pulses. We skip the fake food that amplifies addictive drives that cause dependency in favor of the freedom that comes from using the sustainable, non-addictive dopamine delivered by Joy Points.

At a follow-up evaluation session for a study of EBT for weight loss conducted by the Washington County Health Department in Hagerstown, Maryland, I met all the participants in the study who attended a post-study celebration. Three Certified EBT Providers, Tammy Thorton, Lisa McCoy, and Paula Ernst had conducted the program.

One participant, a woman in her 40s whose extra weight put her at extreme medical risk, left a lasting impression on me.

She greeted me warmly, with a huge smile on her face. She shared how she had lost weight for the first time in decades and was not even dieting.

Then, with tears in her eyes, she said, "I have counted calories my whole life. Now, I count Joy Points. Thank you for EBT."

That's all I remember: her tears and her smile.

Joy is that powerful. Sometimes just telling a person that they deserve joy is enough to inspire them to lose weight. Other times joy changes people because they make it a game of "'How many Joy Points do I need to stop wanting chips?'"

Anyone raised in chaos and trauma is at risk of their brain extracting from that experience a "truth" that they cannot have joy. Joy isn't in the cards for them. They sense that even if they stood in the "joy line" for days, by the time they arrived at the front of the line, the person doling out Joy Points would say, "Sorry, the person before you got the last one."

By using EBT, you can create joy, and not only experience a dopamine hit on demand, but adopt the practice of creating joy as a way of life. The approach is risk-free as nobody can "overdose" on joy.

How many Joy Points do I need?

Once the Reward Glitches have been cleared, many people find that the floodgates open, and they start bingeing on joy.

When that happens for you, consider having a "Joy Challenge." Collect 25 Joy Points per day for three days. Most people are surprised at how effective it is in resetting their brain to create joy as a way of life.

Meredith, a school counselor from Texas, loved her job but she merged with her clients as she had not yet rewired her relationship circuit ("Love Circuit"). She "over-gave" to her clients, which drained her of dopamine so that by evening needed to use the brute-force slug of dopamine from external sources just to feel normal. She binged on technology, internet shopping, and food. I suggested a Joy Challenge to get her unstuck enough to rewire her merge circuit and stop this self-defeating cycle.

She agreed.

When I saw her a week later, she said, "The first day I forgot all about Joy Points. That shows how much of my work stress has been stored in my brain. I started again, and on Day 2, I did 25, on Day 3, I did 18, then I added another day, and on that day, I did 25 again."

Then she let out a giggle.

I said, "Meredith, I'm not sure I have heard you laugh like that."

She said, "I do feel different. I feel more buoyant, lighter! I didn't over-give to my clients on the fourth day."

By using Joy Points intensively, she was at a higher brain state, which naturally deactivated her merge wire. That experience of being at work with her joy chemicals surging gave her the motivation to roll up her sleeves and roust out of her amygdala that problematic merge wire and crush it. The stress and joy tools work together.

The "What's my reward?" Joy Point

Although I like variety in my Joy Points, the "What's my reward?" is the most powerful for me. First, it's a simple way to make decisions about eating. If I look at a food I'm about to eat, I can say to myself, "What's my higher-order reward for eating this?" If no higher-order reward comes to mind, then most of the time, I don't eat it. I always reserve the right to say 'freedom' when it comes to eating a wickedly obnoxious ultra-processed food when I need it. Deprivation is stressful! However, that brief 'reward check' can help. One new provider, Shelby Killion, said, "Asking the question has a huge benefit for me. If I can't identify an earned reward for doing something, then I do not do it. If I do identify a reward, I get a pulse of dopamine and endorphins and feel great."

Jessica had no trouble adjusting to this joy practice as her set point was 3 and she had used EBT vigorously from the start. Charlotte and Kevin struggled more as they had more Stress Circuits to clear which caused their set points to be in the 4-to-5 range. The stress that caused their set points differed. One had mainly chronic stress and the other had reactive stress.

Charlotte's stress was mainly chronic as she had been in stress overload since age eight, and her Stress Circuits were firing almost continually. She was almost always in Brain State 4 or 5, in the dissociative continuum, and numb.

On the other hand, Kevin's primary sources of stress were his glitches, his reactive circuits. Often, he could be in all five brain states and would move through each state rather quickly.

However, when a strong Stress Circuit fired, he would go to a Brain State 5 and could be stuck in stress for several hours or even a day. He was on the hyperarousal continuum, so he was raging, eating, or drinking.

I asked Kevin how his joy practice was going.

He said, "The Joy Points are helping me. The Happy Memories option is the easiest for me, and I've had some luck with the Love and Kindness and Spiritual Connection options. It's already had an impact. Things are going better with my wife, mainly because I'm not raging anymore. I feel a lot of compassion for her in what she has put up with for the last few years."

I said, "Wonderful! Keep using Happy Memories. Have you tried the Sensory Pleasures option?"

"That's what I have been working on."

Kevin was training his brain to differentiate internal sources of dopamine with their subtle dopamine waves from the external sources with their big blasts of neurotransmitters.

He said, "I was overdosing on sensory pleasures, the artificial kind. I did a Cycle and found my Reward Glitch: 'I get my safety from big bolts of dopamine regardless of their source.' That was encoded when I was 13 and a very out-of-control young man, so I'm rewiring that expectation and also, clearing the clutter, the fear memories from that time. Accessing sensory pleasure will be easier after I rewire that Reward Glitch."

I asked him about his experience with the option: What's my reward?

Kevin responded immediately and said, "That is a killer technique. I have it down now. If I cannot come up with a higher purpose for what I'm doing, it's dangerous to do it. I stop in my tracks."

Kevin was now in the thick of rewiring. He had mastered the How to Rewire skills and now understood why I say that if it is not fun, it is not EBT. This was fun, as he was proficient in EBT and having a good time rewiring any circuit that blocked his joy.

I said, "Keep on experimenting and only go on to Step 3 Change Habits when boosting rewards has worked biochemically and you look at the food and alcohol and say, 'A change would be sensible for me. I am ready.'"

He said, "I got it. I don't want to push forward until my emotional brain is ready,"

Kevin was on target to repair his nucleus accumbens after years of stress. Charlotte's experience was equally challenging but more moving.

Charlotte said, "I think my reward center is beyond repair. Genetically, I'm not a happy person. I'm shy. I overthink, and I am not a good candidate for joy training."

At that moment, Charlotte was at Brain State 5, and her brain chemistry was activating negativity. In allostasis, we cannot see light at the end of the tunnel, in fact, there is no light at all. Add to that isolation and the distorted thoughts make life seem hopeless. That's one of the reasons people love our Spiral Up Groups and why they are available daily. A person can feel 4ish when they drop in, but within a couple of minutes, they are running at Brain State 1 or 2. Joy is catching.

Joy is catching: the power of voice and connection

I wanted Charlotte to catch my joy. My goal was to use my voice and words that came from a higher brain state to deactivate her Stress Circuit and activate a Joy Circuit.

I said, "When you're stressed, joy sounds preposterous, but I've heard you spiral up numerous times now, and when you do, I hear one thing: JOY."

It worked. She let out a sigh of relief and said, "Actually, that's true."

"Charlotte, all you need to do is focus on the present moment. Create just one flicker of joy. You never know when the next flicker can lead to a breakthrough. Try all five ways of creating joy and find one or more that please you, then use them. Which one do you like best so far?"

Charlotte responded, "No question about it. I like 'What's my reward?'"

"How would it be for you to launch your joy practice focusing on purpose?"

"I'd like that. That gives me hope."

As you begin training your brain to create joy, see it not just as a way to make yourself happy, although happiness matters, too. See it as a way to get a dopamine hit, which makes it easier to change your habits. Habits account for 50 percent of the variation in health, so use joy to feel better but also to adopt healthy habits naturally and be healthier.

Start your day by saying, "I am creating joy in my life." Then collect massive amounts of joy. Keep creating joy until the thought of eating healthier sounds like a nurturing act. Then you will be ready for Step 3. Changing Habits.

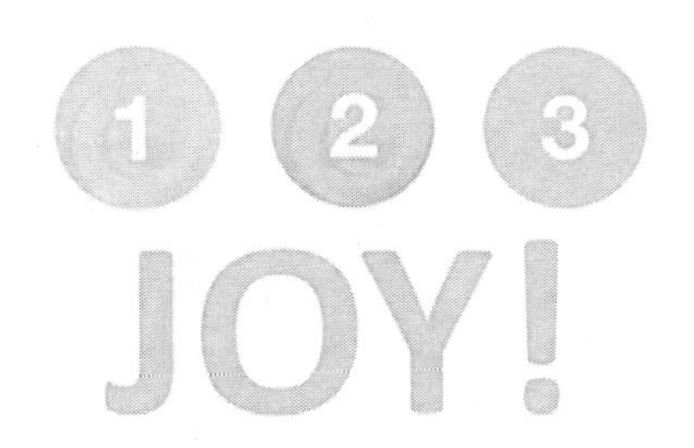

Step 3: Change Habits

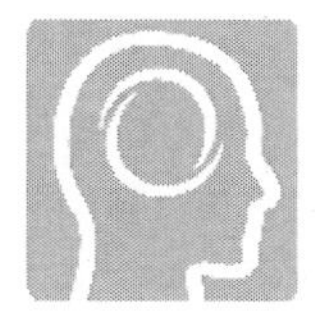

15

Your Habit Center: Coax Your Hypothalamus Gently (It's Sensitive!)

The EBT journey begins by trusting that your emotional brain is amazingly powerful, and you can teach it how to create joy.

That's just what Mattie did. She was in the EBT training for people for whom weight-loss surgery had proven unsuccessful. She told me on the first day of the course: "I have no joy. I am not capable of joy. I have no tingle of joy in my body."

Trusting our brain's capacity to create joy

In the first couple of weeks, Mattie learned to spiral up. Then she discovered her Food Circuit. It was "I get my love from food." She used the app to negate the expectation encoded in the circuit, saying "I can NOT get the love I *really* need from food. That's ridiculous! Even if I ate all day and all night, food would not give me the love I need." Then she replaced it with the expectation, "I *can* get my love from connecting to my personal strength and the goodness inside me."

I instructed her to hold herself accountable for saying this "grind in" by using the app before eating, always finding the earned reward for eating healthy.

That would be challenging, but even more difficult was stopping the tyranny of judging her food. She was more important than what she ate and it was by clearing that glitch and staying connected to the sensations in her body that, over time, she would learn how to feed herself. She would discover when, what, why, and how to eat in a way that no formula could deliver.

The "golden rule" of habit change is that if you can't make a behavior change that lasts for 30 days, the habit change is not accurate. That might work for habits like brushing teeth or taking vitamins, but not for behavior driven by Survival Circuits. Even "successful" habit change, on average, does not last more than six months. Mattie's challenge was to move to the new brain-based paradigm and measure her success by observing changes in her desire for food or drive to overeat, and watching for spontaneous, effortless changes in her eating, as they are rooted in reconsolidation of the offending circuit, the glitch.

At the fourth weekly session, Mattie reported her progress to the group.

She said, "I usually eat dinner, then after that, I have a sandwich. I stopped needing the sandwich. I had no interest in eating it."

Then she laughed and said, "Just saying that, I have a tingle."

I was totally delighted. She was beaming.

I asked the group, "Do you see the difference, everybody? Mattie shifted gears and focused on changing the circuit!"

Sarah, another participant said, "Yeah, and a couple weeks ago, she was saying she couldn't feel the tingle."

Mattie was amused and said, "I am getting more tingles. In a couple of days, I'll be a bundle of tingles!"

Caroline responded, "In a couple of days, your husband won't recognize you."

Mattie chuckled and said, "That's my goal."

The other group members chuckled, too, however, the essence of Mattie's comment is why EBT is effective. In the past, she had lost, then regained 100 pounds on her surgical program with medical supervision of her recovery. More importantly, the treatment had not changed her brain. Now she was using her brain to change her biochemistry and electricity and she was radiating joy. It is magical. That is the power of the method.

Ready for Step 3, a new approach to habit change

When you have cleared stress and boosted joy enough to notice some changes that are not "logical," do not rush to Step 3. Trust that your emotional brain will guide your way and continue spiraling up to be sure the joy of releasing weight has kicked in and you are aware of your higher purpose for releasing weight.

Also, take a little extra time to separate from your previous ways of approaching food and weight. If you have been using a diet program, do not go back to "eat less" and "exercise more." If you finished using weight-loss drugs, do not worry. Bradley Olson, who was coming off weight-loss drugs, wrote in an article published in the *Wall Street Journal*, "I had traded one kind of anxiety for another. I had to learn to eat just the right amount at just the right time."

Eating in a way that is right for you is not a problem, because you have the skills to connect with yourself and know what you need. That "internal compass" that was missing before because the Stress Triangle was spinning out of control is now at your beck and call. All you need to do is begin using that compass more and more effectively, rewiring a few Habit Glitches, and continue with the program until you are Wired at One.

Jessica reached that point of feeling the joy of releasing weight after six weeks in EBT, with 280 spiral ups and 349 Joy Points collected on the app. She was in a weekly group and had her support circle in place. She was very clear that she was more than eager to change her behavior out of self-love and joy. Her purpose was Freedom.

Kevin reached the point of joy of releasing weight at nine weeks in EBT, although his joy was wobbly, and he was still inconsistent with spiraling up. He was in the habit of dropping into two Spiral Up Groups per week, one with Angie and the other with Michele. He had hit 240 spiral ups and 272 Joy Points. His purpose was Sanctuary.

Charlotte knew that the right path for her was a slower one. She had experienced so many "loops" of losing and then regaining weight that she wanted to "declutter" her brain thoroughly of wires before she tampered with habit change.

She watched the videos of the program, came to the weekly Spiral Up with Dr. Laurel meetings, and dropped into the Sunday Spiral Up Group led by Shelby. Charlotte reached the joy of releasing weight after 11 weeks in EBT, with 419 spiral ups and 580 Joy Points. It was a Joy Challenge that she did during her 10th week, collecting 20 Joy Points a day, that tipped the balance in her brain toward the joy of releasing weight. Her purpose was Vibrancy.

The crown jewel of EBT: Fixing Habit Glitches

The scientific aspect of the third step in The EBT 1-2-3 JOY Program was shepherded by the program's Medical Director, Dr. Michele Welling. She is an Internal Medicine physician, has completed an Integrative Medicine Fellowship, and is currently serving as medical director for an addiction treatment center. She specializes in brain-based health and has a special interest in the role of stress on chronic disease and pain management.

Dr. Welling has been certified as a Master Trainer in EBT for a decade. Out of her work treating primary care patients in underserved populations, including those with addiction, mental health disorders, and chronic pain, she quickly recognized how much difficulty people have in changing their habits and how these habits fit into the framework of brain-based health. She proposed reconceptualizing the Limbic Triangle, and specifically the hypothalamus, as the center for "metabolic detection errors," called Habit Glitches in EBT.

In subsequent meetings with Dr. Welling and Clinical Research Director Dr. Lynda Frassetto, a metabolic research specialist, we sharpened the definition of Habit Glitches. They are the brain changes resulting from the body's metabolic adaptation to the stress-induced habits we are forced to embrace because of today's extreme and ubiquitous stress overload. It is these glitches, not the individual's self-will, that block behavior change, and clearing them is a brain-savvy way to promote easy and lasting changes in our habits. The concept of Habit Glitches is also consistent with the work discussed in a previous chapter by Robert Lustig and Michele Mietus-Snyder, outlining how the Limbic Triangle is affected by stress.

Rewiring Habit Glitches is an essential skill that we need to learn for modern life. National statistical data show that health-damaging habits are increasing over time. In fact, our habits account for 50 percent of our risk of mental health problems and chronic diseases, the predictable consequence of the stress pandemic without the widespread availability of appropriate tools to switch off the Stress Triangle.

Our mission at EBT is to bring these skills – stress skills and the tools to rewire circuits as a prelude to successful habit change – to people across the nation and across the globe. You are now part of that movement as you are reading this book. The EBT mission does not ask people to change their habits, as research shows that habit change at the level needed to prevent and treat health problems is next to impossible if you don't deal with your stress. We need to do better than that, and you are already a part of that as you are learning this new paradigm.

No diets, no drugs, no measuring, no rules

As the EBT approach is not to toggle our behavior but to wipe out the offending circuit that drives the behavior, there are no diets in this program. Nobody will tell you what to do or how to eat. What's more, there is no "food guru." The method is based on science and can be replicated. It is solid, so you become your own guru. You are using your brain to make the many important daily decisions needed to change eating and weight with grace and ease.

A big part of creating that grace and ease for yourself is completing the part of the program of fixing Habit Glitches. I think of this step as paying dues. You ask your brain to deal with your bad habits, but as it does, you then have to ask it to end the love affair with your bad habits and start a new romance with new and better habits.

Break-ups always include a little discomfort. We recommend making the break-up easier. Instead of the drama of a dietary fast or paying for a fancy diet spa for a week (how stressful), you ease into it. Keep it fun. Yes, there may be a little discomfort, but not as much as you expect because the process creates immediate joy from clearing stress and boosting rewards. Then you find it easier to weave in new habits that are challenging but still achievable in the long term.

As your brain warms up to this new way of living, you'll notice that new healthy habits come more easily. Once these habits transition into the "commitment" stage where you feel secure because the new behavior is the norm, the glitch is fixed and the benefits are huge. Just as your old set point caused weight gain cycling combined with stuffing and starving yourself, the new set point fights back when you have an occasional food binge, keeping you safe with new healthy habits, and doing it with a touch of grace.

The hypothalamus is quite sensitive to change, but there are no blood tests, brain scans, or tried-and-true formulas for how quickly you can change your habits or the precise foods and amounts to eat that keep it from getting riled up. Only you know the perfect pathway to changing your glitches. It's a matter of listening to your body, personalizing the process, and then trying out the changes you make.

The EBT Program, including this book, will share the science and provide a scaffolding for you to build upon, but the art of EBT involves noticing what you are drawn to changing, what tools feel good to you, and then doing the work. Nothing takes the place of you trusting your own body, being playful, and discovering what is right for you – step by step.

Kevin did not find these ideas welcoming. He said, "If you tell me what to eat, I can do that. I need the specifics."

"That would be out of integrity for me, Kevin, and disrespectful of your intelligence."

"Why?"

"Your food needs vary widely from moment to moment, and you already have the most powerful processor on the planet, your emotional brain. Now that your thinking brain is in charge, you can apply a few concepts and make better decisions than any nutritionist, psychologist, or physician could suggest."

Kevin sighed and said, "Okay, then tell me the concepts."

Be gentle with your hypothalamus

Let's look more closely at the brain structure that we are changing. The hypothalamus is the structure that ultimately decides how to respond to our stress. It is the regulator of our metabolism and controls our hunger, attachment behaviors, body temperature, thirst, sleep, and fatigue. It "pulls the trigger" of the stress response and all our basic bodily functions. Because our responses become habits (neural connections), the hypothalamus decides which habits to drive based on the perceived needs of the stress triangle of the brain and the activations of its other centers. It adjusts to both our Stress and Reward Glitches by normalizing deleterious behaviors as habits, creating an entire web of neural, biochemical, and cellular changes that cause adaptation to bad habits (Habit Glitches). These bad habits can include those associated with eating, energy, relaxation, relationships, the expectations we have about ourselves, safety, and the emotions we generate based on internal and external stimuli. In addition, when we change the way we eat in terms of food quality and quantity, our body adjusts its energy metabolism to adapt to what it now perceives as the new normal. This also becomes a Habit Glitch, which continues to drive our abnormal eating.

Who doesn't have stress? If we have stress that goes unfiltered by the emotional brain, we have some Habit Glitches. They are extremely important to clear, as without clearing them individually – and as a national health priority – we'll continue to have skyrocketing rates of chronic diseases, mental health problems, inflammation, immune system problems, and accelerated aging.

Habit Glitches cause those accommodations to our health because both the amygdala and the nucleus accumbens are compromised in their functioning. The nature of allostasis (changing to stay the same) is to sacrifice short-term biochemical and behavioral health to try and maintain a semblance of civil functioning in the body and brain when chaos is reigning in the structures of the Stress Triangle. Think of the activities of the hypothalamus as trying to maintain this functioning and "mopping up" to prevent chaos.

Change habits gently and consistently

We change Habit Glitches by changing our behavior and maintaining that behavior for long enough that the brain perceives it as the new norm.

To change consistently but not rigidly takes being at a sustainable Brain State 1 more of the time. That means keeping your higher purpose in mind and avoiding reactivity.

We are reactive (trigger a Stress Circuit) when the change is too extreme. A good rule of thumb is to notice that you are a little hungry, at Brain State 3, but not hungrier. Allowing yourself to be at Brain State 3 with challenges is productive. For example, Walt is dealing with pain after his back surgery, and is learning to tolerate Brain State 3 pain, but not let it get to 4 or 5. First, he uses EBT (the Anger Cycle and Joy Points). He hopes they will return him to Brain State 3. If they don't, he uses ice or distraction. If that still does not work, he uses medication. Changing habits with EBT is much like that.

When you feel a little hungry (Brain State 3), reassure yourself that being slightly hungry is not the worst thing, and there is no need to immediately react and eat. Use EBT. Take away the stress by using the Instant Boost (Spiral Up #1) or collecting a few Joy Points. Great Joy Point options are What's my reward? and Nurturing Inner Voice. If that isn't enough, try taking the edge off the hunger with a small amount of food. Eating protein works best, or consuming a liquid such as water, tea, or broth. Some people quiet their stomach with an antacid. Another option is to distract yourself with a rewarding activity, such as collecting more Joy Points or taking a break for five minutes to do something physical or fun ("play").

What about finding yourself at Brain State 4 and 5? That's not helpful. It can reinforce a relationship with yourself and food that feels depriving. Set a limit with habit change: you do not tolerate a Brain State 4 or 5 caused by changing habits too quickly. Changing faster than your emotional brain will tolerate is counterproductive as only sustained changes rewire the Habit Glitch.

Learning about yourself through habit change

Changing habits reveals a lot about our early training. The same parenting styles that cause the emotional bypass cause overreaction to pain at the level that is needed to change habits, either underreacting or overreacting to stress. Children raised with permissiveness (expectations "too easy") do not learn to tolerate moderate discomfort for long enough to feel proud of themselves, so they do not persevere. They give up, often encoding a Mood Circuit of depression or false highs (everything is "fine" when it is not).

Those raised with deprivation (expectations "too hard") learn to tolerate too much discomfort, so they persevere at a level that is exceedingly uncomfortable until they give up and return to old habits that are permissive. The Mood Circuits that are associated with this pattern are anxiety, hostility, and numbness. Scarcity panics and rebellion are common.

Even if habit change was difficult for you, it will not be difficult now because you have expanded your skills. First, your practice in spiraling up has strengthened your brain's resiliency pathways and you have rewired a fair number of Stress Glitches and Reward Glitches. All that is left in healing the Stress Triangle is fixing any remaining Habit Glitches. That takes making significant but non-triggering and consistent changes in food. Like Walt learning to deal effectively with physical pain, responding effectively to the modest stress ("essential pain") of changing your food intake is just a matter of skill. Use the process: 1) spiral up, 2) take the edge off, and 3) distract with joy. If that 1-2-3 process leaves you at Brain State 4 or 5, eat food until you are just satisfied, wait 20 minutes, and you will be full, without being overly full and uncomfortable.

Brain States and Changing Habits

Some stress is good, but not too much.

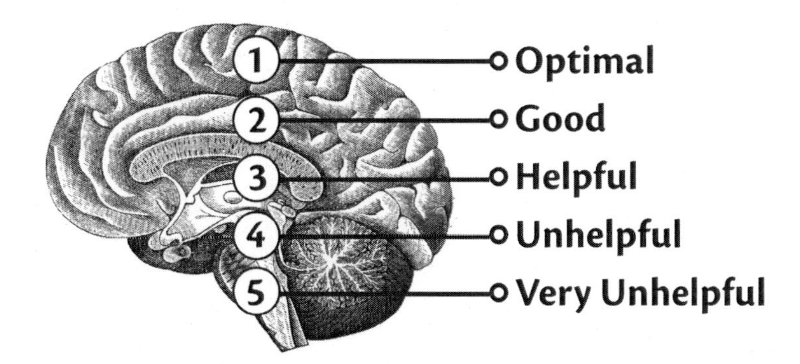

Kevin said, "I understand the merit of Brain State 1 and that Brain State 2 is good. You can't always be at Brain State 1, but how do I know if Brain State 3 is not really Brain State 4 or on the way to 5, and I will be eating or drinking in a nanosecond?"

I responded, "You must be vigilant in a relaxed way."

"Now I'm baffled."

"If it is not fun, it is not EBT, and if you were always at Brain State 1 and 2, there would be no sense of victory. You like to win, right?"

He scoffed, "Of course!"

"When you are at Brain State 3, you enjoy the challenge and stay present to the sensations in your body, allowing yourself to be slightly uncomfortable for a higher purpose."

"My higher purpose is Sanctuary – peace and power from within."

"Your thumbprint of signs that a helpful Brain State 3 is at a tipping point and about to turn into an activated glitch, needs to be figured out experientially."

"Learn by doing."

"Exactly."

The concept of using self-regulatory strength at Brain State 1 to stay above the fray of glitches is important to Kevin's success. Also, his circuitry is still quite brittle. My father had Type 1 diabetes, but his physician called it "brittle" diabetes, and if he missed a rapid decline into hypoglycemia he would be in danger. Similarly, anyone with a history of trauma, like Kevin, would be particularly vulnerable to a near-instantaneous decline into higher levels of allostatic stress arousal. The 4 and 5 States can reactivate any unhealed trauma circuits and an array of glitches that launch strong drives for consuming ultra-processed foods that block Sanctuary.

For Kevin, mastering the skill of identifying his Brain States and feeling relaxed and secure that he has a reliable procedure (spiraling up) to help him win at rewiring are important. He can fix his Habit Glitches and experience more lasting peace with food and healthy weight by knowing his limits, how long he can stay at a productive Brain State 3, and when to pull the plug and spiral up.

When Kevin returned for more coaching a week later, he had learned a great deal. He said, "Early in the week, I realized my brain bypasses Brain State 3. I can be at Brain State 1 or 2 in one moment, then at Brain State 5, and be mindlessly eating."

"What happened next?"

"I started noticing times I was at 3 and shifted gears, so I monitored how long I was hungry, but not starving, before I went into severe stress."

I was curious, "How long did it take?"

"When I was triggered at work it was almost immediate, but I started using the tools at Brain State 3, not to get to One, but to help sustain my productive Brain State 3."

"What were your signs of Brain State 3?"

Kevin replied, "Negative thoughts, blaming myself."

"Sensations in your body?"

Each time Kevin reflected on the sensations in his body and related them to his emotions and brain states ("interoceptive awareness") he boosted his ability to differentiate helpful from unhelpful stress.

Kevin said, "Feeling lethargic with a slight burning in my stomach. It lasts anywhere from one to eight minutes. When I stopped blaming myself that I was hungry or rushing to stop the productive Brain State 3, I could stay in that state for 20 minutes or so without scaring myself that I would starve to death."

"How did it work for you, Kevin?"

"It worked great. I lost two pounds in the last week and did not diet."

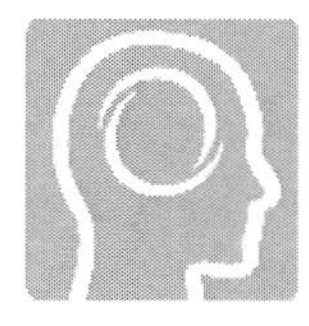

16

Check Your "Body Joy Meter" for Releasing Extra Weight

The magical joy of releasing weight typically occurs when the wires of the Big 4 Circuits, which include the Body Circuit, have been thoroughly done in. To accomplish that, use the Spiral Up Grind-in numerous times until the drives of the circuits cease. It's a beautiful feeling when that happens and well worth the effort.

A physician in one of my telegroups had been working on clearing the clutter from the trauma of her father's rejection, which continued through her college years in relationships with men who were abusive. When she told me she was ready to crush her Body Circuit, I advised her that it might take 100, 200, or 500 repetitions to do that, as there are many other circuits from past trauma wired into her Body Circuit.

A few weeks later, she came to the telegroup and announced, "I did it. I cleared my Body Circuit." She sounded like a different person. Our voices are attached to our emotional brains, so you can literally "hear" a person's set point going up via their vocal tone.

I said, "Your voice is different. Clearing the Body Circuit might have changed your set point."

She answered, "If changing my set point means I have a completely new mindset on life, then it did!"

When your joy of weight loss kicks in, the evidence of that will be heartwarming. Your set point will go up, and you will notice spontaneous changes in your eating. When this happens, watch for leaving food on your plate. You are not connected to the reward of food anymore. You are connected to your emotional and spiritual core. Chewing on salami, swallowing donuts, or giving your body more food than it needs becomes unappealing. It's no longer fun. What IS fun is the joy of releasing extra weight.

3 activities to boost weight loss

Regardless of whether you have that joy of releasing weight in your psyche yet, consider trying one or more of the following activities that we have been using as part of EBT for over 20 years. Even completing one of them can tip the balance in your set point toward experiencing that joy.

Activity #1. Using Words, Not Weight

It's normal to express ourselves wordlessly through the appearance of our body, and body size speaks volumes. If we are stressed, particularly if our way of coping with emotions is to overthink or stay busy, we don't know what our weight is expressing to ourselves or the world. We can find those words by using this activity. Then, when we say them, often the drive to stay at that body size eases or even disappears.

Complete this Imagine to identify the words you most need to say so you can stop using weight to express yourself. Not everyone is able to find these words, but if you do, expressing them can boost your joy.

To prepare for this Imagine, identify if you have extra weight and, if you do, how much. Do not use government standards. Use your own standard of what you would like to weigh. First, record your current weight. Next, subtract what you believe is your healthy weight, the weight you would be if you had healthy habits and lived life at Brain State 1 without stress wires. Subtract that healthy weight from your current weight to identify your "Extra Weight." Use that number as you complete this activity.

Estimating Your "Extra Weight"

Current weight		____________
Healthy weight	(minus)	____________
Extra weight	(equals)	____________

■ ■ ■

Imagine: Using Words Not Weight

Relax: Begin by relaxing. Turn your attention to your body and your breathing and breathe in through your nose and out through your mouth, or in any way that feels comfortable and comforting to you. Then, when you are ready, begin to imagine.

Imagine: See yourself sitting in your home on a chair next to a backpack. Bring to mind the extra weight you are carrying and see yourself putting that weight into the backpack, then putting it on.

See yourself arising from your chair, walking out your front door and onto the street with the backpack on, then walking around the block. Notice the weight of the backpack as you walk the first block. See yourself walking the second block. Be aware of the sensations in your body as you carry that extra weight in your backpack. Next, see yourself walking the third block . . . then the fourth block, and arriving back home. See yourself walking through the door, sitting on your chair, and not taking off your backpack.

Say lovingly to yourself, "What are the words I need to say aloud so I do not need to carry this extra weight? If I say these words, it becomes safe for me to release this extra weight. If I do not say these words, I may continue to try to lose weight, but my emotional brain will force me to hold onto it."

Bring to mind those words and say them aloud as many times as needed so you naturally feel safe releasing the extra weight.

■ ■ ■

When Jessica used this Imagine, she identified words that surprised her.

"Jessica, what words came into your mind?"

She said, "It was shocking. The words were, 'I need help.' I am carrying 35 pounds. Why don't I just tell people that I need help? Why don't I allow myself to need help? This was amazing for me."

When Kevin identified the words he needed to say to release extra weight, they contrasted starkly with Jessica's. Kevin said, "I am carrying around 50 extra pounds. When I arrived back home and sat down on the chair, the words that came to mind were 'I need love.' I won't admit that to myself, and I never tell my family I need their love. If I tell them their love means everything to me, perhaps I can stop trying to get love by being big."

Charlotte used the Imagine technique. She realized that she was holding onto 80 extra pounds. She had been shaming herself for her weight, so I suggested she see the extra weight as four butter cubes per pound. She liked the idea.

She said, "There were a lot of butter cubes in my backpack, about 320 of them. I was hardly able to get around the block, so I was surprised when I did not naturally drop the backpack as soon as I arrived home. The words I needed to say were: 'Stay away from me.' That's so sad. I'm lonely and using my body fat, my butter cubes, to keep people away and sabotage my chances of feeling safe in a relationship."

The Imagine activity was beneficial to Charlotte, as she began clearing emotional clutter by saying the words to herself that weight was saying for her. That lightened her emotional load, making it easier for her to find safety in releasing extra weight and even beginning to see the start of the joy of weight loss.

A history of trauma is so common in obesity that Dr. Vincent Felitti, whose seminal research in adverse childhood experience changed psychotherapy, wrote an article: *Obesity: Problem,*

Solution, or Both? His clinical research on patients showed the unexpected psychological benefits of maintaining a large body size. Extra weight can serve as body armor for emotional or physical safety.

Activity #2. Getting My Love from People, Not Food

A common cliché is that people use food for love. A great way to test how true this is for you is to try out this activity. I was astonished when I first tried it over 30 years ago. Here's the activity:

Plan to have lunch with a friend or family member in a private location, either in a car or someone's home. Have two sandwiches on hand, one for each of you. Sit opposite each other, face to face. Have one person be the feeder and the other the fed. The fed must tell the feeder how big the bite will be each time they want a bite of food, and then wait for the feeder to bring the food to their lips, take a bite, and swallow it. The feeder pays attention to each chew and swallow. The participants continue to feed or receive bites until the fed says they are satisfied. Then, you reverse roles.

When I first did this activity, I felt full, even stuffed, after consuming less than a half sandwich because I realized that what I really needed was the loving connection I was receiving. When I received it, my appetite faded away. I met my actual need and consumed less than half the food I normally would eat.

Activity #3. Freedom from Body Size Clutter

When I was pregnant with my third child, I gained 45 pounds as I had an unstoppable appetite for Saltine crackers and cheddar cheese. That combination quieted my nine months of nausea. I was already at high risk due to my medical history and age, so gaining weight rapidly made that worse, and my physician requested that I be seen in his office weekly. I was happy to have the support and showed up to each appointment.

One week I stepped on the scale, and when the nurse read the number, she put her hand over her mouth and said, "You gained seven pounds." Then she started laughing. There I was at my most vulnerable, and she was laughing at me. Our wounds about body size can cut deep. A wave of sadness still comes over me when I tell that story. I could do a few more Cycles on it, but some hurts leave behind emotional scars that never completely go away and can be non-toxic and even beneficial. At this point in clearing my clutter from this incident, I do not blame the nurse, I do not shame myself when I gain weight now, and I appreciate that this hurt has helped me boost my empathy and compassion. I will let this cluster of wires, which is largely cleared, stay where it is. I don't have to be perfect to be wonderful and neither do you.

For this activity, bring to mind a particular hurt that resulted from your body size or weight. Use a new skill, the Anger Cycle, to weaken that cluster of wires. It is a variation of the Cycle Tool that encourages the safe, productive expression of more profound anger to clear away clutter and train the brain to activate and weaken 5 Circuits.

The Anger Cycle is a version of the Be Positive Tool that removes access to sadness, fear, and guilt. It holds us in a safe place while strongly protesting the hurt. The stress melts away and turns into a spiritual high of gratitude. It's a beautiful tool. (To be guided using this tool, see the EBT app.)

Choose the number of spiral ups you will do to weaken this circuit cluster. A very productive habit in your EBT Practice is to become accustomed to clearing clutter routinely. It is like mowing the lawn. For this activity, select a number of spiral ups, using Spiral Up #1, and process your emotions. Begin gaining freedom from that clutter.

Freedom from Body Size Clutter

How many spiral ups will you do now?

5 10 15 20 25

Jessica selected five spiral ups. I asked what she learned from doing this cluster of spiral ups. She said, "The Anger Cycle helped me overall with my EBT Practice because anger is my missing feeling, the emotion most difficult for me to express. I learned that I have let weight define me. How outrageous! I will never do that again. I need at least another five spiral ups to clear more of this clutter."

Kevin mainly used both Body Size Clutter Removal and the Anger Cycle to express anger at himself for neglecting his body for so long. He said, "I did 10 spiral ups about being so stuck with weight and how stubborn I have been. The best part of the Anger Cycle is it makes me get to the 5 Circuits at the bottom of my brain and always leads to gratitude. I feel proud that I am doing something about it now!"

Charlotte chose 25 spiral ups. She said, "I did five spiral ups per day for 10 days. My anger was directed at all the lies I have been told about weight and how much people have judged me for my weight. I blew off enough anger that I don't feel angry anymore. I feel grateful to be alive and releasing extra weight."

The Body Joy Meter

As you clear your Body Circuits, the joy of releasing weight will naturally increase. At some point that joy becomes so strong that you may feel somewhat emotionally and spiritually "transported" and not sure you are the same person. Your relationship with your body and food can change radically. That is the nature of rewiring the emotional brain. Good things happen that surprise you.

At that point, your brain will begin releasing weight and you will feel more peaceful inside as you release that weight out of self-love and personal power.

Look at the following Body Joy Meter and decide which of the five choices best describes your emotional brain's drive for changing your weight and the pride you feel in your body.

The "Body Joy Meter"

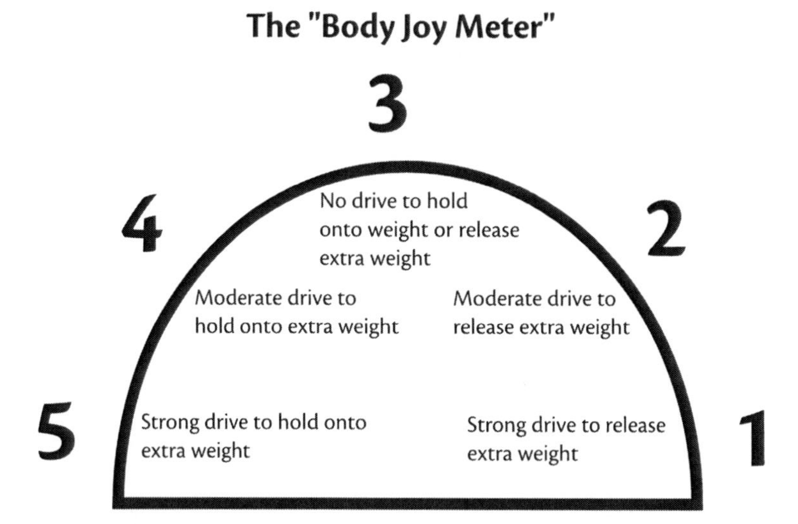

Setting yourself up for easy, natural weight loss starts with recreating your relationship with yourself and your body. Each spiral up brings you more self-love, body pride, and confidence to take action and release weight that feels "extra," out of alignment with who you are now.

Whether it takes you one month or several months to get to the Body Joy Meter, you are on the pathway to releasing weight with joy. You are giving yourself the skills that you have needed all along – skills that will change your life.

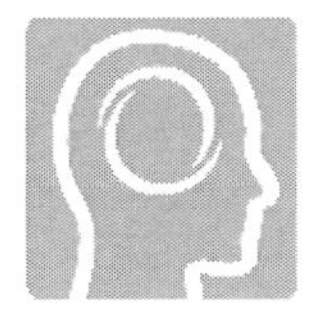

17

Food Rebellion and Scarcity Panics: How to Regain Control

What's so hard about switching from eating a muffin for breakfast to eating a couple of scrambled eggs?

It's not hard unless you have some emotional clutter and most of us do. Our Habit Glitches are not just unhealthy habits but circuits that were encoded in a moment of terror and so, changing habits can unleash a firestorm of suppressed emotions. It is like playing with fire. Fire is dangerous, and in EBT we fight fire with . . . fun and joy.

Even as you change your habits gradually, every now and then you will activate a circuit that takes you right to Brain State 5. Changing eating is like going to the county fair, with the chaos of Ferris wheels, jugglers, dunking contests, bull riding, and a house of mirrors.

It can be a fun, but also scary adventure because traces of trauma wires often become activated when we fiddle with changing food. That's why making it a standard practice to spiral up before eating is so powerful. It's a self-nurturing act. We clear the stress associated with our food wires at that moment. They are activated when we eat, and their synaptic connections between neurons are fluid, so It's a perfect time to rewire.

Scarcity panics and food rebellion

These trauma activations can show up as scarcity panics, sudden experiences that we are not going to get enough. It's not that we will be slightly hungry physically, but that not having enough food will annihilate us. The reaction can be that strong.

Raymond was in his mid-40s, and was coming to terms with his childhood trauma. He had a scarcity panic every time he made the slightest change in his diet. Even thinking about eating differently could send him to Brain State 5. I coached Raymond through a Travel Back and he brought up an image of standing in front of the refrigerator in his kitchen at age four. His two brothers were standing next to him and when he opened the refrigerator door, there was no food. His Travel Back led to updating those wires, so he could change his food habits without setting off a scarcity panic.

Most often, scarcity panics are triggered by emotional abuse or sexual, rather than physical, deprivation. These panics at not having access to the food that will keep us physically or emotionally alive are three to four times more common in people with obesity who report a history of childhood sexual abuse. Of course, changing behavior becomes the focus, because it is so hurtful, but that is not the problem. The problem is the trauma of that moment, not the circuit the brain encoded to escape from that pain.

The brain is survival-driven, and that primitive drive doesn't care about what we ate. It is directed at healing the moment of abuse. Without our permission or awareness, that experience stores memories that were never filtered by the prefrontal cortex. Most of these stored expectations are completely ridiculous and cause us more stress. Yet the healthcare system identifies the problem as the response that is at the tail end of the circuit.

That lack of recognition of the biological root cause of the unwanted behavior causes us to try to change the behavior or categorize the drive as psychopathology. Something is wrong with us. Nothing is wrong with us! The problem is that we are not identifying the root cause of the symptom, which is a wire. A simple reset of seeing the problem as a cluster of circuits that are begging us to do the emotional work of clearing the emotions and adjusting the unreasonable expectation does the trick. It's about changing the paradigm, so these wires don't terrorize us over the decades.

A radical approach to unconditional love

Although habit change seems rather innocuous, consider any persistent and extreme behavior to be encoded in a trauma circuit ("5 Circuit"). As mammals, love is a survival need, and the trauma circuit activation causes the reliving of the experience of feeling abandoned, terrified, or abused. Implicit in that experience is loss of love, suggesting that rewiring the brain for unconditional love of self is foundational to treating obesity. I learned how to think differently about unconditional love during an EBT session with university faculty members.

I was guiding a psychiatrist known for her sensitivity to patients through a challenging Cycle. The Cycle brought up circuits encoded in early childhood when she experienced chaos and violence that left her feeling abandoned and unloved.

I told her, "Even if everyone on the planet rejects you, you must make a personal decision not to reject yourself."

Immediately, she corrected me, saying, "No, It's more than that. A secure connection to the deepest part of ourselves requires that we make a personal decision that even if everyone on the planet rejects us *for good reason*, we will not reject ourselves."

At that moment the other faculty members in the room fell silent. They sensed the deep wisdom in her words. We must love ourselves no matter what, particularly when nobody else does. That love scares away any self-judgment that comes from rogue wires that are activated when we begin to change our eating. It gives us a foundation for taking action when these circuits activate. That action is spiraling up.

Switching off the old circuit is only half of the ultimate solution. We need to encode a replacement circuit of how to eat in a new way. Most of us who have struggled with eating and weight have been raised in a stressful environment and have learned to be indulging (too easy) or depriving (too harsh) of ourselves, unable to find ways to eat that are responsive to our needs. So, encoding a new circuit can be challenging, but ultimately rewarding.

This chapter and the next will touch on finding that balance of rewiring old circuits and encoding new ones. We begin by focusing on avoiding self-deprivation and how it shows up in our habits: scarcity panic and food rebellion.

The neural anatomy of a scarcity panic

After Jessica cleared her glitches and her drive for buttered popcorn binges after the children went to bed faded, she had a new challenge. She knew how to stuff and starve herself. Also, she knew what she "should" eat based on various diet plans and eating systems. But these things were all external solutions and a new love affair with herself had awakened by clearing her glitches. Jessica cared that she did not deprive herself. She was on her way to "acquired secure attachment," which happens at Set Point 1.

EBT Director of Emotional Health, Judy Zehr, speaks eloquently about developing a loving relationship with ourselves. EBT mirrors the spiraling up between parent and child that encodes a secure attachment and optimal resiliency pathways. EBT gives us a way to take the baton from our parents and accomplish that on our own. That process brings us inner security.

Jessica was looking to me for rules about food, but I said, "I cannot give you rules, recipes, or plans. What you eat is far too important to leave to the wisdom of your emotional brain. Get to Brain State 1, as that's the state in which you eat for higher purpose. Feel the glow of that, then your brain will slip down to Brain State 2. Use the tool for that state which is: 'How do I feel?', 'What do I need?', and 'Do I need support?'"

She said, "How do I know the answers to those questions?"

I responded, "You must not rush or answer them from your thinking brain. You have security from your emotional brain after you switch off the noise from glitches and the allostasis they cause. However, in a homeostatic state, emotions still take a while to sort themselves out. During that time, you must tolerate not knowing the answers. When you have processed the emotions, a wise answer will appear."

Jessica said, "You mean I must face my inner void?"

"Yes, face it for as long as it takes to feel your feelings until they fade, which they will, and then you will know precisely what you need. Even before you meet that need with whatever you decide to eat or not eat, you will be at a magnificent Brain State 1."

"How could that be? I haven't even had the food yet."

I shared, "Our deepest need is not for food. In evolution, our physical and spiritual survival is based on whether we can tolerate not knowing, trusting ourselves, and waiting for our deepest emotions to arise. Then the corresponding need appears in our mind, and we are saved physically and spiritually by knowing precisely what we need."

Jessica responded, "What if I don't do that?"

"Many things could happen, but a common one is a fear that you will not get what you want or need – we call that a scarcity panic. When you deprive yourself of a morsel of luscious food you believe you really need, that food deprivation triggers cortisol and epinephrine release from a traumatic experience in the past, and you end up eating ultra-processed food that is toxic to your body and brain. Or, you may just sabotage your joy of releasing weight.

She said, "When you say scarcity panic something lights up inside me. It rings true from the past, but not since I rewired my glitches. I don't have that panic anymore, but I do need to find out how to eat."

"As your set point rises, new worlds open up and you need new skills. That's the purpose of the last months of EBT: the courses clear emotional clutter and build new skills for how you want to live your life."

Jessica said, "I understand. The procedure is not to look at a list of foods I can eat, but to go inside, face my inner void, allow it to pass, and dig deeper to know how I feel and what I really need. When I ask, the answers will appear."

"Ask, and the answers appear. You can trust the tools and yourself."

The special drama of a food rebellion

If you have scarcity panics, they typically arise from clutter encoded in trauma when you could not get the emotional or physical sustenance you needed. Rebellion is another common response to deprivation. Instead of being panicked by scarcity, we protest that someone did not see, hear, or feel us and instead tried to control our food in ways that made us feel emotionally or physically violated.

Our rage is suppressed from deprivation and turns into a fire-in-the-belly drive to rebel against food limits and can ignite strong drives to binge eat. The aggression we experienced from others we now apply to ourselves.

Charlotte had a food rebellion wire. She had no idea that she was rebelling, even though she realized that her eating episodes revealed a side of her that was agitated and aggressive, in contrast to the calm and passive person she presented to the world.

Charlotte was disturbed about her eating. She said, "I eat junk foods, stuffing them into my mouth or binging on sweets as fast as possible."

I said, "There must be a lot of clutter at the bottom of your brain. If so, It's not reasonable to expect you to do something other than eat aggressively, but that won't heal you. It will wear you out. Then you will return to being passive and passionless when the binge ends."

"I'm so sick of unpacking emotional clutter. There is so much of it."

"It takes as long as it takes. If you short-change yourself and do not do all the spiraling up you need to do to clear it, you'll meet that trash again at your next attempt to heal, or use drugs and surgery and try to bypass it. It never goes away until you process it. Never."

"What do I do until then? How do I eat?"

I said, "Spiral up before eating. That is your commitment to your emotional and spiritual core. Do not commit to changing how you eat. Commit to spiraling up before you eat, then eat in any way that is responsive to you."

Charlotte replied, "It's not responsive to me to binge."

"The pain of the binge comes from the perfection of your emotional brain. If you need the food, then have it. Your essence is joy, and each time you bypass clearing the emotional blockade to that joy, your emotional brain will give you grief, and part of that grief is the binge. Own it!"

"My emotional brain will punish me?"

"Not at all! It will give you a tap on the shoulder and say, 'Hey, sweetheart, I will remind you by overeating each time you ignore your joy and shut down your magical capacity to heal. You will experience a natural consequence – bloating, nausea, or a 'bad feeling' in your body. I hope you listen to it, but if you do not, I'll have to tap a little stronger in other ways until I get your attention. You matter that much to me.'"

"Like high blood pressure, diabetes, my family badgering me to lose weight . . . so I need to fix my glitches."

"You like fixing your glitches."

Charlotte laughed, "Yes, the aha moments."

"Of course, it is fun because the survival of the species depends on each person doing their 'emotional wisdom' work. Each spiral up provides a kernel of wisdom. Nobody can opt out of that evolutionary force to become their best selves without a major loss to the quality of their lives."

Charlotte chuckled. "I had hoped I could duck out!"

"You have gifts to give the world. Imagine the drives for passion, energy, and love you will uncover once that clutter is cleared."

Charlotte smiled, "So EBT is not about the food. It is about me reclaiming my joy?"

I said, "Yes, your joy and purpose."

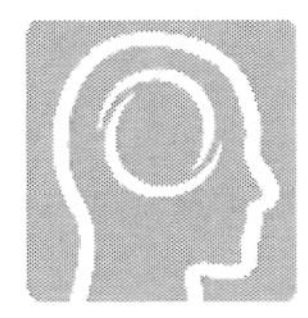

18

Rock-Solid Boundaries: Eat Only What You Want to Store

Kevin was in the hospitality business, which made eating healthy next to impossible. He asked me, "How can you be so good when it comes to food? I am so bad."

"I'm not good, Kevin. I like avoiding pain. I can't stand the cravings, weight gain, and nausea when I overeat. I don't diet either. I wouldn't do that to myself."

Kevin has stopped overeating but is still "white knuckling it" some of the time.

I said, "Kevin, you will only be entirely free of the drive to overeat once you have raised your set point. Meanwhile, it's important to have compassion for yourself as our food environment is toxic, and to create some boundaries for yourself to make losing weight easier.

He said, "I don't know what my set point is."

Set your goal at Set Point 1

The set point is the brain's stress habit, the brain state that is its home base or default state, and Kevin was raising his. He had already rewired his Big 4 Circuits, the reactive wires that triggered him.

However, he still had some drives to overeat, late at night or in the middle of the afternoon. At Set Point 1, he wouldn't want the larger portions, or his brain would be activating natural chemicals so he would feel rewarded without overeating.

The set point goes up when we repair the wear and tear ("allostatic load") caused by stress. He could not undo the injuries to his knees from playing varsity football in college or his back pain from the fall off a horse when he was in his 20s. Yet he had been rewiring circuits, clearing clutter, and in general, moving through the courses of the EBT Program.

I said, "Kevin, you can take some chemical tests to estimate your set point and the body signs of your stress load."

Kevin's physician could guide him through appraising his set point and his allostatic load. A 2022 review of measures of allostatic load conducted by researchers at Washington State University showed that clinicians use 26 different biomarkers in 18 different ways. Yet, there has been progress in measuring allostatic load quantitatively. Recent research by Daniel Mauss and Marc Jarczok confirmed that five biomarkers are reliable indicators of allostatic load: 1) diastolic blood pressure, 2) hemoglobin A1c, 3) low-density lipoprotein, 4) heart rate variability, and 5) waist circumference. They are all associated with a validated questionnaire, the Cohen 10-item Perceived Stress Scale.

I said, "Kevin, you can use the EBT Set Point One Self-Test that's on our website. As you complete the EBT Program, you can get readings about whether your set point is at One. The test is based on: 1) normal values for all five biomarkers, 2) a Set Point 1 score on the EBT Inventory Scale, and 3) optimal stress based on the Cohen Perceived Stress Scale, a validated measure of physiologic stress."

Kevin said, "I'll do both: talk with my physician and take the Set Point One Self-test."

I strongly recommend that you take laboratory tests and record your medications as you start EBT and every three to six months after that. Your physician may be surprised that you need fewer medications over time and your laboratory tests show improved health.

Dopamine deficits and ultra-processed foods

Apart from set point, food intake is the strongest predictor of weight loss. Marion Nestle, my mentor early in my career, later became a world-renowned food politics expert and a founder of the field of food studies. She is a champion of calling out the food industry and government as creating today's obesity crisis.

According to Dr. Nestle, "The whole purpose of a food company is to get people to eat more of its products." The combination of packaging, advertising, and ingredient manipulation is aimed at lighting up the reward centers, so we can't get enough of them. Who can take only one bite of a chocolate chip cookie or pluck one potato chip from a bag without downing the rest?

The fast-food industry peddles artificial food that sparks appetites. The more highly processed the food, the faster it delivers dopamine, the bigger the dopamine wallop, and the more addictive it becomes. Dr. Nestle explains ultra-processed food this way: "Corn on the cob is unprocessed, canned corn is processed or minimally processed, and Doritos are ultra-processed." No matter what the nutrition education or food labeling, people are eating more of it, in part, because sales are well-funded. For every dollar of product, 19 cents go to the food, but 81 percent goes to marketing. In a recent University of California talk on her latest memoir, *Slow Cooked*, Dr. Nestle said that if people ate healthy, "nobody would make any money. The food industry's billion-dollar ultra-processed products wouldn't sell."

How culpable is the food industry for the obesity crisis? The science is quite condemning. In a review of reward by Paul Kenny of Scripts Research Institute in *Neuron*, compared to non-obese people, the obese overshoot dopamine in response to highly palatable food. The stronger the dopamine, the more addictive the wire. Obese people may automatically encode more 5 Circuits that trigger overeating than non-obese people. Not fair!

What do you do when you overeat? You over-restrict. It turns out that either one – depriving or indulging – boomerangs back to cause overeating. On a cellular level, obesity is associated with low dopamine and reduced dopamine receptor levels. Low dopamine is more common in the obese than the non-obese, so just the people who need a neurotransmitter boost the most are the most negatively impacted by it.

An obesity study conducted by Dr. Kenny made the sinister nature of ultra-processed foods for those of us who are obese clearer. He compared tolerance, the hallmark of addiction in rats, for highly palatable food, cocaine, and heroin, and to his surprise, all three substances showed similar patterns of the reward value of the chemical diminishing with time. The impact of the relentless promotion of these artificial foods falls most on the obese. Given that ultra-processed foods are legal, cheap, and ubiquitous, the obese pay the highest price for the pushing of ultra-processed foods by the food industry.

Put up a firewall or eat smarter?

What can we do to protect ourselves from the toxic food environment? One option is to put a firewall between ourselves and ultra-processed food. It is to abstain from them, a common strategy for drug treatments. Weight-loss programs that promote deprivation are widespread, as we forget that obesity is a "stress symptom" and restrictive diet programs do not teach patients stress resilience or how to create joy and have only fueled the rise in the prevalence of obesity and disordered eating.

I said to Kevin, "In EBT, changes in eating come naturally after stress is cleared and the brain's reward centers light up flush with dopamine and endorphins. You could make ultra-delicious, processed foods off-limits, but I don't recommend it."

He said, "I know. Once I know I can't have something, I want it more."

Obesity treatment appeared to be taking a step forward when more organizations shamed people for "fat shaming." Unfortunately, they offered a half-truth, which is that nobody should ever be judged for their weight, but that doesn't mean that a high weight promotes health. Inadvertently, the trend in society went from one extreme to the other without first, promoting that anyone has the right to weigh whatever they choose, and second, providing information about the risks to some people of high levels of obesity.

The effort to destigmatize weight was well-intentioned, but any extreme increases the risk of negative consequences. One policy originating from Brain State 5, such as judgment of obesity, can easily be replaced by an equally "5ish" policy that there are no health consequences of even extreme obesity.

I would never suggest that a person release extra weight, as it is a personal decision. However, without getting a dopamine rush from the idea of releasing weight out of self-love, how many people would push back from the table or say "no" to seconds, particularly because the foods deliver just the rush that dopamine-deficient people not only want but need? The sensible plan is body pride for all sizes and awareness of the risks and advantages of releasing weight versus holding onto it.

Our hunter-gatherer genes do not like change, suggesting that the gentle, natural approach of the EBT 1-2-3 Joy Program makes sense. Coax the amygdala, nourish the nucleus accumbens, and make food changes at Brain State 1, in which the chemical cascade fades and the brain can integrate competing needs. We can relax into eating in a way that is right for us. The emphasis is on spiraling up and raising the set point to One, at which food is just food, not a fix, and eating in response to our desires, healthy but not perfect, occurs quite naturally.

The lower the set point, the more obesity behaviors are like an alcohol use disorder. Just the way some people cannot take a sip of wine without finishing off the whole bottle, some of us with histories of obesity and disordered eating prefer to abstain from ultra-processed foods. Once we start, it's too hard to stop. A "firewall" of a boundary may be needed. However, the higher the set point, the more an "eat smart" approach is effective. Bite into a piece of candy, and if there are no errant glitch wires, a few bites are enough now and then, and it can all be part of preventive deprivation and deactivating excessive restraint, and a well-lived life.

How do I apply this in my own life? I start with activating the joy of releasing weight, as without that dopamine surge weight loss is depressing. I wait until it feels nurturing and even a little exciting to release weight, like clearing away something I don't need anymore. I eat to prevent cravings and to keep my blood sugar strong for long periods, so the protein, healthy fat, and some fiber approach works well for me. I don't do well with artificial chemicals, so I stopped using Splenda, in favor of a teaspoon of sugar on my Greek yogurt. I still have a Diet Coke now and then and if I need some rather disgusting ultra-processed food, I have it – without guilt. My needs matter. I absolutely eat for hunger, and don't think much about food, but more about spiraling up to One, the brain state that makes sensible eaters out of all of us.

I asked Kevin, "What approach to food do you want to use?"

Kevin said, "Everywhere I go, there are comfort foods, even at work. I live and work in an ultra-processed food swamp. My wife is not dealing with her sugar addiction, and I have no safe zone for food, even at home – none."

I said, "How difficult."

He replied, "I know."

"Let's go back to talking about your set point. The lower your set point, the more what you eat is stored as fat, and you'll need to set limits. Ultra-processed foods may be disproportionately counterproductive for you."

Kevin said, "I was at Set Point 4 when I started EBT. Now I'm at Set Point 3."

I said, "That's fantastic, but you are still in the stress zone, so chemical cascades can sometimes turn your body into a fat-storage machine. It is not your fault, and the problem is universal. Your reward centers light up to the thought, taste, or smell of ultra-processed foods, then the calories are stored in your fat cells. Set some limits. Do not eat what you do not want to store."

Kevin caught on very quickly.

"So, you're saying not to blame myself or others but to start creating boundaries?"

I said, "Big boundaries."

Kevin asked, "What do you mean?"

"Don't let the environment or people control your food. Love your body and yourself enough to eat what works for you, even if other people don't like it."

"I'm not sure I can do that. I never set limits with my children – or myself."

"It all starts with self-love. Bring up a loving voice of your own or borrow one from someone who was loving, but encouraged you to do hard things and to succeed."

He said, "That's my Grandpa Harry. When I was seven years old, I spent the summer at his house. We planted raspberry bushes, and he taught me how to ride a bike."

"Bring up that image of yourself at age seven, with Grandpa Harry, and feeling loved."

"I've got it."

I asked, "How do you feel?"

"Safe. Loved. Powerful."

"What would Grandpa Harry tell you to do to set boundaries?"

Kevin laughed, "He was strong. He would never cave to the wishes of others. He always did what he thought was the right thing."

I said, "Can you bring to mind Grandpa Harry when it comes to food?"

Kevin responded, "I am having a hard time imagining that."

"Then let's do an Imagine. Are you willing?"

Kevin said, "Yes, I'd like that."

▪ ▪ ▪

Imagine: ME with Rock-Solid Boundaries

Relax: Begin by relaxing. Turn your attention to your body and breathing and breathe in through your nose and out through your mouth, or in any way that feels comfortable and comforting. Then, when you are ready, begin to imagine.

Imagine: See yourself waking in the morning and bring to mind a person who loved you and encouraged you to do hard things and succeed. Take a moment to identify that person . . . Use their loving, powerful voice throughout the day, particularly when it comes to food.

Now, see yourself getting out of bed and going about your day. What are you doing with your day? You are creating joy, aware of your forcefield of love, safety, and power.

Next, notice that your friend is knocking at the door. Answer the door. He is bringing you coffee and pastries. See yourself welcoming him in and the two of you settling into the kitchen chairs. See the cups of coffee and the bag of pastries between you.

See yourself chatting. Then notice your friend is eating a pastry. A small trace of an old Food Circuit activates briefly, and so does your Merge Circuit. Just for a moment, you have an urge to eat.

Next, you become aware of that special person's safe, loving, and powerful voice. You say to yourself, "I do not put any food in my mouth that I do not want to store. The more ultra-processed food I eat, the faster my fat cells vacuum it up, and make my fat cells bigger. That food blocks my joy" or whatever encouraging words you need to hear.

Then, see yourself speaking to your friend and saying whatever you need to so that you create a rock-solid boundary and do not consume any food that you choose not to eat.

Last, feel a wave of compassion for yourself and pride in setting limits. You realize that you created rock-solid boundaries, and it was so easy. Pause and savor the image of you connecting to yourself and creating healthy boundaries, and when you are ready, share with me what you imagined.

■ ■ ■

Kevin said, "Okay, I have it."

I asked, "What did you imagine?"

He said, "I imagined having Grandpa Harry's voice and attitude. I felt safe and loved, and I was accountable to myself."

I asked, "What do you mean by accountable?"

Kevin said, "That the buck stops with me. The fast-food industry is not going to back off. My wife is not going to stop her sugar problem. It's up to me. I have to protect myself."

"What did you say to yourself?"

"I said to myself, 'I matter. My food and weight matter. I have boundaries.'"

Kevin paused.

Then he said, "I felt closer to my friend. I was emotionally honest with him, and said, 'I appreciate your bringing the coffee and pastry, but I'm not eating pastries these days. Thanks for thinking of me, though.'"

"How was that for you?"

He laughed, "It was great. I tapped into my personal forcefield of safety, love, and power. Grandpa Harry was right there with me. I had boundaries that were rock solid."

I smiled and said, "Nicely done," and thought: Kevin's set point is going up!

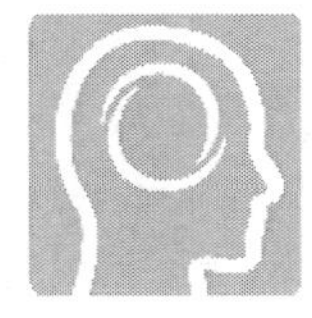

19

The Special Joy of Eating for Body Hunger

In one of our early studies of EBT, 134 adults used the method for three days straight. We learned a lot about how bursts of intensive use of EBT improve health outcomes. In the follow-up comments, these two were typical:

"I've finally found what I've been looking for my entire life: the power to stop overeating." Ann from Salem, Massachusetts

"It feels like a light has been turned on inside my body. I have more energy and vitality than ever." Lyssette, Los Angeles, California

People lost up to six pounds, and most importantly, they saw how using EBT in an intensive way can improve their emotional and physical health. We extended the experience to five days (the "5-Day Cortisol Detox"). Many people use the 5-Day Detox the first five days of each month as a way to reset their body and brain for optimal health.

One of the benefits of the 5-Day Detox is that the brain gets into the habit of being at One, and, in that state, it is easier to eat when hungry and reset one's relationship with food.

Think of a time when you were stressed and eating.

In a way, it is easy to become "merged" with our food, eating automatically rather than intentionally. Use the following activities to reset your relationship with food, so that you're more apt to experience the joy of eating when hungry and to gain more pleasure from what you eat.

Activity #1. The "Joy of Body Hunger" Experience

Evolution gave us genes that make food taste better when we are hungry. A fundamental pleasure in life is eating when hungry when almost anything is tasty. Much like all survival needs, such as putting on a jacket when cold, drinking water when thirsty, or having sex in response to desire, fulfilling that drive brings a burst of pleasure initially. When the need is satisfied, the drive for the behavior stops.

If we cross the line to eating when we are not hungry, we lose that joy and that clarity. Once eating becomes a source of entertainment or as a stop-gap measure to fulfill needs for safety, love, sex, comfort, or pleasure, there is no clear indication of when to stop. This puts us at risk of issues, problems, excesses, and missed pleasure. Eating a hamburger when not hungry does not replicate the experience of salivating in anticipation of that first bite, feeling the food in your mouth as it delivers life-sustaining nourishment, swallowing that bite, and noticing it fill up your stomach and ease your hunger. Nothing replaces that exquisite sensory experience.

If we eat when we are not hungry, the clean, simple, healthy approach to food ceases, and the problems begin.

When I presented these ideas to Jessica, she had a lot to say.

"I am not sure when I crossed that line and started using food as a substance, a way to get high. Well, actually, it was when my brain encoded my Food Circuit, but then the other problems I was having made it worse."

"What happened?"

"I was depressed as a teenager, and food made me feel better. It became my best friend. I had friends, but I never felt that they really liked me. Then I got into social media, which was a distraction and another addiction. I controlled my weight with overexercise – another circuit of mine – but when the twins were born, I had no time to exercise, so I gained weight. I applied my 'I have to be perfect' wire to judging my body."

"So, it wasn't about food."

"No, it *was* about food. Food was my 'lead addiction,' the one that caused my health problems, and the one that is #&%@ impossible to change when the entire food industry is making money off of it and making me addicted to food – and sick – and fat!"

I said, "I understand."

Jessica was close to being in a rage.

"I hate it that I have done this to myself, and I am going to shift gears and learn how to eat for body hunger. I want to feed my body, not my addiction."

For Charlotte, that fork in the road – eating for health vs. addiction – was sobering.

She said, "I can't remember eating for hunger. Ever."

Charlotte was raised with parents who both used food for a dopamine rush to anesthetize themselves with a false high. This is using food as an addiction. Then, as her body size moved from overweight to obese to extremely obese, her thinking brain disconnected from her emotional brain. She could not access the sensations in her body to inform her when she was hungry, satisfied, or overly full, and her Stress Triangle was biochemically driving her to overeat. The body fat itself was a stressor and amplified the biochemical drives.

Charlotte said, "I have a new reason to release weight. It's not physical or psychological, but spiritual. I want to reconnect with myself. I lost that little girl . . ."

She stopped speaking, and I could feel her looking back, trying to discover when she lost herself. When she spoke again, her voice was soft and calm.

"I may have lost myself in my mother's womb. I may never have had a chance to connect with myself . . ."

She went on to talk about the "lost years" and her desire to begin again. Then Charlotte returned to the topic that started our conversation: food.

"It will take a lot of spiral ups for me to find body hunger and to experience grounding myself and my eating in sensations in my body, but I will never find and nurture that little girl until I set an intention to honor my body and eat for hunger."

For Kevin, bringing up the idea of eating for body hunger had broad meanings.

"I could gloss over what you just said, but I'm feeling it in my chest."

I asked, "What do you mean?"

"Part of my 'big guy' personality is that I am always trying to game the system. I do not eat when I am hungry. I eat if I can justify eating, which is all the time. I convince myself that the rules don't apply to me."

"What makes you judge yourself for that? Maybe you are just trying to make the best life for yourself."

Kevin responded, "Not really. In my gut, I know that I am not in integrity."

"Is that the reward that motivates you to release weight?"

"I thought it was Sanctuary, but now that I am changing my habits, it is Integrity. I want to be straight about food and everything else. Eating for the joy of body hunger sounds like the perfect place to start."

Compare the experience of eating when hungry to eating in the absence of hunger. Most people find the experiences so different that they are more likely to want to eat when hungry, stop when just satisfied, and then discover feeling full, but not overly full, about 20 minutes later.

The "Hungerless Eating" Experience

Below is a list of common experiences of eating in the absence of hunger. Consume a meal when you are not hungry, then check off the experiences that were true for you:

- ☐ A blunted sensitivity of the taste and smell of food
- ☐ Mouth is watering from sensory or emotional hunger
- ☐ Eating rapidly, swallowing food without savoring it

- ☐ A sense of disconnection from my body
- ☐ A fear that the food will be gone, my needs will not be met, or I won't be able to stop eating
- ☐ An "afterburn" caused by meeting my pleasure drive but not being sensitive to my body's needs or aware of higher purpose
- ☐ Other ________________________________

The "Joy of Body Hunger" Experience

Below is a list of common experiences of eating when hungry. Consume a meal when you are hungry, then check off the experiences that were true for you:

- ☐ A heightened sensitivity to the taste and smell of food
- ☐ Mouth is watering from physical hunger
- ☐ Eating slowly, enjoying each bite
- ☐ A sense of connection to the body
- ☐ A deep security, knowing that the body will signal when satisfied
- ☐ An "afterglow" caused by relieving the stress of hunger, meeting my biological need for food, and being aware of higher purpose
- ☐ Other ________________________________

Activity #2. The "First 3 Bites" Experience

There is no need to avoid all ultra-processed foods. Eating a great cupcake, even though it is processed, is still wonderful in its own way and gives you pleasure. Choosing what food to eat is based on tradeoffs. The higher your brain state, the more likely you will be to be rational about the tradeoffs between the pleasure of eating ultra-processed foods and the pain of overeating or sabotaging goals for weight loss. Amounts count. Often the first few bites provide most of the pleasure from the food and subsequent bites have diminishing benefits.

Discover the pleasure you derive from eating ultra-processed foods. Select a portion of an ultra-processed food, such as a candy bar, a slice of cake, or a large cookie. Cut the food into bite-sized pieces. Eat each one, enjoying every bite: looking at the food, putting it in your mouth, chewing it, swallowing it, and feeling the food go down your esophagus and into your stomach.

Rate the experience on the following pleasure scale, circling your pleasure number on the scale below after each bite. Continue eating and rating until you have learned enough from this activity to stop.

The Pleasure Scale

	Low pleasure		Moderate pleasure		High pleasure
Bite #1:	1	2	3	4	5
Bite #2:	1	2	3	4	5
Bite #3:	1	2	3	4	5
Bite #4:	1	2	3	4	5
Bite #5:	1	2	3	4	5
Bite #6:	1	2	3	4	5

Activity #3. The "Eating for Body Hunger" Experience

As you eat healthier and release extra weight, eating for physical hunger becomes easier. Most people realize that they were eating much more food than their body needed, and that extra food, especially non-protein foods (particularly ultra-processed foods) increases perceptions of hunger. They cause "self-created hunger" as well as cravings. However, a discrete skill that is fundamental to eating in a way that is responsive to our needs is reading signals of hunger and satiety.

This activity is designed to boost your awareness of how to use hunger cues to gauge how much to eat. The topic of foods to choose to improve the accuracy of hunger cues will be addressed in the next chapter.

For three meals: breakfast, lunch, and dinner, do not eat unless you are hungry or very hungry. Pause and put down your utensil after every bite. Stop eating the moment your hunger is gone and you feel satisfied. This might be stressful, as a slight scarcity panic may arise. Stop anyway and set an alarm for 20 minutes, the time it takes for our gastric and intestinal chemicals to signal satiety.

Use one or more of these techniques to stop eating: 1) brush your teeth, 2) spiral up, or 3) engage in a physical activity (go for a walk, stretch, do yoga, lift weights, or dance). Then, continue with your daily activities.

After 20 minutes, check the hunger scale. Notice that you are full, but not overly full. Use this as your guide for deciding on how many bites of food you need to release weight and promote optimal health.

The most common observation from people completing this activity is that they have been eating until they were full, which caused them to feel overly full (overeat). The consumption of excessive food promotes weight gain, hyperglycemia, insulin resistance, and hyperinsulinemia.

The Hunger Scale

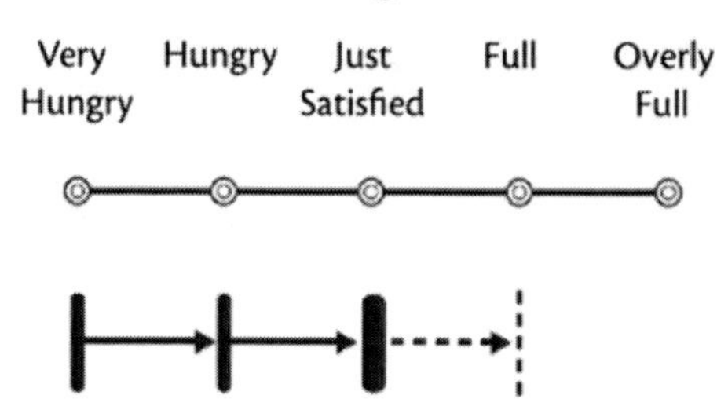

Start eating only when hungry. If not hungry, do not eat.
Stop when just satisfied, and 20 minutes later you will feel full.

Breakfast

☐	Started when hungry or very hungry:	☐ YES	☐ NO
☐	Stopped when just satisfied:	☐ YES	☐ NO
☐	Waited 20 minutes. Felt full, not overly full:	☐ YES	☐ NO

Lunch

☐	Started when hungry or very hungry:	☐ YES	☐ NO
☐	Stopped when just satisfied:	☐ YES	☐ NO
☐	Waited 20 minutes. Felt full, not overly full:	☐ YES	☐ NO

Dinner

☐	Started when hungry or very hungry:	☐ YES	☐ NO
☐	Stopped when just satisfied:	☐ YES	☐ NO
☐	Waited 20 minutes. Felt full, not overly full:	☐ YES	☐ NO

The Joy of Eating When Hungry

I will do my best to:

- ☐ Be sensitive to the joy of eating when hungry
- ☐ Be aware of diminishing pleasure when eating processed foods

- ☐ Eat slowly, savoring every bite
- ☐ Start eating when hungry or very hungry
- ☐ Stop eating when just satisfied
- ☐ Wait 20 minutes. Feel full, not overly full

With a commitment to honoring the special joy of eating when hungry, the next step is to consume foods that meet your needs. Having a simple system for making choices about the foods to eat – one with no forbidden foods – will complete the basic training on eating.

Right now, we focus on changing food, not other habits, such as sleep and exercise. If you concentrate on training the brain past these Stress Circuits, your set point will go up, and sleeping well and exercising regularly will be easier. Exercise supports neuroplasticity, but it can be stressful. If you exercise, consider it "play" and have fun. Using your major muscle groups for 30 minutes daily (e.g., brisk walking) increases brain-derived neurotrophic factor that supports your new learning (changes in the brain from spiral ups) to lock that new learning into existing neural networks rather than being sloughed off. Sleep is very sensitive to stress, and eight hours per night is recommended. If you lie awake at night, use this time to practice EBT. Calm yourself by spiraling up, using the Ladder Tool, or listening to the Relax audio tapes of the seven rewards.

As food intake is the most important predictor of weight change, focus on that aspect of lifestyle. The EBT "Vibrancy Plan" and other information about lifestyle as part of the program are available on the EBT Spiral Up Community website.

Let's take a look at the EBT 1-2-3 JOY Eating food system.

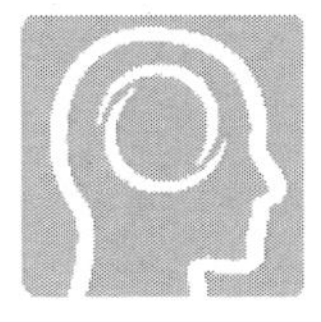

20

Food? Keep It Simple and Scientific

Food is simple. Eating whole foods that contain all the complex chemicals that have nourished humans over the eons is a good thing. Also, nutrients matter and to cover all the bases takes consuming foods from more than one group. Nutritional contributions do cluster together based on food types.

Perfect nutrition is not required for weight loss, so it helps to keep it simple and avoid cognitive overload. For example, Doug, an attorney, was newly single after a very difficult divorce that added 25 pounds to his already substantial frame. He came to EBT to prepare to start dating, both in mood and body size.

He told me, "I don't know what to eat. Is it farm-raised, free of trans fats, organic, or locally sourced? Besides, everything has sugar in it. So, I eat whatever tastes good to me."

To keep it simple, we've addressed the top needs for anyone wanting to lose weight and keep it off. The first need is to avoid pain, and pain for "weight releasers" is cravings, bad-tasting food, and hunger. The second is to make it flexible, so you can choose foods, combine them in any way you want, and have plenty of ways to make food taste great. Third, there are no forbidden foods, just a way to figure out the cost and benefit of what you eat. One group of foods increases stress in the longer term and the other one releases stress and promotes joy. Sometimes you don't mind having that stress. It's worth it. The choice is always yours.

To address all three and keep it simple use the EBT 1-2-3 JOY Food List. It is a simple, scientific way to decide what chemicals you want to put into your body. It is based on two parameters:

Simple: Is it a Stress Food or a Joy Food?

Are the foods you are considering real with high nutrient density? If yes, they are Joy Foods. If they are not Joy Foods, then are they low nutrient density or ultra-processed? These are Stress Foods.

Stress Foods are ultra-processed and artificial. When consumed in excess, they cause spikes of cortisol and trigger abnormal highs and lows in dopamine, cravings, chronic hunger, and they fail the "Is this tasty?" test. They also increase insulin, which blocks leptin signaling by fat cells, causing increased hunger and blocking weight loss.

Joy Foods do the opposite. Their overall impact on chemicals is positive. They promote decreasing cortisol, insulin, cravings, and chronic hunger, and they balance dopamine. By decreasing insulin and thereby enhancing leptin signaling, the fat cells can more effectively message the brain to say, "I am not starving. It's time to stop eating."

Scientific: Is it a Protein, Healthy Fat, or Fiber Food?

Although micronutrients (vitamins and minerals needed by the body in small amounts) are important, deficiencies in them do not cause obesity. Macronutrients (nutrients that provide energy and are needed in larger quantities) are strongly linked to weight-loss success. Beyond differentiating real foods ("Joy Foods") from ultra-processed and low nutrient density foods ("Stress Foods"), we keep it simple by dividing food into three groups based on macronutrients. These groups are Protein, Healthy Fats, and Fiber.

The EBT 1-2-3 JOY Food List is designed to show you the comparable balances of eating various foods, as only you can determine which foods meet your needs. No foods are forbidden, and no portion sizes are given. If you really need to eat 100 percent Stress Foods, then eat them.

The basic premise of this program is that how you feel is more important than what you eat or how much you weigh. Never deprive yourself of any food but use this system to be sure your needs are met without judgment but based on nutritional realities. If you really want cookies and don't eat them, that's stressful, and creates scarcity panics and food rebellion. Use this plan not only to release extra weight, but to change your relationship with food so that you have Freedom.

#1 – The Protein Group – The major finding based on the scientific literature concerning macronutrients and weight loss over the last decade has been that high-protein diets deliver a metabolic advantage over other patterns of eating. EBT does not include a diet, as the goal of the method is to enable people to be at Brain State 1 more of the time. At that optimal state for human functioning, they can make their own cost-benefit analysis. However, the role of the program is to convey scientific information to participants, so they make informed choices.

The list of advantages is exhaustive, including one I learned decades ago studying nutrition at UC Berkeley as an undergraduate: the thermic effect of protein, as it gobbles up 20 to 30 percent of its calories through digesting and metabolizing them. The protein leverage hypothesis proposes that as the body's need for protein goes unmet, satiety signals are dampened, and consumption of carbohydrate and fat increases.

Although this "drive" has not been proven, the trends support an interaction between the macronutrients. In a study published in the *American Journal of Clinical Nutrition* based on the National Health and Nutrition Examination Study, nearly all segments of the population are eating more UPFs. Meanwhile, average protein intake has plummeted to 18.4 percent. Ultra-processed foods contribute an average of 57 percent of calories.

Meanwhile, research on the benefits of eating with meals centered around protein has grown. As protein takes longer to digest than carbohydrates, high-protein meals suppress appetites as well as boosting GLP-1, the chemical that weight-loss drugs mimic. High protein intake also increases Peptide YY, which sends messages to the brain to stop eating and decreases ghrelin, a hormone made in the stomach that tells your brain that you are hungry, both of which reduce food intake. High protein intake during the day, especially at breakfast, decreases calorie intake and cravings in the afternoon and evening.

The 1-2-3 JOY Eating was initially developed in 2012, with fiber foods as the #1 macronutrient and protein taking third place. However, in 2022, the science was so convincing that we flipped the order of the macronutrient groups to promote planning meals with a "solid base" in protein. Protein foods became Group #1.

#2 – Healthy Fats – Adding a small amount of healthy fats to meals has multiple benefits. Dietary fat displaces carbohydrates in a meal. This is beneficial as the more carbohydrates you consume, the more your insulin levels rise. Excessive carbohydrate intake can cause the overshooting of insulin, followed by a blood sugar low ("self-created hunger"), which increases stress and promotes overeating. Excessive insulin can block leptin signaling, so the message from fat cells to the brain that you have eaten enough, and your fat stores are sufficient to prevent starvation is impaired. Even small amounts of foods in the healthy fats group add flavor to food without increasing carbohydrate intake. They boost dopamine enough to prevent drives for more extreme highs of dopamine from ultra-processed foods that block weight loss and foster food addiction.

#3 – The Fiber Group – Foods high in fiber prevent overeating by increased signaling from the intestine to stop eating, caused by "gut fill." Dietary fibers prevent obesity by reducing hunger and prolonging feelings of satiety. Some of the impacts are mechanical, and others are biochemical. Fiber supports gastric distention ("feeling full"), and it delays gastric emptying. On the biochemical side, fiber activates GLP-1 and Peptide YY, which decrease hunger and prolong satiety. Support for the role of fiber in weight loss is strong, but it does not match the power of relying on protein as our primary macronutrient, principally because of the high carbohydrate content of many high-fiber foods and less clinical evidence that high-fiber foods alone produce weight loss. When consumed as part of the 1-2-3 JOY Eating Program, the Fiber Group of foods adds to the overall feasibility and effectiveness of the plan.

EBT 1-2-3 JOY! Eating

Joy Foods

These foods switch off the Stress Triangle and increase joy. They decrease cortisol and insulin, balance dopamine, and boost GLP-1 to suppress appetite without promoting obesity, diabetes, anxiety, depression, or Alzheimer's Disease. Eat Protein Foods to decrease stress, Healthy Fats to feel rewarded, and Fiber Foods to decrease hunger. Eat mainly Joy Foods.

1. The Protein Group

Fish & Shellfish*
- ☐ Albacore
- ☐ Anchovies
- ☐ Bluefish
- ☐ Calamari
- ☐ Catfish
- ☐ Clams
- ☐ Cod
- ☐ Crab
- ☐ Halibut
- ☐ Herring
- ☐ Lobster
- ☐ Mackerel
- ☐ Mahi-mahi
- ☐ Ono
- ☐ Prawns
- ☐ Red snapper
- ☐ Salmon
- ☐ Sardines
- ☐ Scallops
- ☐ Sole
- ☐ Shrimp
- ☐ Trout
- ☐ Tuna

Poultry & Meat
- ☐ Beef round steak
- ☐ Beef round steak, ground
- ☐ Beef tenderloin
- ☐ Chateaubriand
- ☐ Chicken, ground
- ☐ Chicken breast
- ☐ Chicken drumsticks
- ☐ Chicken thighs
- ☐ Flank steak
- ☐ Hamburger meat
- ☐ Pork chops
- ☐ Pork tenderloin
- ☐ Sirloin tip roast
- ☐ Turkey breast
- ☐ Turkey drumsticks
- ☐ Turkey, ground
- ☐ Turkey sausages
- ☐ Turkey breast
- ☐ Veal cutlets
- ☐ Veal, ground
- ☐ Veal scallops
- ☐ Veal steak

More
- ☐ Beans and legumes
- ☐ Egg whites
- ☐ Eggs, whole
- ☐ Milk products**
- ☐ Plant-based burgers

2. Healthy Fats

Nuts. Seeds, & More
- ☐ Almond butter
- ☐ Almonds
- ☐ Avocados
- ☐ Brazil nuts
- ☐ Cashew butter
- ☐ Cashews
- ☐ Flax seeds
- ☐ Guacamole
- ☐ Hazelnut butter
- ☐ Hazelnuts
- ☐ Macadamia nuts
- ☐ Olives
- ☐ Peanut butter
- ☐ Peanuts
- ☐ Pecans
- ☐ Pine nuts
- ☐ Pistachios
- ☐ Poppy seeds
- ☐ Pumpkin seeds
- ☐ Sesame seeds
- ☐ Soy nut butter
- ☐ Soy nuts
- ☐ Sunflower seeds
- ☐ Tahini
- ☐ Walnuts

Oils
- ☐ Canola mayonnaise
- ☐ Canola oil
- ☐ Canola oil margarine
- ☐ Flaxseed oil
- ☐ Margarine, trans-fat-free
- ☐ Olive, regular
- ☐ Olive oil, extra virgin
- ☐ Peanut oil
- ☐ Safflower oil, high-oleic
- ☐ Sesame seed oil
- ☐ Soy oil
- ☐ Sunflower oil, high-oleic
- ☐ Walnut oil

3. The Fiber Group

Fruit
- ☐ Apples
- ☐ Apricots
- ☐ Bananas
- ☐ Blackberries
- ☐ Blueberries
- ☐ Cantaloupe
- ☐ Cranberries
- ☐ Cherries
- ☐ Grapefruit
- ☐ Grapes
- ☐ Guavas
- ☐ Figs
- ☐ Honeydew melon
- ☐ Kiwis
- ☐ Lemons
- ☐ Limes
- ☐ Mangoes
- ☐ Melons, other
- ☐ Nectarines
- ☐ Oranges
- ☐ Papayas
- ☐ Peaches
- ☐ Pears
- ☐ Persimmons
- ☐ Pineapples
- ☐ Pomegranates
- ☐ Plums
- ☐ Prunes
- ☐ Raisins
- ☐ Raspberries
- ☐ Strawberries
- ☐ Tangelos
- ☐ Tangerines
- ☐ Watermelon

Vegetables
- ☐ Acorn squash
- ☐ Artichokes
- ☐ Arugula
- ☐ Asparagus
- ☐ Bamboo shoots
- ☐ Banana squash
- ☐ Bean sprouts
- ☐ Beets
- ☐ Bok choy
- ☐ Broccoli
- ☐ Brussels sprouts
- ☐ Butternut squash
- ☐ Cabbage
- ☐ Carrots
- ☐ Cauliflower
- ☐ Celery
- ☐ Chard
- ☐ Chayote
- ☐ Corn
- ☐ Cucumbers
- ☐ Eggplant
- ☐ Endives
- ☐ Fennel
- ☐ Green beans
- ☐ Green onions/scallion
- ☐ Hubbard squash
- ☐ Jicama
- ☐ Kale
- ☐ Leafy greens
- ☐ Leeks
- ☐ Lettuce
- ☐ Mushrooms
- ☐ Okra
- ☐ Onions
- ☐ Parsnips
- ☐ Pea pods
- ☐ Peppers
- ☐ Pumpkin
- ☐ Radishes
- ☐ Snap peas
- ☐ Snow peas
- ☐ Spaghetti squash
- ☐ Spinach
- ☐ Sprouts
- ☐ Tomatillos
- ☐ Tomatoes
- ☐ Water chestnuts
- ☐ Yellow summer squash
- ☐ Zucchini

Whole Grains
- ☐ Whole grains, 100%

Stress Foods

Everything Else (Ultra-Processed and Low-Nutrient-Density Foods)

These foods can activate the Stress Triangle and increase stress. They increase cortisol and cause dopamine extremes, cravings, and chronic hunger. Stress Foods increase insulin, which blocks weight loss. They increase GLP-1 to suppress appetite but also promote obesity, diabetes, anxiety, depression, and Alzheimer's Disease. Do not "diet." Eat Stress Foods if you really need them and always, without guilt.

* The amount of mercury and other toxins in these foods vary.

** Combining protein group foods with calcium from milk products boosts the rise in GLP-1.

To personalize your plan, consult a Certified EBT Provider (Stress Eating Specialist) at EBT.ORG

1-2-3 JOY Eating

- Before eating, spiral up and identify your reward for releasing weight.
- Check your hunger level. If you are not hungry, do not eat.
- If you are hungry, select foods you enjoy from these groups:
  1. Protein Group (a protective base)
  2. Healthy Fats (for tastiness)
  3. Fiber Group (to fill you up)

  Add Stress Foods as needed (do not deprive yourself).
- Eat slowly and enjoy every bite.
- Stop eating when just satisfied.
- Enjoy the afterglow, the joy of body hunger satisfied.
- Be aware of your reward. ("I did that! My reward is ________.")
- In 20 minutes, you will feel full without the "afterburn" of being overly full.

Consider eating as a procedure, much the way you approach downloading an app or doing an online search. Much more is at stake with food than with your computer. By performing the procedure correctly and consistently – even if that means eating a lot of ultra-processed foods sometimes – you will train your brain for easy, lasting weight loss. Your 1-2-3 JOY Eating will become spontaneous and automatic with practice.

Fix the Habit Glitch

- **The first 30 days: "The Vibrancy Reset"** – It takes about a month to train your hypothalamus to adjust to healthier habits and about one year to raise the set point so the new habits stick. During the first 30 days of your Vibrancy Reset, experiment with ways of eating until you both enjoy your food and experience the rate of weight loss you want. Perhaps you try eating eggs for breakfast and, at first, eggs sound revolting, however, you have more energy all morning and begin to release weight. As the brain changes by associative learning, by pairing eating eggs with these benefits, soon those eggs begin to taste fantastic.
- **During the Vibrancy Reset, experiment** – The best way to find a way of eating that both promotes your vibrancy and releases extra weight is to try different approaches and check your weight daily to see the impact. This strategy works best when the joy of releasing weight is strong, and you have rewired both your Food and Body Circuits. You are not passionate about food and do not activate scarcity panics or food rebellion. You can be rational and see what works for you. Be gentle with yourself during this phase as you "reset" your brain for eating differently. Stick with the general rule of staying present to the stress of Brain State 3 but setting limits and not tolerating a Brain State 4 or 5 caused by habit change.

- **While fixing that glitch, nibble wisely** – During your Vibrancy Reset, the hypothalamus takes a while to reset. It is used to your old way of eating, and resetting it takes small waves of hunger now and then. See hunger as a sign that you have been successful in making progress toward fixing that glitch. You may even find that a little bit of hunger starts feeling good to you, a new way of having a "lightness" of being. When you are hungry and decide to eat, notice how effective it can be to just "take the edge off" your hunger. Have a few mouthfuls of chicken, drink some water, sip hot broth, eat raw vegetables, or eat a few nuts. Experiment until you find a few ways of nibbling when hungry that work for you. Keep in mind: you are taking 30 days to retrain your hypothalamus and this will pass. Your higher reward will make it all worthwhile.
- **Boost dopamine and oxytocin naturally during these 30 days** – Make these 30 days "a party" for yourself. Post the 30th day on your calendar as your "I fixed my glitch" day. Drop in more often – even daily – to Spiral Up Groups to boost your oxytocin, the "love chemical," a natural appetite suppressant. When a craving hits, laugh out loud! Then reach for the app and use this "Conquer the Craving" combination: 1) the Anger Cycle, 2) the Ladder Tool, and finally, 3) the Compassion Tool. That will not only quiet your hunger but bring you to a state of bliss and transcendence.

More Tips for Success

- **Check the effect of meals and choosing 1-2-3 Foods** – Although nibbling or snacking throughout the day is one way to transition to resetting the hypothalamus, feeling hungry every couple of hours means thinking about food a lot. Each thought of food can activate insulin and increase appetite. If you eat every two hours, your brain will create "hunger" every two hours. Eating less frequently, typically three times per day, can prevent your thinking about food and the burden of having to decide what, when, and how to eat throughout the day. Thoughts of food are problematic because they can switch on ghrelin, the hunger hormone. Adjust your food intake so you feel satisfied for four to six hours. Check if the EBT approach of eating from all three groups – Protein, Healthy Fats, and Fiber – plus any needed Stress Foods works for you.
- **First course? Fiber foods** – When fiber-containing foods arrive in the colon, the "I am satisfied" chemicals (GLP-1 and Peptide YY) activate. That takes about 20 minutes. Most people consume their entire meal much faster than that. So, when the situation allows, most frequently at dinner, consider eating Fiber Group foods first, especially greens and other high-volume (water + fiber) foods. By the "second course" (Protein Group, Healthy Fats, and whatever else you need), you will probably feel more satisfied with less food, and not overload your body with food you do not need. This is a bit of a "hack," so if it interferes with your enjoyment of food, do not use it.

- **Take a food rest** – Intermittent fasting has become popular, but research has shown that it is not associated with weight loss in the long term. The idea of fasting is appealing, giving the body time to metabolize glucose first, then body starch (glycogen), and finally, triglycerides, burning up fat. It takes eight hours of fasting to induce gluconeogenesis, making glucose, so this food rest is appealing. The conflicting research on this practice highlights that losing weight and maintaining weight are different processes. This is why using the 30 days of the Vibrancy Reset to find a new "groove" for eating that results in weight loss is so important. For some people, skipping breakfast, then eating a very high-protein lunch and dinner can support weight loss. Again, the cost-benefit ratio can only be determined by you.
- **Conclude eating by 7 p.m.** – Research shows that eating earlier in the day promotes weight loss, with the most convincing research based on eating a high-protein breakfast. Eating early decreases ghrelin levels, eases hunger, and increases evening leptin to promote less fat storage. Nurturing yourself in the evenings without reliance on food pays off. When you feel a little hungry in the late evening, that is your decision time. If you eat a meal then (and It's hard not to because energy and dopamine are low in the evenings), chances are you will not lose weight. If you have a cup of tea or nibble on some nuts or a few bites of chicken, you will be likely to lose weight. There is no one right way to do this. The choice is yours.

What if you have special dietary needs? If you do, or you need more personalized support in improving your nutrition, consult a health professional who is EBT Certified in the specialty of Stress Eating. Visit EBT.ORG for more information about coaching by Certified EBT Providers. If you look locally for a nutritionist or dietitian, ask if he or she is certified in EBT. Always, be sure that your physician approves any changes in your food intake.

EBT as a Natural Alternative to Drugs

EBT is a natural alternative to weight-loss drugs or can be used in combination with them to reduce their side effects and promote lasting weight loss.

These weight-loss drugs are mostly diabetes drugs that are used for weight loss as they boost GLP-1 (glucagon-like peptide-1), which decreases appetite and promotes satiety. While drugs, as well as surgery, provide the right choice for many people, even if just for the short term, they can come with a price.

With these medications, nausea, constipation, and diarrhea are common. If you want to avoid these problems, use EBT, but even if you do use weight-loss drugs, EBT can help by addressing the root cause of the problem: stress, and when you feel nauseated, use the EBT tools.

Katie had 140 pounds to lose and she had decided to take weight-loss drugs. After two months, she had lost 14 pounds, yet she was nauseated often. She announced in her telegroup session that she was using the Ladder Tool and it saved her.

I asked, "From what?"

Katie said, "From nausea from the weight-loss drugs. I use the Ladder Tool (on the app as "Climb the Ladder" on the Progress page). This tool takes about seven minutes and guides you through using all the tools in order from the 5 Tool all the way to the 1 Tool, finishing with feelings of compassion for yourself, others, and all living beings.

She said, "The nausea vanished."

What do GLP-1-mimicking drugs do? They can improve appetite, satiety, and weight loss. However, they have significant side effects for many people, particularly nausea and pancreatitis. These drugs also cause your body to feel as if it is in starvation mode, leading to possible headaches and fatigue, and eventually metabolic adaptation. If your physician prescribes a GLP-1 agonist drug for you, be sure to ask about possible side effects.

As described in Keep It Simple: Create Joy, EBT does more than change one chemical. It activates and rewires the neural Stress Circuits of allostasis (health harming) as homeostatic (health promoting). The tools support you in improving the broad range of biochemicals that directly and naturally impact hunger, satiety, and weight and make it easier to eat healthy and use food to increase GLP-1 naturally. As drugs are an artificial source of GLP-1, the risks posed also include downregulation of the system, lessening the impact of the drug, and when treatment is stopped, weight is regained. The EBT Program includes natural ways to amplify and boost GLP-1 based on these research findings:

- **Protein is effective in increasing GLP-1** – The emphasis is on protein as it boosts GLP-1 the most. Build your meals around protein, choosing a hand-sized portion from the Protein Group at all meals. Add foods from the Healthy Fats and Fiber Group based on your appetite. Never deprive yourself, so add Stress Foods as needed.
- **High protein is more effective** – The EBT Program encourages using protein as your natural, affordable "drug." Research has shown that a very high level of protein is the biggest boost of GLP-1 when protein contributes 50 percent of calories per meal. In fact, the higher the dose of protein, the more the protein load may reach the distal parts of the intestine where GLP-1 is secreted. Our research shows that people consume about 33 to 40 percent of their calories as protein, so consider how much protein you are getting in your meals and whether or not you need more.
- **A high-protein breakfast enhances GLP-1 levels** – As described above, eating a high-protein breakfast translates into a boost of GLP-1 that promotes spontaneous decreases in food intake for the rest of the day. This finding builds on a large body of research showing that a high-protein breakfast promotes weight loss, primarily from increasing GLP-1 and decreasing ghrelin after meals, which signals satiety.

- **Olive oil boosts GLP-1 more than butter** – The EBT Food System promotes eating healthy fats. Consuming olive oil increases GLP-1 response greater than a butter-rich meal, which further supports the value of consuming olive oil for health and as well as making foods tastier.
- **Fiber-rich foods enhance GLP-1** – Choosing foods in the Fiber Group, specifically those high in fermentable fiber found in beans and legumes can increase both Peptide YY and GLP-1 in the gut. Other high fermentable fiber foods such as apples, artichokes, asparagus, berries, cabbage, carrots, onions, and citrus give a boost to feeling full, too.
- **Calcium amplifies the impact of protein on GLP-1** – As someone who has gravitated to eating chicken for lunch with Greek yogurt spiked with a teaspoon of sugar and some vanilla extract because that keeps me satisfied and my energy strong for about five hours, I wasn't surprised when this research was released: Calcium (e.g., yogurt) can help boost GLP-1. Consuming protein foods (e.g., chicken) with calcium-rich foods increases GLP-1 markedly. See if that synergy of protein and calcium supports you in feeling more satisfied and releasing weight more easily.

1-2-3 JOY Eating: The process works!

Yesterday, I went out to lunch with my husband, Walt. It was New Year's Day and our first trip out of the house since his recent back surgery. Both of us were a little rattled (running at 3 rather than at 1).

When we arrived at the restaurant, the mood was festive. Walt ordered a drink that was a blend of cream, sugar, and a little alcohol, like a milkshake for adults who are celebrating.

I thought, "That looks delicious." Instead of my habitual process of 1-2-3 Eating, I said, "I'll have one of those!"

Instead of focusing on my process – 1-2-3 JOY Eating – I was on a false high, which is not bad. We all need a few false highs in daily life. However, I paid the price.

By the time we left the lunch, I had an "afterburn" from the cream, sugar, and alcohol, and I felt a little nauseous and bloated for the rest of the afternoon. Allow yourself to abandon the process periodically, because it only serves to confirm that life goes better when we stick with the process.

After aborting 1-2-3 JOY Eating, get the most from the experience by forbidding self-judgment. I did a quick Cycle to be fully present to how bad my body felt from overeating. Then I did another Cycle about having gone "off process." I learned from both Cycles, and I kept with the basic premise of EBT: give yourself unconditional love no matter what!

If you do one thing – do your best to use the process of 1-2-3 JOY Eating – the outcomes of feeling great, losing weight, and keeping it off will take care of themselves.

Change your food preferences naturally: Spiral Up!

The choice to make it a habit to spiral up before eating is a great "hack" to the system.

We all have five "eaters" inside us, one food preference for each brain state. The person inside you who likes chocolate cake and vanilla milkshakes will always be there. Love that part of you! However, when you spiral up before eating, your biochemistry and food preferences change. A different area of your brain is in charge and a different kind of circuit. As your set point goes up, the more you always reserve the right to consume as many Stress Foods as you like, the more your body will start enjoying healthy foods. It's natural and biochemical.

Natural Food Preferences and Brain States

Spiraling up before eating encourages healthy eating.

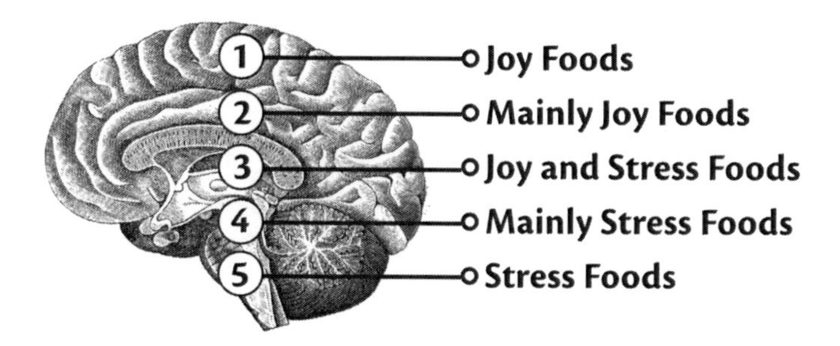

Keep it simple and scientific. Spiral up and eat foods that support you in shifting away from stress eating, reward eating, and habitual overeating. Bring out the Brain State 1 "eater" in you naturally by connecting to the deepest part of yourself and spiraling up before eating.

It's important to eat foods you enjoy and plan out a program that goes at the pace that is right for you. The last part of Step 3, Changing Habits, is to identify foods you enjoy and set out your intentions for releasing extra weight.

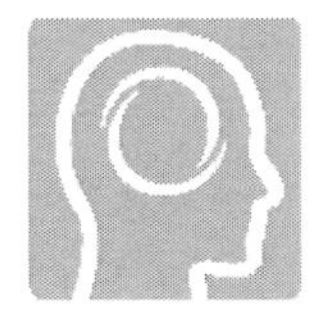

21

Make It Easy: EBT 1-2-3 JOY Eating

A few years ago, a psychologist, Kathleen Wilson, was trying to determine if she wanted to seek certification in EBT and dropped into one of our three-day retreats. After the retreat, she called me and reflected on her experience.

She said, "EBT is human development on steroids."

Your brain is changing quickly, and often you will find yourself in what is called "asynchronous development." This is when one part of you evolves before another, or one lags behind the rest.

Raising your set point in a year is full of these zigzags. For example, you may have a drive to eat healthy, but then when the weight comes off, you may feel scared, or you might have a strong drive to drink a milkshake, but your body awareness of how you will feel afterwards sends up red flags.

Rewiring the Brain for Healthy Eating

The purpose of this chapter is to make it easy to eat healthy without triggering a scarcity panic or rebellion, and still fast-forwarding your eating and weight progress.

There are two treatments integrated into one process. The first is to use the "Healthy Boundaries Tool" to switch your mindset for habit change.

The Healthy Boundaries Tool

- **In the past, I did this:**
- **Now, I do this:**

- **My higher-order reward for doing it is:**
- **Collect a Joy Point.**

Example:

- In the past, I dealt with stress by overeating.
- Now, I clear stress by creating joy in my life and eating the Protein Group Foods I like: chicken, Greek yogurt, and eggs.
- My higher-order reward is Vibrancy.
- Collect a Joy Point.

The prefrontal cortex requires that we tell a story, and if we do not supply an inspiring one, it will fill in the blanks with one that holds us back and creates stress. The strategy is to prime your thinking brain to tell a new story about how you eat. Use this tool to tell a story about what you used to do, why you did it, what you do now, and your higher-order reward for embracing the new way you want to be in this world and living your life with purpose. Complete the process with a dopamine surge by collecting a Joy Point. Notice slight sensations of lightness, relaxation, or tingling in your body. Do this for each of the three food groups and weight.

Planning Easy, Natural Weight Loss

What about your weight goals? I recommend losing weight slowly to make it easier and keep it from coming back. Every pound of weight you lose has a biochemical, emotional, cognitive, relational, spiritual, and behavioral impact. If you do not process your emotions and give your body time to adapt to changes, your weight loss "gets ahead of" and sabotages your emotional brain's capacity to process it.

What if you do not like to weigh yourself? You don't have to, but weighing yourself daily gives you evidence of trends in your weight based on biological variables.

When Walt and I took our brand-new puppy Tammy for training, we asked the experts at the facility how much to feed her. They responded that there is no set amount to give her because each dog's needs differ. They said the general rule is to watch how her body changes. If she is eating too much or too little, we would know. We are all puppies. As most of us have "wires" about our weight, we are at risk of continuing to overeat and convince ourselves that we are releasing weight, and of undereating and taking weight off so quickly that our body and brain cannot sustain the weight loss.

Be sure the joy of weight loss has kicked in, as that alone can deactivate a lot of Stress Circuits. If checking your weight is triggering, consider that fascinating, and do five Spiral Ups. If you need another five, it's well worth the time and effort. You are not your weight any more than you are your circuits. You have made a personal decision to release weight, so consider clearing clutter until checking your weight becomes a nurturing act. The essential pain may be to check your weight, but the earned reward is Freedom from counting points, measuring portion sizes, or writing down what you eat. What if you decide that checking your weight is not right for you? Then do not do it.

To complete this plan, please create a healthy boundary for each type of eating and select foods you will consider eating to meet your goal, with a focus on which area of the brain is closely associated with that goal, both the brain structure and the primary chemical.

Only eat foods you like, eat only when hungry, stop when just satisfied, and wait 20 minutes and notice that you are comfortably full, but not overly full.

1. End Stress Eating with Protein Foods

- Why: Stop Cravings
- Brain Structure: Amygdala
- Primary Chemical: Cortisol

Create a Healthy Boundary

In the past, I dealt with stress by:

- ☐ Overeating
- ☐ Eating Stress Foods
- ☐ Binge Eating
- ☐ Other __________

Now, I clear my stress by creating joy in my life and eating Protein Foods that I like.

My reward is:

- ☐ Sanctuary
- ☐ Authenticity
- ☐ Vibrancy
- ☐ Integrity
- ☐ Intimacy
- ☐ Spirituality
- ☐ Freedom

Collect A Joy Point.

1. The Protein Group

Fish & Shellfish

- ☐ Albacore
- ☐ Anchovies
- ☐ Bluefish
- ☐ Calamari
- ☐ Clams
- ☐ Cod
- ☐ Crab
- ☐ Halibut
- ☐ Herring
- ☐ Lobster
- ☐ Mackerel
- ☐ Mahi-mahi
- ☐ Ono
- ☐ Prawns
- ☐ Red snapper
- ☐ Salmon
- ☐ Sardines
- ☐ Scallops
- ☐ Shrimp
- ☐ Sole
- ☐ Trout

Poultry & Meat

- ☐ Beef round steak
- ☐ Beef round steak, ground
- ☐ Beef tenderloin
- ☐ Chateaubriand
- ☐ Chicken, ground
- ☐ Chicken breast
- ☐ Chicken drumsticks
- ☐ Chicken sausages
- ☐ Chicken thighs
- ☐ Flank steak
- ☐ Hamburger meat
- ☐ Pork chops
- ☐ Pork tenderloin
- ☐ Sirloin tip roast
- ☐ Turkey breast
- ☐ Turkey drumsticks
- ☐ Turkey, ground
- ☐ Turkey sausages
- ☐ Veal cutlets
- ☐ Veal, ground
- ☐ Veal scallops
- ☐ Veal steak

More

- ☐ Beans and legumes
- ☐ Egg whites
- ☐ Eggs, whole
- ☐ Milk products
- ☐ Plant-based burgers

2. Quiet Reward Eating with Healthy Fats

- Why: Increase Pleasure
- Brain Structure: Nucleus Accumbens
- Primary Chemical: Dopamine

Create a Healthy Boundary

In the past, I rewarded myself by:

- ☐ Overeating
- ☐ Eating Stress Foods
- ☐ Binge Eating
- ☐ Other ___________

Now, I clear my stress by creating joy in my life and eating Healthy Fats that I like.

My reward is:

- ☐ Sanctuary
- ☐ Authenticity
- ☐ Vibrancy
- ☐ Integrity
- ☐ Intimacy
- ☐ Spirituality
- ☐ Freedom

Collect A Joy Point.

2. Healthy Fats

Nuts, Seeds & More

- ☐ Almond butter
- ☐ Almonds
- ☐ Avocados
- ☐ Brazil nuts
- ☐ Cashew butter
- ☐ Cashews
- ☐ Flax seeds
- ☐ Guacamole
- ☐ Hazelnut butter
- ☐ Hazelnuts
- ☐ Macadamia nuts
- ☐ Olives
- ☐ Peanut butter
- ☐ Peanuts
- ☐ Pecans
- ☐ Pine nuts
- ☐ Pistachios
- ☐ Poppy seeds
- ☐ Pumpkin seeds
- ☐ Sesame seeds
- ☐ Soy nut butter
- ☐ Soy nuts
- ☐ Sunflower seeds
- ☐ Tahini
- ☐ Walnuts

Oils

- ☐ Canola mayonnaise
- ☐ Canola oil
- ☐ Canola oil margarine
- ☐ Flaxseed oil
- ☐ Margarine, trans-fat-free
- ☐ Olive, regular
- ☐ Olive oil, extra virgin
- ☐ Peanut oil
- ☐ Safflower oil, high-oleic
- ☐ Sesame seed oil
- ☐ Soy oil
- ☐ Sunflower oil, high-oleic
- ☐ Walnut oil

3. Tame Hunger Eating with Fiber Foods

- Why: Feel Full Longer
- Brain Structure: Hypothalamus
- Primary Chemical: Insulin

In the past, I was chronically hungry from:

- ☐ Overeating
- ☐ Eating Stress Foods
- ☐ Binge Eating
- ☐ Other __________

Now, I switch off chronic hunger by creating joy in my life and eating Fiber Foods that I like.

My reward is:

- ☐ Sanctuary
- ☐ Authenticity
- ☐ Vibrancy
- ☐ Integrity
- ☐ Intimacy
- ☐ Spirituality
- ☐ Freedom

Collect A Joy Point.

3. Fiber Group Foods

Fruit

- ☐ Apples
- ☐ Apricots
- ☐ Bananas
- ☐ Blackberries
- ☐ Blueberries
- ☐ Cantaloupe
- ☐ Cranberries
- ☐ Cherries
- ☐ Grapefruit
- ☐ Grapes
- ☐ Guavas
- ☐ Figs
- ☐ Honeydew melon
- ☐ Kiwis
- ☐ Lemons
- ☐ Limes
- ☐ Mangoes
- ☐ Melons, other
- ☐ Nectarines
- ☐ Oranges
- ☐ Papayas
- ☐ Peaches
- ☐ Pears
- ☐ Persimmons
- ☐ Pineapples
- ☐ Pomegranates
- ☐ Plums
- ☐ Prunes
- ☐ Raspberries
- ☐ Strawberries
- ☐ Tangelos
- ☐ Tangerines
- ☐ Watermelon

Vegetables

- ☐ Acorn squash
- ☐ Artichokes
- ☐ Arugula
- ☐ Asparagus
- ☐ Bamboo shoots
- ☐ Banana squash
- ☐ Bean squash
- ☐ Bean sprouts
- ☐ Beets
- ☐ Bok choy
- ☐ Broccoli
- ☐ Brussels sprouts
- ☐ Butternut squash
- ☐ Cabbage
- ☐ Carrots
- ☐ Cauliflower
- ☐ Celery
- ☐ Chard
- ☐ Chayote
- ☐ Corn
- ☐ Cucumbers
- ☐ Eggplant
- ☐ Endives
- ☐ Fennel
- ☐ Green beans
- ☐ Green onions/scallions
- ☐ Hubbard squash
- ☐ Jicama
- ☐ Kale
- ☐ Leafy greens
- ☐ Leeks
- ☐ Lettuce
- ☐ Mushrooms
- ☐ Okra
- ☐ Onions
- ☐ Parsnips
- ☐ Pea pods
- ☐ Peppers
- ☐ Pumpkin
- ☐ Radishes
- ☐ Snap peas
- ☐ Snow peas
- ☐ Spaghetti squash
- ☐ Spinach
- ☐ Sprouts
- ☐ Tomatillos
- ☐ Tomatoes
- ☐ Water chestnuts
- ☐ Yellow summer squash
- ☐ Zucchini

Whole Grains

- ☐ Whole grains, 100%

JOY! Release Extra Weight for Higher Purpose

My current weight is: ____________________
My healthy weight goal is: _________________

My reward for releasing extra weight is:
☐ Sanctuary
☐ Authenticity
☐ Vibrancy
☐ Integrity
☐ Intimacy
☐ Spirituality
☐ Freedom

I expect myself to release weight:
☐ At the rate that is right for me
☐ Averaging 1 pound per week
☐ Averaging 2 pounds per week
☐ Not sure
☐ Other _________

To assess my weight change, I will:
☐ Weigh myself daily
☐ Clear clutter about checking my weight daily
☐ Ask health professionals to check my weight
☐ Not sure
☐ Other _________

I will continue using The EBT 1-2-3 JOY Program until I have:
☐ An abundance of all seven rewards of a purposeful life
☐ All the EBT skills through completing the program
☐ A new set point of One
☐ Freedom from stress eating

- ☐ Freedom from reward eating
- ☐ Freedom from chronic hunger
- ☐ A healthy weight
- ☐ Not sure
- ☐ Other __________

Experimenting with 1-2-3 JOY Eating

I asked Jessica what she learned from the first weeks of her Vibrancy Reset.

She said, "When I started thinking of food based on what it would do for me, it was motivating and . . . fun. I looked at a piece of chicken. It looked more appealing because it stops cravings and reduces my cortisol. It calms my amygdala."

"Then what happened?"

"I started eating healthy as a way to nurture myself, and the weight started coming off. I did some spiral ups about the scale – I have never liked weighing myself, but it didn't bother me this time. I saw that I had lost a few pounds, but I saw some big fluctuations."

"Tell me more."

"I had a big argument with my husband, and the children could hear us yelling. He went to bed. I went to the kitchen and ate. The next morning, I had gained two pounds and had a food hangover. That's when I decided I wanted a partner who was EBT literate. After that argument, he was motivated, and now he is a couple of weeks into using the method."

"When couples do this together, the benefits for both increases. Walt and I listen to each other spiral up nearly every day."

"We're already closer because we communicate when we are at Brain State 5, so we prevent difficulties. The food part of this has been pretty easy. Most of my eating is triggered by stress, and I now use protein as medicine. When I start getting anxious and have a craving, I nibble on some chicken or tuna. I eat stress foods a couple of times a week, sometimes only one, but I think I have reset my hypothalamus. I'm excited. I'm releasing weight, sometimes two or three pounds. I'm now in Advanced EBT, the course on Sanctuary.

Kevin had been combining EBT with weight-loss drugs and had a very different experience.

He said, "The commitment to eating healthy is what my physician had asked me to do when she gave me the prescription, but I was still eating and drinking and thinking that I could use the drugs to avoid dealing with my issues."

I smiled, "Did you talk with your physician about EBT?"

"Not yet, but I have made a reset, which includes cutting down on alcohol as well as stopping the Stress Foods. By eating only when hungry, it was clear to me that I was habituated to eating about twice what my body needed."

Then he laughed, "I trained my body to overeat, and now I am training my brain to eat what my body needs. I'm rarely hungry now and had no idea that the foods I was eating were making me hungry, angry, and shut down."

Charlotte's journey was somewhat more complicated.

She reported, "The moment I committed to changing my food for purpose, I started binge eating. It was too soon for me."

"I'm so happy you listened to your body."

"But I have done that before, and I knew I had the skills to get past my reptilian brain's hissy fit."

She was on her way!

"What did you do?"

"I arranged for more help. I got an EBT Provider as a coach and am meeting with her regularly. I realize that even though the problem is food, not drugs, I am still addicted. I need daily support, so I drop into the Spiral Up Groups for 30 minutes each day, watch the weekly video program with you, and have three Connection Buddies: my neighbor, my sister who lives in Cleveland, and my ex-boss, who has become a good friend. I have plenty of support."

"What have you learned about your food?"

"If I eat protein, healthy fats, and fiber, I am not hungry. Doing all three works like a drug. It suppresses my appetite."

"What about sugar binges?"

"I know I'm addicted enough to sugar after 40 years of it that it works better for me to eat for purpose and not eat sugary foods."

"If you over-restrict . . ."

"Keep in mind that I am in this for the long haul. When my set point goes up, I'll start experimenting again, but for now, this is working for me."

All three participants had changed their food and weight, but they were still on a journey. As their set points rise, they will see food and weight differently, and as they release the extra weight, they will see themselves differently.

They had accomplished their Vibrancy Reset and rewired the Big 4 Circuits. However, establishing a lasting set point requires clearing more clutter and training the brain to achieve spontaneous resilience and to access an abundance of the seven rewards of a purposeful life.

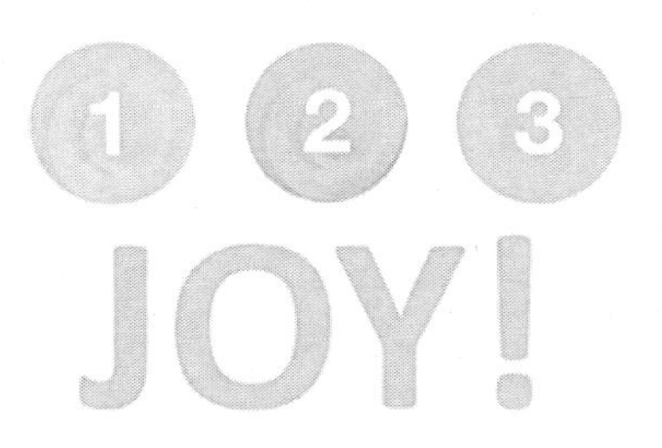

Profound and Lasting Results

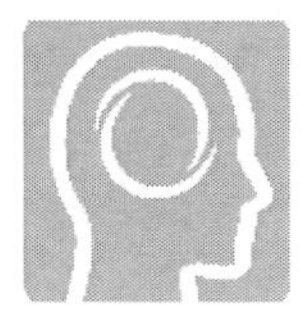

22

No More Glitches: See Miracles Everywhere

After the Vibrancy Reset, Jessica, Kevin, and Charlotte settled into easy, natural weight loss.

They each had learned to think about eating and weight based on neuroscience. They knew that they weighed what their emotional brain told them to weigh and ate what it told them to eat. So, instead of dieting, they updated their wires and went on to complete the EBT 1-2-3 JOY Program to raise their set point for lasting results.

People stay with the program because the tools work. Last week in a Spiral Up with Laurel Zoom session, Jennifer spoke up and said, "Your program works. I've been using it online for a year and I've lost 30 pounds." Yet, I believe the more powerful reason is that after the drive to overeat fades, the program gives us what we really need, which is transcendence.

As the set point rises, a new life unfolds

Brain State 1 is more than a powerful appetite suppressant, it is the state that gives us immediate access to the deeper meanings and goodness of life. In the age of social media, texting, and video games, the daily experience of seeing small miracles everywhere makes most people want more EBT.

It's not a religion and there is no guru. We rely on science to shape the skills. When I first started hearing participants share that they "feel different inside" and that the world looks so beautiful to them since learning the skills it made sense. The emotional brain is the seat of the soul.

During a telegroup this morning, I was explaining to the participants that as the set point goes up, they should expect to see miracles large and small. A young woman who came to EBT to treat anxiety and binge eating said, "I don't believe in miracles."

I said, "That's a term used in EBT, but feel free to use another one, such as unexpected welcome gifts, perfect coincidences, or happy surprises."

Miracles in everyday life

There are two types of miracles: large and small. I think of big miracles as the things that happen to us, when out of the blue something surprising and wonderful occurs that is not explicable by science or nature. Small miracles are neuroscientific. We can explain them by brain state as at Brain State 1 our beautiful homeostatic wires color our perceptions of ourselves, others, and life, and attract into our orbit other people, places, things, and events that radiate Brain State 1, too.

As the set point rises, the brain is running "1 Circuits" most of the time, and it's not unusual for people who are finishing up the EBT Program to say that they "see miracles everywhere." What about those big miracles? When our brain is weighed down by stress chemicals, a real bona fide miracle could occur in our living room and we may just shrug and say, "Pass the remote."

In contrast, the smooth workings of our brain and body ("neural integration") that come with our rising set point can boost our sensitivity to big miracles, causing us to tremble with delight and revere the deeper meaning of our lives.

For me, the big miracles always have arrived at my most vulnerable and grittiest of times and given me precisely what I needed, at the perfect time and in the perfect way. One of them happened a few years after my beloved father had passed away when he not only protected me from some real and present danger but also comforted me on a soul level.

Early one morning, I awoke and noticed an odd sensation on my shoulders. It felt like wooden planks. I could see them. They were dark brown. Then a strong male voice said loudly, slowly, and urgently: "Do Not Quit." That statement struck me as bizarre as I was expecting a day of celebration. Half a minute later, in a slightly softer tone, the voice said, "Be Proud of Yourself." I realized it was my father's voice, he had visited me.

Then, the next morning, the bad news came. What would otherwise have left me feeling dead-in-the-water humiliated left me calm. In fact, I was at One and almost welcomed the news with a sense of wonder, as it was proof that I was loved and cherished. My father was still with me, and still loved me, and was even still doing his part to protect me. My soul was pulsating with gratitude and awe. On a practical level, his gift enabled me to get through the situation well because, on a spiritual level, I was at One. I could feel my dad's forcefield of love around me. I soon forgot the bad news and saw its bright side, but the good news of that morning will stay with me forever.

Apart from these big miracles, as the set point rises, small wonders start entering our world. The stressed-out brain that early in EBT training was beleaguered with all that cortisol becomes a free agent, able to open up to the beauty of life. Every single dopamine surge counts in the brain, as it switches off the HPA Axis and the chronic cortisol secretion and acts as a gentle anesthetic for the pain of transforming our lives. Each of the participants we are following came to EBT to achieve lasting weight loss, but toward the middle of their journey realized that the method was about far more than weight loss and stayed with it for the larger transformations that using the skills can bring.

Kevin was a dabbler: several common excesses

As Kevin began the advanced work to raise his set point, I worried about him. He was a "dabbler," a person who had multiple external solutions that were not all that extreme but taken as a whole kept him chronically disconnected. The classic pattern is starting the day with coffee addiction, then phone excess, overworking, overspending, overeating, and the list goes on. These circuits often clear in the first three months of the program, but the early positive results can camouflage the greater need which is to train the brain to be securely connected, thinking brain to feeling brain, by raising the set point.

The basic rule in EBT is not to bore or scare the reptilian brain, and in service of not boring Kevin, I asked him if he was starting to see "miracles everywhere," the neural sign of being nearly Wired at One.

At the time, he was bringing a hot cup of coffee to his mouth, and promptly dropped the cup and spilled coffee down his shirt.

Wiping his shirt, he said, "Did you say miracles everywhere?"

I said, "Absolutely."

Kevin said, "I'm at One more, and I'm happy. Isn't that enough?"

"Actually, no. You are the owner of an emotional brain that is the most powerful processor on the planet, and it is set for survival, which means it will not let up and stop your stress symptoms until you are wired for joy."

"I am not a joy person, Dr. Laurel."

This man was so endearing, as he was now quite sure that he didn't have to conform to the rules of human genes.

I told him, "Kevin, you don't have a lot of choice in the matter. We can't choose our genes and all of us have 23 pairs of chromosomes, each made up of long strands of DNA that all point in one direction: Brain State 1, the state in which we are drenched in the biochemically-based and electrically-fortified drives to give back, be of service, and find deeper meaning in our lives."

"That's ridiculous. What about all the people in jail or who commit terrible crimes or just numb out . . . like I used to?"

Now he was chuckling, "Okay, you got me on that one. What do I have to do?"

"I want you to recommit to the program, that you will dig deeper into your beautiful unconscious mind and move through the courses until you can say that you have an abundance of all seven rewards of a purposeful life – all of them – and Set Point 1. The last part of the journey has some beautiful unfoldings that are not just nice, but necessary. Will you stay the course?"

"What does that have to do with miracles?"

Now I was laughing. I said, "That's for you to find out. When you start seeing miracles everywhere, that's a sign that you are Wired at One."

Kevin said, "I commit"

I said, "Great!"

Jessica had a serial circuit and was miracle-insufficient

Although Jessica started her EBT journey to treat her binge eating, she also had diabetes and a smattering of other circuits – social media, overexercise, and more.

Now that her Food Circuit had been transformed, she was at risk of having a serial circuit, stopping one excess only to take on another. As a person who "thinks too much," all the mental space crowded with analyzing, planning, deciding, and then redeciding blocked what her genes required: to let go of over-control and receive the goodness of life. I had already shared with her my standard explanation, the one my children still tease me about because I must have told them the story 1000 times. You can do this "tight fist of over-control" exercise right now.

First, turn the palm of your hand to the heavens and cup your fingers together as if you want to collect rainwater. Next create a fist, digging your fingernails into the palm of your hand until it hurts. That's the tight fist of over-control. It's not effective in collecting rainwater. Last, turn your hand over and let it dangle. That is the limp wrist of under-control. It is not effective either. Your job is to open your hand to the goodness of life, palm up, fingers together, collecting the rainwater you can and letting go of the rest.

What would make Jessica willing to let go of over-control and surrender to experiencing the goodness of life? It would be through the portal of alleviating her pain, which centered around Jeremy. Rewiring not just any 5 Circuit, but one so dear to her heart that it felt more like a 10 Circuit, could help her make the shift.

That strategy appealed to me because it could help her in three ways. First, the natural neurotransmitter surge would bring her so much rapture and bliss, that her attitude toward clearing clutter would shift. She would lean into her emotions rather than push them away.

Second, she would find that she not only had no desire to binge eat but she also had a strong adverse response to the idea of it. This is extremely important because the transcendent experience is a sacred one. When at Brain State 5 is the time to spiral up to experience it. If instead, she ate bowls of buttered popcorn, she would block her capacity to transcend. One cannot serve two Gods: the food wire and the spiritual circuit. If she chose the addiction pathway, her inner peace wire would short circuit in that moment. As her set point was already on the high side, she had the brain function ("self-regulatory strength") to execute either option. The choice was hers.

Third, although she stayed so busy with the twins, her son Jeremy who had special needs, and her work, the ache in her heart about her son's challenges was so painful. Dismantling that knot of wires would take dozens of Cycles, but if she could orchestrate a moment of transcendence, it could potentially clear away all that pain in a "pop." The underbelly of trauma circuits sparkles with the potential for miracles. All we must do is the work. For Jessica, I thought the Transcendence Tool could help.

Another pathway to bliss: the Transcendence Tool

The Transcendence Tool is pretty simple. Like most EBT, the secret of the tools is to unravel the emotional blockade caused by Stress Circuits, with their toxic feelings, and once cleared, stand out of the way, and allow the healing powers that be to take charge. Even the prompts of the Cycle Tool are guided by our genes. The next step that is most healing is guided by interoceptive awareness ("body feel") as to which would feel most rewarding. The emotional brain is that perfect.

The process can be used during a full-blown stress response, with the equivalent of a five-alarm fire offering the best impact. It does not matter whether the circuit is activated in real-time by the situation or cognitively activated by thoughts, images, or sensations of that experience. Jessica had cleared a lot of emotional clutter at the Brain State 4 level, but less at Brain State 5, and it is clearing the 5 Circuits that produces physiological and spiritual results.

I said, "Jessica, we need to do some 'brain surgery' here, and that means unlocking the emotional brain and clearing circuits, with the goal of finding your 'pain point,' what bothers you the most. Any way we can amplify your stress in the moment can increase our chances for a moment of transcendence, and what can follow is a more rapid and lasting reconsolidation of that cluster of wires."

She said, "I think I know the answer. No one pushes my buttons the way Jeremy does, and I am so stressed at work as we have been acquired by another company and a lot of the transition work falls on my shoulders. I might be able to activate a 5 Circuit – going on a 10 Circuit –naturally. If not, I'll do the regular approach and do five spiral ups a day until I activate a really strong wire."

"I love that idea. Let's go for it."

I explained to Jessica how to use the Transcendence Tool:

When you are at Brain State 5, with a little kerosene added to the fire for good measure, as evidenced by plenty of harsh judgments and unhealthy drives, use this tool. Notice that a stress-induced time warp makes you sure there is no hope. All is lost. Be brave. Connect with your body. Do not think. Enter your emptiness, and stay present to the void we all have, without fear. It is part of the process. Pause again. Then, feel the shift. Notice an expansive awareness that you are part of a world in which you are separate and alone, however, what is inside you is inside everyone. You are part of something that is more. Love abounds, and you feel present, in awe, and fully alive. You may notice a desire to ask for help. If so, ask for support from the spiritual, God, or the universe. Stay present to your emotions until you feel complete.

The brain strongly remembers the emotional experience, so it is no wonder that using this tool is apt to change the emotional architecture of your brain, strengthening what you might think of as your "God Circuit" or "Source Wire." After each use, be aware that you are more inclined to love, not judge, trust life's goodness, and open that tight fist of overcontrol. You cup your hand palm up ready to receive yet another amazing blessing of that day.

For me, once I make that spiritual shift, the weight of the world falls away. I appreciate that I am this tiny speck in a much larger system, and my only job is to be of service. Sometimes, it ends with little fanfare. I think, "Well, I tried my best to stay emotionally connected through that ruckus and get to Brain State 1. That's all I can do." Other times, I transcend the boundary of time and body and have some epiphany that may not arise any other way or a sense of direct knowledge that everything is connected to everything, and I have nothing to fear. I am safe.

As using this tool can be a practice – reaching for it in those 5 PLUS moments – I often combine it with what EBT Master Trainer and genius in applying the method, Deanne Hamilton, calls the "Dig Deeper Tool." That is doing one Cycle after another, going deeper into the pile-up of circuits blocking our joy until we hit the spiritual "pay dirt" of feeling peace inside. Ahhhh, it feels so good! Typically, within moments or hours, not days, of using this tool, even though I often cannot even remember what I was so upset about, gifts come out of the blue through no effort of my own. Consistent with neuroplasticity research, the stress of the 5 PLUS state may jar something loose in my brain, or perhaps the stress gives my soul a wake-up call. I have learned to trust that things work out when I am in a brain state in which I make a spiritual request without being attached to whether I receive it. When I am in overcontrol, a sign of Brain State 5, not so much. Those stress chemicals raging give a scientific explanation for the common adage that when "self-will" runs wild, we are doomed, and if we open our hearts to surrender to "thy will," the coffers of life's bounty open up to us. At Brain State 1, that is easier to do.

Consider watching for patterns of "after the 5 comes the 1." Notice if within 24 hours of an otherwise debilitating 5 Moment when you stayed emotionally present and rode it out, something that delights you beyond your imagination occurs. If it does, consider it one of those everyday miracles and start seeing them everywhere. For instance, last week, Walt had a setback in his recovery from "mega" spine surgery, not able to sleep for several nights with the pain medications flat-out ineffective, when out of the blue, my daughter-in-law Ana called, giving love, empathy, and some astute advice about pain strategies, drawing from her expertise as a pharmacist. Her choice to call strengthened the deep peace circuits in my brain – and was a small miracle.

A week after Jessica mapped out her plan, she returned for a session with good news. She said, "The day after we met, Jeremy had hand-to-hand combat with one of the twins, pulling her hair. The other twin started hitting Jeremy back, and the whole room exploded with screaming and crying. My boss quit the company that day, leaving me with all his work, and I got COVID for the fourth time. I went into 'poor me' mode and 'how could it get any worse?' Immediately, I asked my husband to take over. I went to bed, pulled the sheets over my head, and hit such a 5 PLUS that my mind went blank. There was no way out. I had no hope, then I surrendered. I stayed present to my emptiness. Then something shifted, and I felt very calm – incredibly calm. All the weight of Jeremy's challenges lifted. All I could do was love him. I was part of this sea of parents all over the planet who worry about their children and find that whatever they do is never enough. I felt unconditional love for Jeremy, myself, and all of us – in our family and worldwide."

"Jessica, how beautiful. How was that for you?"

"Liberating. I put so much pressure on myself to be a perfect parent, and it's so exhausting. Something shifted because that evening, I put Jeremy to bed, and for the first time in years, he curled up next to me, his body finally relaxed, and he cried. I became a safe haven for him, just what he – and I – needed."

Like Jessica, it is when we are so miserable that it feels like all is lost that we are closest to the divine. Often, we are just one spiral up or one Transcendence Tool away from seeing ourselves, others, and life in an entirely new and empowering way.

Charlotte: Freedom from Food Circuits

What if the circuit is encoded at Brain State 5, and at the time of encoding, a myriad of fear memories, trauma circuits, and Core Circuits were encoded along with it? Often, it leads to being a "One Circuit" person whose "go-to" is always the same. This was the case for Charlotte. Nothing else worked for her. She had several Food Circuits, however, she would discover one, rewire it about 50 percent of the way, then drop it and find another wire. Her amygdala did not want her to give up food.

Charlotte's Joy Circuit to connect with herself had to be stronger than her Stress Circuit to connect with food. In psychological terms, she had to love herself more than she loved food. To encode that love, she needed Precision EBT, which would help her replicate the loving connection of a "perfect parent." In our coaching, she was clearing clutter about being raised in a family in which she did not matter. If she could feel the intense love for herself that responsive parents feel toward their children, she would strengthen her Joy Circuit and the drive to connect to herself rather than food. As Charlotte was in the advanced courses of the program, her brain was effective in staying present to her tender, loving sadness and aware of a healthy fear of not rewiring that self-harming wire. Our relationship had deepened enough that her emotional brain would trust me, and our two brains connecting could bring her to Brain State 1 and rewire trauma.

We didn't even get to fear. The circuit broke at sadness.

She started by stating the facts, saying, "After my sister Maddie was born, I didn't matter, my weight didn't matter, my life didn't matter. I was alone, abandoned, and lost." Then, she settled on the topic of I didn't matter.

After a robust Anger Procedure, Charlotte said, "I feel sad that I didn't matter."

This was the critical moment of coaching that made all the difference.

I said, "I didn't matter is your topic. The sadness statement is about how that changed your inner life. You are grieving the loss of being treated by others as if you did not matter. Our hunter-gatherer genes perceive that rejection as inflicting the same level of pain you might be in if a lion were biting into your arm."

Charlotte was minimizing her pain. That was damaging because healing takes bringing that reality front and center, with the emotions blaring, if only for a nanosecond before it turns into bliss. We only heal what we can feel.

I said, "That experience for you as a young child of your sister coming into the family and vacuuming up all the love and attention was shocking at the time and is now a gaping wound. I feel so sad that happened to you, but the most powerful next step is not for others to appreciate how hard that was for you, but for you to be present to that pain for a moment, and then, release it. When you do that, your suffering will stop, and you will spiral up to a state of transcendence."

She listened quietly.

"Your brain is so resilient now that you can have freedom from that wire, the one that has been stored in your emotional brain since . . ."

Charlotte said, ". . . since age four."

Charlotte understood, perhaps for the first time, and when she spoke again, it was a whisper.

She said, "My one deepest sadness is the loss to me of treating myself like I don't matter . . . how that feels inside me is . . . that the life is sucked out of me, and I feel like I have no right to be alive."

As Charlotte had stated two sadnesses, not the deepest one, I could easily coach her to circle back around and use that lead-in again. The purpose of it was to guide her to really listen to her body and to her most primitive and strong emotions. That would reconnect her to herself.

I said, "Again, the deepest sadness, the one that is closest to your heart."

She said, "My one deepest sadness for the topic I do not matter, what happened inside me living with that . . . I feel sad that . . . I feel like I do not have the right to live."

Although Charlotte could effectively rewire 4 Circuits on her own with the app, it was far more challenging to stay present to the wild and woolly emotions of her 5 Circuits, the ones that hold more possibility for transcendence and trauma. I knew that if I could slow her down so that instead of dodging her feelings, she stayed fully present to them, she could heal on the spot. The part of her that was still four years old, that lost little girl, had been waiting and hoping for decades that someone would see her pain and rescue her from it. Now, she was seeing her own pain, articulating it for a whole brain and body experience, thereby rescuing herself.

I said, "You feel sad that you felt you did not have the right to live. Feel your feelings . . . stay with it . . . extract as much healing as possible . . ."

Charlotte was silent, completely absorbed in feeling her feelings, until they disappeared.

I sensed that I had witnessed a healing.

When she completed her Cycle, I asked her, "How do you feel?"

She said, "I'm in wonder. I never thought to ask myself how it was for me . . . because I didn't matter. If I don't matter, then I do not advocate for myself and I have no bliss. That's outrageous! I don't want to do that anymore!"

An image arose in my mind of Charlotte at four years old, sitting in the corner dejected, but now running, skipping, and dancing around the room. She, too, could have joy. That is the perfection of the emotional brain, the ultimate love organ. Until we give ourselves the intense love that a "perfect parent" would have given us, the circuit does not budge. That single, profound loving experience led to Charlotte crushing her last Food Circuit and ushered in the transformations that followed.

The story of all three people from diverse walks of life who came to EBT was remarkably the same. They came to EBT with a desire for freedom from a few circuits and stayed with the program because the method solved their problem, but more importantly, gave them the power to see miracles everywhere.

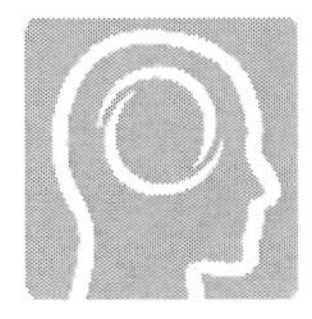

23

Lasting Weight Loss: Celebrate Your Joy

What did we just accomplish? We mapped out a method that is based on brain science, one that puts us in control of our physiology and promotes lasting weight loss that is easy and lasting.

We've harnessed what is free and accessible to all of us – our emotions – and have kept it simple:

Say what is bothering you, protest feeling hurt, and unravel the negative emotions that crop up.

Then, any errant messages from the wires that moments before were hidden in your unconscious mind reveal themselves – they become conscious.

Now you have power. You change those messages, so they reflect who you want to be and how you want to respond in your daily life, including what, when, and how much you eat.

Last, you lock those new messages into your unconscious mind, so they spontaneously govern your responses, and you can move forward with joy and purpose.

In about two to three minutes, you have meaningfully impacted the chemicals in every cell of your body without the use of food, drugs, or medications. You feel connected to the deepest part of yourself, your emotional and spiritual core, and have pride in who you are and how you live your life.

In a world of artificial food, artificial intelligence, artificial friends, and artificial bliss, you have used the most potent "real thing" you have – your emotions. You have changed your physiology, so that even if moments before the ultra-processed foods looked appealing and you might have mindlessly consumed them, now you ask, "Do I really want to put that material in my body?" More often than not your body answers, "I don't really need that."

What I know for sure

Using emotions to treat obesity is the right idea at the right time. Twenty years ago, I sat on stage next to Oprah Winfrey at Harpo Studios as her guest. It was a program on *The Pathway*, a best-selling book I had written on an early iteration of EBT.

During a commercial break, we discussed her "What I Know for Sure" magazine column, which that month proposed asking two questions: "How do I feel?" and "What do I need?"

It was an amazing coincidence that she had invited me to be a guest on her show that month and that she shared those two questions with me, as those same questions are fundamental to EBT.

After our interchange, there was silence. I did not speak, keeping to the basic rule to not say anything unless you have something to say. Then, with her signature tone of authenticity deepened with empathy, Oprah remarked, "I feel for you. It is hard to ask people to feel their emotions."

People haven't wanted to feel their feelings because they have not had a way to make feeling them feel safe. The skills of EBT provide that safety.

Back then, there was no pressing need to process emotions. There was still hope that people could eat healthy for life without harnessing the power of their emotional brain. Why step over the thinking-brain barrier and enter the world of the emotional brain if you didn't have to?

However, times have changed. Based on the National Health and Examination Study, a survey that examines statistics on national health and nutrition, obesity has increased by 39 percent, and severe obesity has increased by 82 percent since then. Oprah's insight was perfectly attuned to those times: going on a "diet" was all you needed to do. Now we know that skipping over the emotional brain, the controller of eating and weight, is not enough. In order to heal our relationship with food, we must feel.

The world changed, so we have to change

Obesity rates rose so dramatically because the environment was more hostile to our health, with food becoming more tempting and the "portion sizes" bordering on obnoxious. The structures that gave us a sense of safety – religion, government, corporations – were feeling the stress and not always behaving well.

Even then, we could have gotten by with the old way of processing our stress, but then there came a perfect trifecta for avoiding emotions. First, there was the release of the smartphone. Next came texting. Finally, there was social media. We could distract ourselves from our otherwise pressing problems and avoid connecting with our own emotions and with the emotions of others.

One evening, Walt and I took the ferry from Larkspur, near where we live, to the San Francisco Ferry Building. It was a beautiful night, reminding me of Van Gogh's Starry Night. We were huddled in the back of the boat, chatting and feeling the crisp air on our faces, when

I noticed something odd. The dozen or so other passengers were sitting alone and looking at their phones.

All the stress that has been pouring into our brains in recent years is catching up with us. Global stress continues to mount, but if we cannot process our stuck emotions, we'll continue to feel unrewarded, and look for big blasts of dopamine in all the wrong places. If it is not overconsuming food, then it is drinking alcoholic beverages, gambling, shopping, streaming videos, using illegal drugs, or popping pills. Our current pile-up of health crises and epidemics has followed, not only obesity, but diabetes, anxiety, depression, PTSD, addiction, and suicide.

Our fundamental need for joy

What's missing is our joy. We have now arrived at a fork in the road where the losses caused by not updating how we process emotions are not only impacting our health but also eating away at our spirits. Most of us are willing to put up with health issues, but not with stress causing us to lose that connection to the deeper meanings of our life.

To get our joy back, we must bite the bullet and learn how to turn toxic emotions into elevated, flowing feelings. That capacity must become our new priority, the foundation not only for our health but for exerting maximum control over the quality of our lives.

I remember one night when Noah, a friend of my son John's, spent the night at our house. At breakfast the following day, he told me immediately that he had to go outside.

I asked why.

He said, "My mother tells me to go outside every morning, run around the garden, and feel my joy."

At the time I thought, "Do parents really say those things to their children?" However, Noah's mother was right.

What's more, we are all like Noah. We all need to tell ourselves to go outside and play, run around, and create joy.

Noah and John went outside and threw a ball for the dog, played tag, and climbed the mammoth acacia tree with its yellow blossoms. Then, they came inside and ate breakfast.

They put joy before food. They got their dopamine surge from natural pleasures. According to Peter Sterling, intrinsically-triggered dopamine from natural pleasures is released in *small pulses*. They are timed perfectly, right after we make an adaptive choice. If we do something healthy, like run around and play or eat food when we are hungry, there is effort involved. The dopamine surge is modest and helps us learn how to do things we don't want to do because we get the payoff of that small, non-addictive pulse. Children learn healthy habits from countless experiences like these.

According to Dr. Sterling, extrinsically-triggered dopamine from artificial pleasures is another matter. If we do not become accustomed to enduring the small "essential pains" of life to get small but important "earned rewards" of small pulses of dopamine, what do we do? The brain is reward-driven, so it becomes desperate enough to make salient artificial rewards. When it comes to food, the smell of chocolate chip cookies, the sight of golden-brown onion rings, and the thought of a juicy cheeseburger with special sauce all excite us.

Yet all of them provide something dangerous. They deliver a *larger-than-expected surge* of dopamine. That holds us back in two ways. One is that the brain over-remembers the experience, creating a stronger drive to repeat that behavior. The brain becomes dependent on these large surges of dopamine for joy, so it will drive us to continue to use artificial pleasure. The other is that it changes the way cells use dopamine. They "downregulate," decreasing the number of "docks" on cells to let in dopamine and making them less effective. The intrinsically-triggered dopamine from natural pleasures that are released in *small pulses* cannot "out-shout" the dopamine blasts, and with the downregulation of dopamine receptors, more of the big blasts of dopamine are needed for us to feel "normal."

I had many lonely Friday evenings as a teenager when I whipped up, cooked, and consumed meringue cookies. I loved them, but now I see that the damage they did was more than weight gain. They changed my reward system in favor of wanting "big blasts" of dopamine. Even if I started controlling my sweet tooth, my brain would look for something equally extreme to replace it, whether that would be gambling, drinking, taking drugs, tech addiction, or overspending.

Perhaps most concerning, by putting meringue cookies in my mouth, then obsessing about controlling my food intake or my weight, I missed out on evolving. I was too distracted to feel my feelings, such as loneliness and sadness, then identify them as a problem, and then address them by learning how to make friends. Anxiety is now ubiquitous because of missed developmental learnings and the small everyday fears that we didn't pause for long enough to process and thereby extinguish. No medication will treat that problem. In order to heal, we must feel.

Missing out on being rewarded by those intrinsically-activated dopamine pulses that are "evanescent" and quickly fade interferes with our evolution-imbued physiological resilience. The small surprises and discomforts that we endure to experience subtle rewards diminish our need for those major dopamine blasts and the chronic stress they bring. These "little pleasures" do not change the sensitivity of the dopamine receptors, so they do not cause us to burn out or become addicted. Also, those small pulses of pleasure keep us out of chronic stress, and, as it turns out, small bursts of stress are actually good for us. Much like a muscle that is activated, then rested, builds strength, stress that is activated, then allowed time to abate, builds resilience.

Although it would be wonderful if there were a "magic pill" for weight loss, learning how to create joy remains the solution. Recovering from what relying on consuming too much of those abnormally-pleasurable foods does to our brain and body takes staying present to our emotions and delivering to our brain a normal, biologically-health-promoting pulse of dopamine – a sparkle of joy.

How love and joy are intertwined

Last year, I gave a talk on EBT to members of the Collaborative Family Healthcare Association, part of the new movement for integrated care with behavioral healthcare workers, and I asked the participants, "What is the most important emotion?"

One woman in the front row waved her hand enthusiastically and said, "It's love!"

Neuroscientist and psychiatrist George Vaillant agrees with her. In his book *Spiritual Evolution*, Dr. Vaillant writes, "Modern ethology and neuroscience make clear that all mammals are hardwired for love. Of all the fauna on earth, however, *Homo sapiens* is the most radically dependent on love."

We need familial love, as that is rooted in evolution. It evolved due to our protracted need for dependence on a nurturing other to mature. Survival is based on attachment to such an extent that we experience a greater oxytocin (love hormone) burst from giving to others than from receiving. My husband faults me for overspending on our grandchildren, but who receives the biggest oxytocin surge? Me, not our grandchildren.

Yet love and joy are intertwined. According to Dr. Vaillant, "In short, joy is the motivational system that reinforces return." Our experiences in relationships are so central to our survival that our memories of loving experiences and the anticipation of reconnecting with loved ones bring joy, and both are not limited. One loving memory activates another, so love of self, love of others, love of the spiritual, and love of life create a biological inner climate that promotes not only enough reward chemicals to make it easier to eat healthy, but to manifest optimal health.

The trouble is that the opposite is also true. The circuits of judgment, division, extremes, and hate amplify and extend in the same way. They cause the beautiful human brain to encode circuits that attach us to pleasure, not purpose, and ego, not spirit. That is the nature of the brain when we are at Brain States 3, 4, and, especially, at 5.

What we see now is a lowering of the set point that can cause the nation to combust. Applying Bruce Perry's view of brain states to the situation at hand, we can be trapped at Brain State 3, 4, or 5 into functioning like children, toddlers, or infants. Instead of empathy, compassion, cooperation, and finding a middle ground, we throw tantrums and want what we want when we want it regardless of how it impacts others and future generations. The good news is that after Brain State 5, can come Brain State 1. If stress becomes threatening enough, the maladaptive circuits in the amygdala that when triggered put the reptilian brain in charge unlock, welcoming transcendent experiences that rewire the brain for something we can all agree on: purpose. The question is how bad it has to become before there is a national effort to equip our population with the tools to turn stress into joy and hate into love.

The magic of the emotional brain

How do we transform our lives? It all begins with believing that joy is possible for us. That first wave of joy matters most because raising the set point is an act based on hope. It starts by saying that life is good despite what reality tells you. You are not bad, and by believing in your humanity and inherent worth, you can have joy. If you feel it once, you will want it again.

When we have the belief that joy is possible for us, it sparks interest in our thinking brain to learn the ropes of how to use our emotions to create joy. The emotional brain takes notice. Then, we do it again, and the Joy Circuits of homeostasis become stronger and bolder, and the Stress Circuits of allostasis stop bullying us. At some point, the emergent effect takes hold, when the resilient Joy Circuits become dominant and start quashing the Stress Circuits. Everything becomes easier from then on. The emotional brain informs the thinking brain that life is good, we are lovable, and a whole new world of joy and purpose awaits us.

How long does it take for the emotional brain to favor joy? Our data from one study showed that a big shift occurs at month three in the training, or four months for providers in training because their brains are strongly conditioned for the old paradigm. However, when it occurs the shift is dramatic. The telegroup erupts with enthusiasm. It's contagious! Before that time, most of the providers-in-training expressed interest in how to select patients for using EBT. Now their own life has changed so much, they say, "All my patients need this. Everyone needs EBT." This is the emergent effect in action.

The reality of easy, lasting weight loss

How do you learn to turn stress into joy? It's by following the steps in the tools. There are 23 steps required for steadying the brain to rewire what we all have that causes our issues and problems, those 5 Circuits, but learning them is not that hard.

I learned about making difficult things easy from my son, Joe. He majored in physics as an undergraduate. As I caught glimpses of his assignments, which were pages of scribbles of formulas and equations, I marveled.

Joe responded, "Mom, It's not hard. You just have to break it down into small steps and do them one by one."

Spiraling up is like that, and it is that process, done with precision over time, that promotes lasting weight loss and freedom from stress eating. Think of spiraling up as 23 distinct skills that, with practice, convert to long-term memory, change the parts of the brain that store long-term habits, and notice how easy it is to eat healthy and release weight.

Although there is great drama in weight-loss stories, as people sweat bullets, measure food, write down everything they eat, and go on fasts, once we control our circuits and the biochemicals they unleash, It's not hard. You spiral up, get the Big 4 Circuits rewired, then do a reality check, adjusting your food and observing when your chronic hunger abates, the cravings stop, and the number on the scale goes down.

Consider beginning to see joy as your natural state and eating and weight problems as blessings. They are so sensitive to stress and so annoying, distracting, or harmful that overcoming them gives us just the motivation we need to create joy in our lives.

▪ ▪ ▪

Imagine: My Natural State is Joy

Relax: Begin by relaxing. Turn your attention to your body and your breathing and breathe in through your nose and out through your mouth, or in any way that feels comfortable and comforting to you. Then, when you are ready, begin to imagine.

Imagine: See yourself moving through your day, realizing that releasing weight has become rather easy. You have rewired the various circuits, including the Big 4 Circuits, and you feel connected to the deepest part of yourself. Chronic hunger, cravings, and lethargy are gone, and you are in the groove of releasing extra weight at the rate that is right for you.

Notice that you are aware of the love inside you and feel grounded in your body. Others may be stressed, but you don't have to be. Instead, you are aware of your brain state and when you start feeling disconnected from your body or lose the glow that comes with awareness of purpose, you remind yourself: I am creating joy in my life, and in a flash, you have spiraled up and are back to Brain State 1.

Next, see yourself facing a challenge. Perhaps it is a work issue, health problem, relationship stress, or the world situation. All of a sudden, that Food Circuit is on fire. All you can think of is food. All you know is you are back to square one, really hungry, with as strong cravings as ever. You feel as if you need that food, and if you don't get it, you will perish.

See yourself throwing back your head and laughing, then saying to yourself, "What's going on here? This is not joy. I am creating joy in my life!"

Then see yourself not rushing. You can handle anything if you do it in small steps.

See yourself relaxing and reassuring yourself, "Take a deep breath. Put your shoulders back. Warmly observe yourself."

Notice that you can slow down, as your response now defines your life.

Say to yourself, "I can slow down. It takes as long as it takes. I am going to use my brain's natural pathways and return to my joy, my natural state, the state in which I live my life."

Notice that you are aware of that forcefield of joy all around you and inside you. That moment of stress was perfect in its own way as you released control. You surrendered to the goodness of life and became aware of something more. You were in a state of transcendence and at peace with yourself, others, food, your weight, and life.

Hold onto that vision of yourself, knowing you can bring it up throughout the day, and so even when your brain tells you that all is lost, you are never lost.

Your essence is joy, and you can return to your joy anytime, anywhere, just by spiraling up. Finally, you are free. Eating and weight are no longer issues in your life.

▪ ▪ ▪

I asked Jessica what she learned from that Imagine.

She said, "I don't have to try to be perfect. I just have to use the tools."

"How is that for you?"

"Two months ago, when I started EBT, I didn't think I deserved joy. Now I know that joy is natural, and I can create it."

When I asked Kevin about his experience, he laughed.

"It never occurred to me that I could slow down. My whole life has been one triggering experience after another."

He exhaled loudly. I waited.

"So, you are saying that I do not have to worry or struggle?"

"Yes."

"I connect with myself, trust my inherent strength, goodness, and wisdom, and keep spiraling up. But what if I binge or lash out at my wife?"

"What will you do?"

"I'll appreciate that I am not a bad person. My essence is good, and I am joy."

Of the three, Charlotte had the strongest reaction to this Imagine:

She said, "I needed to hear that! So far, I think of EBT as my joy solution. I've started swimming in the local pool again and changed some of my friends. I am releasing weight and more conscious of trying to avoid overeating than trying to see how much food I am 'allowed' to eat. I bought new clothes – colors, shapes, and even a hat."

"How did that Imagine fit in?"

"I had started to lose weight before, and I became hooked on losing weight and disconnected from myself. I get my love from releasing weight."

"Where do you get your safety?"

Charlotte paused for quite a while.

"I am slowly taking off weight, layer by layer, but I have been grinding in: 'I get my safety from . . . the love inside me . . . and creating joy in my life.'"

I asked, "How long will you stay with it?"

"Until I have an abundance of all seven rewards, including the one that is most important to me."

"Which one is that, Charlotte?"

She answered, "It's Freedom."

Lasting weight loss is a matter of surrendering to the immense power of the emotional brain, being grateful for the gift of life, then using the tools to create one moment of joy, then another, and another.

Whatever comes our way – work stress, delicious food, illness, family problems, the world condition – we can rely on our ability to create a forcefield of love around us and spiral up.

It's a universal process, and even if we are at Brain State 5, all we do is slow it down. We go "under" that blanket of stress, tolerate not knowing, just for a moment, and then find ourselves aware of an enormous pool of love. We ask for help not just because of our own needs, but because what we need is in alignment with the greater good. Often, we are surprised soon thereafter at how many doors open for us. After the 5, comes the Brain State 1.

Lasting weight loss is something to celebrate. Friends will notice that your food preferences have changed, and your body is less encumbered by extra weight. Yet they will notice more how they feel around you. Something has changed. Your skin is glowing, your body is charged up with a zest for life. They don't know what has occurred, but you do. You are so connected to the deepest part of yourself that food and weight are no longer issues in your life. Finally, you are free.

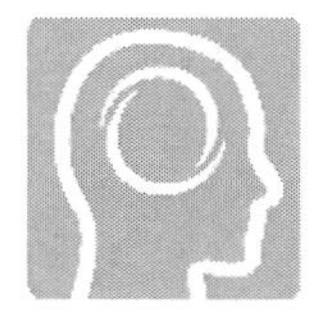

24

Connecting: The Sweetness of Spiral Ups

When I first met my husband Walt 10 years ago, he had never heard of EBT, but he was very interested.

Walt had several stress-induced health problems. As we began dating, he was so curious about the method that I wondered if he was interested in me or EBT.

Walt's excitement about EBT bothered me enough that I finally asked him about his interest point blank.

He paused for a moment, then said, "Both. I'm interested in both EBT and you."

At the time, my brother, Steve, and I were caring for my father, as my mother had passed away and he was in assisted living in a nearby senior residential community.

One day, when I was visiting my dad, I told him that I had posed that question about interest to Walt. My dad was 90 then, and as he aged, he seemed to pause longer before answering questions, perhaps knowing that time was short and wanting to impart only his most authentic opinions.

My father said, "Could you ask for a better answer?"

Soon thereafter, I decided to introduce Walt to my father. I picked my dad up from the retirement center, and we met for dinner at Marin Joe's. This Italian restaurant had been a regular celebration spot for my family since I was eight years old. All the servers knew us, so it was a perfect spot for a cordial introduction over spaghetti, roast beef, and French bread.

It went well.

After the dinner, as I drove my father back to his retirement center, I asked him what he thought of Walt.

He responded, "He is a solid citizen."

I didn't probe further, as any positive comment was the equivalent of an endorsement. My dad was always protective of me, and only years later did I learn that he had told a confidant at the retirement center that "when there was Walt, he stopped worrying about me."

Walt struck up a special friendship with my father, a connection that my dad needed so badly at this time in his life. We first discovered this special connection at Easter dinner. My family gathered around the table and Walt joined in. We were accustomed to my dad not talking much and his hearing aids didn't work that well.

Suddenly, my daughter Haley said, "Mom, look at Papa. He's talking."

I looked across the table. Walt and my dad were in rapt conversation, which did not stop for nearly an hour.

That started a special connection for these two men. When long after restaurants became too much for my dad, Walt would pick him up, and they would swing by the drive-through at the local A & W Root Beer for burgers, sit in the car in the parking lot for long chats, good stories, and heartfelt moments together.

Connection remains the best medicine. That is why EBT is rooted in fostering warm, safe, meaningful connection, both in group sessions and with peer support. The emotional brain is the social brain, and the reward center lights up with those sustainable surges of dopamine and oxytocin, the appetite suppressant, which flow when we use the skills with others.

Making Connections as a couple

Before long, Walt was using EBT, and as a couple, we were relying on sharing our brain states. When I was at Brain State 5 and a little "toxic," I'd say so. Instead of having the standard (and repeatable) couple's quarrel, we had the new language of brain states that was succinct, scientific, and shared. It was so much easier to say, "I'm at 5. I need some time alone. How would that be for you?" than to have a "discussion" that might trigger either of us. So far, so good.

About four months into our relationship, our stress wires started activating, a sign that the relationship was entering its productive stage and doing its job: to rewire each of our gnarly old circuits from early attachment and later hurts from past loves gone awry.

Early one evening, we were chatting before dinner in the den, sitting in chairs across the room from one another. Walt's face looked more like a thick emotional wall than the warm, loving guy I had come to know. It was time to each test the emotional mettle of our relationship that had, up until then, been in the "honeymoon" stage.

I felt a stab of fear in my stomach, wondering if the relationship was another mistake on my part. I clawed my way up to a high enough state (probably Brain State 2 where we can identify our feelings), and proclaimed, "I feel bored and a little lonely."

Walt might have thought something like: "What is this woman saying to me? Is she needy and demanding or just on a mission to criticize and fix me?"

I overreacted a bit, as who knows, he could just have had a headache or been a little distracted because of a work project.

I proclaimed, "If this is how it is going to be, I'm not sure I want to be in this relationship. I need to feel closer to you."

Connections

- Private, confidential, and rapid-acting
- No advice given, just listen or spiral up
- Five minutes, no more than 10
- By telephone or in person, not by texting
- One person uses the skills to spiral up
- The other listens and says kind words
- No chit-chat or wasted time
- The connection ends
- Both people are in joy
- Both people have rewired their brain

This wasn't going well. Was I going to spoil this relationship because all my needs were not being met all the time? Then I realized that we could use EBT together.

I asked, "Would you sit on the couch with me so we can do Cycles together?"

He agreed to try it.

We walked to the living room, both a little "4-ish," sat down on the couch, and turned toward each other. Both of us leaned in and did a Cycle, then said some kind words (gave "Connecting Messages").

It was a little messy and probably took us about 10 minutes, maybe 15, but it worked. Our Stress Circuits calmed down, and those Joy Circuits, previously lying dormant, magically fired. The wonderful man I knew reappeared, and the insecure, borderline demanding woman disappeared. Sparks started flying again, and we had a lovely evening together.

Although using the tools boosted our happiness in the moment, far more important was its longer-term impact. Being in a committed relationship in which both people have the skills to be emotionally honest, and not either avoid conflict or use conflict to avoid growing, we had a process that was scientific and reliable.

When conflicts crop up, instead of pointing the finger at each other, we could Cycle out of our troubles. When the other person appears to be a monster in disguise, the problem is usually those Stress Circuits. However, it is so perfect because the precise circuit that is blocking our capacity for intimacy is activated with its synaptic connections fluid and wide open to being updated by spiraling up. We can engage in our own "relationship therapy" with EBT.

Spiraling up as a couple

Using EBT in relationships takes the mystery out of why that which makes us so happy – loving relationships – can also become our greatest source of stress. In the world of brain functioning, it is the most challenging aspect of life. Each encounter amounts to "Relationship Olympics," as the brain has to perform astonishing gymnastics, toggling back and forth between, 1) awareness of how we feel and what we need, and 2) how the other person feels and what they need.

The stressed brain does not toggle, which is the problem. Instead, it takes sides. If we unplug from ourselves and plug into hyper-awareness of the other person's feelings and needs, called rescuing and people-pleasing, intimacy is lost. Instead, if we unplug from the other person and are only aware of our own feelings and needs, we put up walls, judge others, and end up feeling lonely.

According to Bill Mory, EBT Master Trainer and EBT Director of Relational Health, "There are five levels of stress in the brain, but the only brain state in which we can give and receive love and be intimate is Brain State 1."

Bill often explains the slippery slope that stress creates in relationships, saying, "At Brain State 2, relationships are transactional: you scratch my back, and I will scratch yours. At Brain State 3 or lower, we treat ourselves and others like objects."

Even for couples whose connection is strong, adding EBT skills to their repertoire or even better, participating in our "relationship reset" coaching, can be life changing. All three major aspects of intimacy – emotional closeness, sexual and sensual pleasure, and loving companionship – are all dependent upon the state of the emotional brain.

Molly, who used EBT to improve her relationship, said, "I was considering throwing in the towel on my relationship, and then I used EBT. Now we have more fun and more laughter, we want to spend time together, and the sex is out of this world."

The power of EBT to improve relationships is not surprising as the emotional brain is the seat of attachment. Cognitive control is not a solution. The circuits and the opportunity for transformation are in the limbic brain, so limbic brain skills are the missing link.

Easy, private Connections within a group

Walt had joined Master Trainer Judy Zehr's weekly premium telegroup and began moving through the courses of the method. He enjoyed the groups but initially needed more time to make Connections.

It's a simple, quick process. One person spirals up, and the other listens. Both people end up in joy, and as the brain has no walls, both people rewire their brains. If you are the listener, you experience a "freebie" rewiring. If you are the person who spirals up, you receive the special joy of expressing your emotions so authentically that you are often on a natural high for hours.

We started studying the use of Connections to make the weekly groups more authentic, thinking that If participants relied on each other between sessions the program would be stronger. Also, in those off moments when donuts call, loneliness sets in, or a relationship troubles us, what could be better than someone listening to us as we turn stress into joy?

Soon thereafter, a robust literature developed showing that peer support predicted remission of cancer, and we entered the age where loneliness was as much of a health risk factor as smoking. Still later, a study conducted by Kelly Webber at the University of Kentucky showed that the number of Connections a participant made predicted both weight loss and how much they liked EBT.

Early on, Walt said, "I don't know about Connections. I don't share things with people I do not know."

I listened.

Next, he started to like Connections but preferred to listen to other people spiral up, not spiral up himself, and then give Connecting Messages.

The Connecting Messages fast-forward intimacy training, as they deliver to the other person's brain just the mutuality and loving connection they need immediately after opening up.

There are two "lead-ins" that when used word for word, take us right to that "sweet spot" of intimacy.

The first lead-in is, "When you did your work, the feelings and sensations in my body were . . ." The second is "The way your work was a gift to me (in my own EBT Practice) was . . ."

Using this special formula, the person who did the Cycle is apt to feel seen, heard, and felt. Both people deepen their capacity to be intimate, not just in Connections, but in their other close relationships.

We are in this together: Our common wires

Within a few weeks, Walt was comfortable in the group, learning from Judy and making Connections with all but one person. He said, "I have nothing in common with this one person. We are not at all alike."

The very next week, Walt asked about morning Connections, as he had 10 minutes each morning during his drive to work and thought it would be a great time for a regular Connection. The participant Walt hadn't been connecting with volunteered.

The next day, they made their first Connection. Then, they missed it the next day because of a dentist appointment, but on the third day, they connected again. That evening, Walt said, "I discovered we have the exact same circuit! We both have an 'I get my safety from making people happy' wire."

One of the most rewarding aspects of EBT is discovering our sameness. Although we are vastly different in our neocortex, appearance, interests, and vocations, in the far recesses of our unconscious memory system, the wires are pithy and basic. Our expectations, including our faulty ones, are remarkably similar. When we acknowledge the real issue, a few wires that were implanted in our brain through no fault of our own, we become part of the bigger family of humankind. We expand our capacity to love.

Connections as a pathway to healing trauma

Making Connections is practical. Who can't benefit from someone listening to them without judgment and then offering some kind words? However, the most important reason for Connections is to rewire trauma. It seems as if we might need two emotional brains, not one. To activate a circuit with precision requires keeping the brain at Brain State 1 while activating a Brain State 5 wire. When the wire activates, the entire brain and body are drenched in stress chemicals.

That's a spoiler! The prefrontal cortex must stay flexibly aware and attuned to the emotional activations for long enough to clear the stress and change the message embedded in it from unreasonable to reasonable. How can one brain be at Brain State 1 and Brain State 5 at the same time?

The spiral-up process boosts the prefrontal cortex's capacity to stay emotionally present. However, some of the strong, dominant, and large trauma circuits are more easily rewired if someone else is connecting with us.

Essentially, we "borrow" their brain function just by allowing them to listen to us. Securing support so another person can be a warm presence to us (and us to them) keeps us right on track to rewiring those 5 Circuits. Left to do this work solo, we're at risk of rewiring only 4 Circuits and letting the 5 Circuits continue to activate and become stronger.

Meredith, a psychologist who had joined an EBT group at the university, demonstrated this well. The group came about because of a grant orchestrated by Amy Levine, the director of the Center for Gender Equity and the Chancellor's Council on Faculty Life at the time.

During the first session, Meredith said, "I'm not sure I need EBT. Every time I check in, I'm at Brain State 1."

I realized that she might only be checking in when she is in low-stress states, and I suggested that she set notifications on her phone hourly to discover her "daily profile" of brain states.

At the next week's session, Meredith said humorously, "You can rest assured that I am not Wired at One. I was at Brain State 4 or 5 at least half the time. In fact, I found a circuit that I can't seem to rewire."

The circuits we most want to rewire, the trauma or "trophy wires," activate so much stress that the thinking brain cannot stay present to the emotions. Meredith was using the tools on her own, so I guided her through using the Cycle Tool.

Afterward, she was in awe. "Laurel, I have chills all over my body. That circuit was encoded when I was three years old. I never would have been able to find that on my own."

We are not lone islands. By dropping into groups, connecting by phone, and creating a circle of support among family members and friends, we can clear the 5 Circuits and experience profound and lasting results with EBT.

The most important healthcare problem in the United States is trauma circuits. We all have wires that block us from optimal functioning. Even if the national average number of trauma circuits per person is only 10, we collectively have more than 3 trillion circuits to rewire.

Need for Peer Support and Coaching

Rewiring trauma benefits from more support.

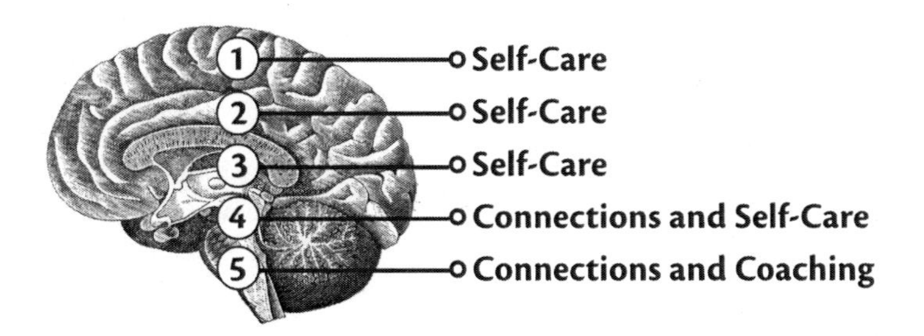

We can all do our small but vital part to clear our own trauma circuits. This is not a psychiatric issue but a public health concern. The first order of treatment is that our population needs access to stress tools that stand up to the intensity of the fight-or-flight response that is chronically activated by them. These wires cause dopamine deficiency, serotonin draining, and a cortisol and inflammation cascade that are breaking our spirits and destroying our nation. Violence and extremism alone are ripping us apart, and that is on top of our chronic disease and mental health crises.

The EBT spiral-up process codifies what exceptional therapists do: make us feel seen, heard, and felt, activate errant wires, and then fix them. We can do that for ourselves and, even better, embrace sharing that experience with others, inspiring them as we delight ourselves.

The EBT resiliency tools give us a way to internalize that great therapist, and bolt on connection with other people listening to us warmly, which helps us to rewire more circuits faster. We can then be present to help heal our nation. We have one of the greatest healthcare systems in the world, yet the foundation for its best use and our overall health is inside of us. Our power to heal ourselves comes from our genes, which gives us the power to experience the healing chemical surge of homeostasis.

In those moments of rewiring 5 Circuits and the sharing of those moments, we experience awe. The hair on our arms stands up, tears come to our eyes, and that sense of both mattering and transcending appears.

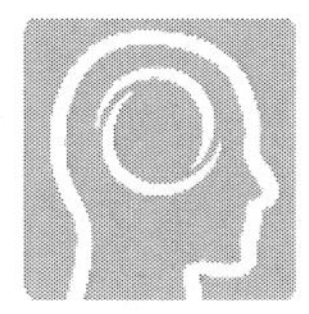

25

Building a Community: A Pathway to Success

In 2012, the method was at a crossroads. EBT is educational, it is based on skills training. We had maxed out in making it attractive based on the pre-technology era.

Our courses started as workbooks, then became a series of journals, and finally, they became "kits." Each course had a journal plus four CDs, a pocket reminder – a small card summarizing the skills. The entire set for each course was enclosed in a colorful plastic case.

Eventually, tech took off to the point that most methods were scrambling to find ways to be more relevant in the age of digital information sharing. Instead, we focused on making the EBT kits more beautiful.

For several years, my son Joe had been very direct with me that we were not keeping up with innovations in technology. He said, "Mom, if this method is not significantly better than the others, then stay home and bake cookies. If it is better, you must be better prepared."

He wanted to protect me if the method ended up disrupting other therapies, as it could result in criticism if we were not up to the standards of the times. Joe had finished a master's program in business design and engineering at Stanford in 2009, right at the time of flourishing start-ups in Silicon Valley and had already begun his first start-up. The energy of Silicon Valley at the time was exhilarating.

When he approached me again, he had a vision.

Joe said, "EBT should be global. People should connect with people across the nation and around the world to use the skills together."

He believed in the power of community and understood the EBT groups firsthand, as he grew up hearing people talking about joy in the groups in our home. He heard people connecting and spiraling up on our front porch. Even his big brown dog Bo was fully accustomed to anticipating the moment when the group would end by participants saying in unison, "We are creating joy in our lives."

Now, he was taking the method to the next level with technology. He wanted people to be able to come together in groups anonymously to do authentic, emotional work without any strings attached – nobody sees your face, knows your last name, or would recognize you on the street.

Joe said, "There is power in a group. Mom, we all need that!"

At that moment, I knew he was right. I felt very old, as if the world I had known was no longer. I realized that the method needed to grow, and so did I.

Joe said, "I'll work for EBT for a year while I'm traveling, and I will create a global emotional connectivity network for you."

He was clear that he would not help me unless I made significant, even painful concessions. We could no longer be "bookbound." The training had to be online and groups would have telephone and messaging connectivity so people could call in anytime, anywhere.

The most painful concession I had to make was "no more pocket reminders." I still have a box of them stashed away in our basement, as they remain contraband. The reason: they were adequate to guide people to get to Brain State 1. However, soon nearly everyone would have a smartphone.

Joe's vision went further. His thesis in graduate school had been about how to optimally employ people, and that goal inspired his first start-up. His interest in EBT, other than helping out his mom, was serving the providers, giving them a portal that performed all their administrative work plus providing them with instant data on spiral ups, Connections, and coursework so they had objective information on how to help participants succeed. Joe also wanted to provide users with a circle of support, allowing them to connect with peers with one touch.

It was an exciting time. For a while, he lived at home and made our garage "tech central." Three tech interns and his business partner in another start up worked from early morning to midnight. They kept the garage door open so that people walking their dog or going for a run could be part of the energy and they took breaks to throw frisbees in the street. Someone would go off to the market and get the fixings for hamburgers that soon found their way to the grill. It was a happy time for me – such energy!

Joe found Dev Singh, a technology master who started building out the new website, and my son John, then at UC Davis, became a master of customer service. The upheaval of changing to a tech-based company kept him wielding two phone lines so he could respond immediately to help new participants find the right group for them. That experience was invaluable, as a decade later, he started his own company in Upstate New York that provided another kind of "survival need" service. Soon after that, Michael McClure joined EBT and shaped the company's communications and Kelly McGrath joined EBT and managed our operations seamlessly and with a smile. A core of committed providers and researchers guided our transition in training new providers and remain cherished leaders in EBT today.

Technology-based EBT was launched.

After the "garage incubation months," Joe traveled internationally, Skyping with the team and with me to complete the design of the new portal. He had set the course and went on to work on other start-ups and now is in big tech.

By then, Walt and I had a committed relationship, and he had his own vision: people helping people help themselves and emotional health for all. EBT had changed his health and his life. As his previous career was in business, then in health and serving the underserved – a company that brought math skills to inner-city children – he was perfectly primed to lead EBT.

We went on to document the method, write handbooks, establish a crash course for rewiring the Big 4 Circuits, and improving the technology. The slowest aspect of the work was finding ways for people to use EBT at work in one minute without feeling their feelings (Spiral Up #1) and creating changes in the skills to make it easier for those new to the method to rewire trauma circuits (The 23 Steps, Spiral Up #3).

Since the launch of technology-based EBT, our whole team and leaders as well as participants have shaped EBT, helping us improve the tools and technology. Then, right when I was convinced that we had fulfilled our task and the precision of the method produced improved medical outcomes more consistently, the heavens opened up. We were ready to disseminate EBT at a level commensurate with its scientific value but did not have the resources to do it.

Then one day, I was coaching a participant who wanted to learn more about people and help us bring EBT out widely to help everyone. He and his wife had studied EBT over time and agreed that their lives had been changed by EBT. They wanted to make EBT affordable for all. Their generosity and vision ignited enthusiasm in our team. Walt contracted with an exceptional team of award-winning individuals in an agency, and "emotional health for all," including funding for producing this book, was launched. Dreams really do come true!

How to build your community

Jessica, Kevin, and Charlotte built their community of support in diverse ways, all of which supported their success.

Jessica went right into joining a group and stayed with it. Kevin dropped into Spiral Up Groups, used coaching, and engaged his wife and one of his daughters in using EBT. Charlotte settled into attending Spiral Up Groups three times per week, as that worked with her schedule, and she recruited friends in her book club to join EBT and watch Spiral Up with Dr. Laurel Zoom sessions most weeks.

All three, however, created plans that shared the basic elements of support: a group, Connections, and community.

1. Groups

Our hunter-gatherer brain loves affiliation and being part of a group. When two or more people gather together to spiral up, the electricity that flows between them garners excitement, possibility, and a sense of being part of something larger than themselves.

All Spiral Up memberships include daily Spiral Up Groups you can join with one touch on your app. Drop in and an EBT Provider will greet you. You need not say or do anything, just listen if you wish. Someone will volunteer to do a Cycle and then several participants will give Connecting Messages.

The joy is contagious. Your brain will change just by listening, and you will leave the session in joy. Drop into as many groups per week as possible, to start. Some people start by participating daily. Others find a couple of sessions each week that they attend regularly. Others stick with participating just once a week. EBT is a new paradigm, so the brain enjoys a strong dose of this connection. The more Spiral Up Groups you attend, the more you will like EBT and the more your brain will change.

Apart from drop-in groups, we offer weekly premium groups, for either one hour or 30 minutes. The key difference between spiral up drop-in and premium weekly groups is that in premium the same eight people get together weekly with a dedicated EBT Provider. The groups work together over time and the relationships deepen. The other people in your group become your Connection Buddies, and you have access to checking in with them for Connections that are private and confidential, with one-touch access on your app. Also, if a special need arises and you want more private coaching from your provider, it is available by telephone.

Both groups include a set structure of an initial check-in of brain states, tracking individual progress with rewiring (choosing one wire per week), and reflections on weekly goals and accomplishments to inspire each person. The 60-minute group includes a provider coaching a participant through a deep Cycle. We also offer 30-day intensives for those who want to jump in, meet on weekdays for four weeks, and do a deep dive into EBT.

My recommendation is to start with dropping into two or three Spiral Up Groups per week and then assessing your needs for additional support.

2. Connections

The one-on-one Connection between two people whose emotional brains are in resonance – circuits connecting with circuits – brings joy and transformation.

Consider recruiting some Connection Buddies who are family and friends as well as your partner, spouse, or best friend. If your relationship is suffering from stress overload, consider requiring your significant other to learn EBT. I have seen hundreds of people make "learn EBT" a requirement, either preventively or therapeutically, seeing their partner or spouse change quite rapidly. EBT is often the "missing link" in relationships. If you are in a committed relationship that is unrewarding but not abusive, consider staying in it for one year while you raise your own set point. Even if the other person is not enrolled in EBT, as your set point goes up you will interact differently with them, and their brain will change whether they want it to or not.

If you are a member of a weekly or daily intensive group, you will have automatically established Connections. If you are not in a group or just want more, it is easy to establish Connection Buddies. Trying EBT is close to free ($1 for the first month), and there are no barriers to checking with others if they want to learn a new way to take care of their health. Anyone can visit EBT.ORG and learn more. A few of the people you mention it to will catch the EBT fever, start using the method, and learn how to spiral up and make Connections.

I recommend establishing a minimum of three Connection Buddies that you use EBT with regularly.

What if you need more time to establish Connection Buddies? That's okay because the emotional brain takes a while to become comfortable with Connections. The EBT Prescription is to make one Connection per day. Start with meeting your prescription in two easy ways: participate in a Spiral Up Group and/or post on the Spiral Up Forum Boards. Both of these activities count as Connections. Then, add a Connection Buddy, then another, and a third, and your basic needs for connection in the program will be met.

3. Community

The community feel of EBT adds to our experience as another way of being part of something larger than ourselves. You can have a sense of community with EBT in the following ways:

Spiral Up with Dr. Laurel

Each week, drop in for a Spiral Up with Dr. Laurel Zoom session. I'll be there to greet you and help you feel inspired to raise your set point. If your Connection Buddies are in vastly different locations, you can meet them there. Join the Zoom session, then afterward check in with them about what they learned. Each session has some important nuggets of information and encouragement.

World at One Day

Once a month, join in celebrating World at One Day. Support the growth of the collective awareness of our individual power to be in joy, to honor our brain's capacity to be at Brain State 1. Put extra energy that day into spiraling up to One and staying in that state as much as possible. Dedicate your effort in doing that to one person or one group, and then send them that loving, healing connection from your mind and heart. It's a wonderful way to start each month.

The 5-Day Cortisol Detox

After World at One Day, your brain will be in a higher state more easily. Much like interval exercise training, continue with interval emotional training. The brain changes with intensive intervals of practice. Do the 5-Day Cortisol Detox, where for five days you continue spiraling up not just 10 times per day, but more – some people spiral up 15, but others spiral up 20 or 25 times. The brain learns to stay at Brain State 1 by practicing doing it.

There are two goals for maintaining this regular practice monthly. One is that the resiliency pathways in your brain become dominant and fire automatically earlier in your EBT 1-2-3 JOY Program. The other is that during the 5-Day Cortisol Detox, you focus on self-regulation only. Use Spiral Up Pathways #1 and #2 on your app, not Pathway #3. Do not address trauma. Many participants report that after the detox, their prefrontal cortex is able to stay at a higher state more readily and doing trauma work becomes far easier.

Build your community slowly and share Connections as well as highlights of your EBT 1-2-3 JOY Program with them. The relationships you make may last a lifetime.

As you receive support, continue to move through the program videos and courses as each is designed to be your "medicine."

Each course in the program is in its fourth edition and includes only the tools, insights, and techniques that participants have rated as highly impactful. Complete one each month or take longer if you prefer to savor the experience.

The program's courses each build on the success of the previous courses and guide you in enjoying the journey as you raise your set point until you are Wired at One and have an abundance of all seven rewards of a purposeful life.

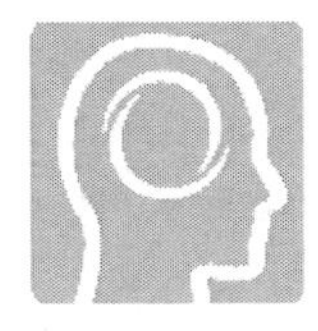

26

Spiraling Up: A Solution for Life

When you picked up this book, you may have been looking for a turning point in your relationship with food.

My turning point in my relationship with food was when I couldn't face dieting anymore. My body was storing some 40 extra pounds. I was bloated and puffy, with a fresh red caesarian incision on my belly. That's when I faced my aloneness, released control, and decided to trust my body and myself.

Freedom: Healer, heal thyself

I've never looked back. My emotional brain was telling me that I could not tolerate living the other way. I knew I had to change.

After that, my emotional brain did the work for me. Although the tools were less precise than they are now, my brain changed. My Food Circuit was the easiest to rewire, as I had already weakened it, but the other ones held on for a while. My Mood Circuit was depression ("I get my nurturing from feeling depressed with a little self-pity thrown in"). When I discovered that wire, I was shocked. How could my unconscious mind see depression as nurturing? However, I did rewire it into the message "I get my nurturing from the love inside me."

For the Love Circuit, I had both merging and distancing circuits, but the merging was definitely the most painful ("I get my security from making sure you are happy all the time, because if you have any pain, I will die.) I stayed way too long in relationships. My Body Circuit was "I get my security from staying slightly overweight, so I don't make you feel bad." That fit in nicely with the merge circuit. If I get my security from pleasing you, I won't even give myself the respect to weigh what I want my body to weigh, not what pleases others.

My emotional brain's capacity was like everyone else's, perfectly capable of creating a force-field of love around me, that is, when I managed to use the skills. It dished up more and more misery when I did not listen to my body, being courteous enough to keep reminding me of the benefits of staying connected to myself. Always, bringing to mind "purpose" worked for me.

My personal EBT journey was linked to my professional life. When the mother of that 10-year-old girl shared that her daughter stopped overeating and I experienced that in my own life, there was no question in my mind that I would not stop working to find out why.

After the Brain State 5 comes the Brain State 1

The years went by – quickly – and I learned that when the worst things happen, if I just stayed the course and connected to the sanctuary within me, the good things happen. Yet, so much of what I thought I would achieve, I have not. I wanted to circle back to teaching EBT to children, making EBT a part of all couples counseling, and turning around the obesity epidemic. My son Joe texted me about a year ago, a time when I realized that some of my dreams for EBT – once again– might no longer be realistic. He consoled me, "Mom, zero percent of this would have even been a thought without you." Sometimes a few kind words from a loved one make all the difference. Soon after that, our wonderful participants gave EBT resources, and right now, those dreams just may come true.

What about eating and weight? Weight and food stopped being issues in my life a few years after making that switch to choosing Freedom and getting to Brain State 1 over dieting or staying stuck. That sensitivity to my body made life easier. When I went through menopause, I knew that I would need to be more careful about listening to my body. I noticed that I felt satisfied with less food, so I ate less food. I did not gain weight. I ate and still eat healthy, out of self-preservation. I really dislike cravings and anxiety.

My father, who had type 1 diabetes, called his disease the "crud" in private, but in his later, more contemplative years confided in me that the best thing that can happen to a person is to develop a "chronic condition" early in life, so they learn to take really good care of themselves.

The Food Circuit that was encoded when I was 11 turned out to be that "condition" for me, and a motivation to learn how to stop judging myself and clear stress so I could discover who I really was and how to make my dreams come true.

Purpose as a process, not a goal

Once I stopped focusing on solving my problems (food and weight) and started connecting to the deepest part of myself, I recouped so much time and unleashed so much energy to live out my purpose.

A participant once said to me, "You're lucky. You have EBT, so you have purpose."

I said, "EBT is not my purpose. My purpose is to get to a brain state where I can follow my spiritual path."

This was an important distinction, because seeking purpose can become its own external solution. We may be apt to search for a goal that will save us, but I see seeking purpose as a process: the transition from wanting power to searching for purpose to surrendering to the greater good. For me, those gritty "5 moments," when I am knocked down a few pegs, is when I let go of the outcome and, instead, open my heart and say with curiosity, "You tell me. How can I be of help?"

That moment of surrender brings me the "golden nugget" of inner peace. Whenever I have willed EBT to get out, I have just made matters worse. That spiritual shift stops my overthinking and being attached to having it my way. Once that switch from power to service takes hold, the answer may be "stay home and bake apricot pies" or "find the cure for cancer." They are the same, as they both lead to transcendence.

How perfect that the best thing that can happen in our lives is radically accessible to all people at all times. It is a brain state, that is, being at One.

Our own stories and crossroads

As you begin your EBT journey, you may have a story to tell about what brought you to EBT, and what it will do for you.

In Jessica's case, her story was that EBT could help her medically. She wanted to prevent prediabetes. She had no idea that by engaging her emotional brain, she would stop binge eating, resolve her judgments about her body, and release weight. Even early in her training, she could see that her relationship with her seven-year-old son was changing dramatically, and that her choice to engage her emotional brain would help him.

Kevin had been so ambivalent about starting EBT that he set aside both his eating and drinking problems and, rightly so, focused on what mattered to him: his family.

He later said, "I almost lost my marriage, but I'm happy that I didn't. I owe that to EBT."

His eating, drinking, and work life moved out of the allostatic range back into the functionality of homeostasis, all because he created a forcefield of love and surrendered to the purpose of creating joy in his life.

Charlotte was facing a grave situation according to her physicians. The seriousness of her health problems had a silver lining. She had the gift of "health sobriety," a commitment to do the work slowly and very well. No other method had solved her weight problem, and her decline in health gave her urgency.

She said to me, "I don't have time to bypass my emotional brain anymore. I wish I had discovered EBT 20 years ago."

I was about to check if she wanted to spiral up about that, when she said, "It's all perfect! I am having the time of my life trusting my body, being a master of rewiring, and releasing weight in a way that nourishes my spirit – and my body."

Each of these participants used EBT differently, creating the EBT journey that was right for them, but from a neuroscientific perspective, they did the same thing.

First, they became "emotional brain literate." Their prefrontal cortex understood neurophysiology – the 5-Point System – and neuroplasticity. They welcomed those inevitable moments of stress to become masters of personal transformation, fix glitches to grieve losses and change habits, and raise their set point.

Then they started spiraling up, and to their amazement, choosing to spiral up before each meal solved a lot of their distress about food. It works. They all "got" that they could go to their app and get a "hit of dopamine" anytime, anywhere.

They soundly did in their Big 4 Circuits, with an especially enthusiastic demolition of their Food and Body Circuits.

They learned to see Brain State 5 moments as preludes to Brain State 1. All they needed to do was connect to their emotions and many gifts would come their way. They created so much joy in their lives that their maladaptive circuits cleared, and they raised their set points for a life of joy and purpose. The forcefield of love always works.

Start EBT to solve problems, stay for the rewards

People come to EBT to solve problems, but they stay because the tools work and the spiritual rewards bring more meaning to their lives. I see EBT at the intersection of neuroscience-based healthcare and a new spirituality independent of religion, doctrine, rules, or clergy. Many methods have spiritual underpinnings, but EBT goes beyond "thinking-based" methods to produce a brain state in which we are immediately aware of the sacred in life, and the goodness that is inside us.

With stress from the new pandemic and all the unrest in the world, rethinking the role of stress is important because it is transmissible. The peace and power we feel inside is not just our gift to ourselves but to others.

Most of us are aware of our carbon footprint, but we may not have considered our emotional footprint. The more we turn stress into joy in our own brain, the more we radiate out the "clean emotional energy" of love and kindness to others. What an intimate gift. The choice to process our emotions rather than suppressing them manifests as a more robust capacity to encode "Love Circuits" in others, perhaps the ultimate way to pay it forward.

Clear stress and joy emerges naturally

On the health side, EBT speaks to the needs of our time to innovate rather than spiral down into unnecessary complexities of tests, diagnoses, medications, procedures, insurance approvals, and healthcare bills. We're beyond that now. That paradigm of fixing disease was the logical next step after germ theory helped us stop infectious diseases from wiping out large population segments. But as stress levels rose, virtually all health problems – chronic diseases and mental health problems – fell under the same umbrella: stress diseases. What both germ theory and modern medicine missed was not fixing the glitches in the motherboard of humanity – the stressed brain, the magical, unconscious memory systems housed in the emotional brain.

The time is right to bolt EBT onto healthcare so we can use all of the medical treatments we need without the wasted resources and disappointing health outcomes caused by bypassing the emotional brain. Stress is the root cause of most problems. The natural arc of homeostasis – turning stress into joy – is truncated if we remain in emotional bypass mode. By learning the skills to turn stuck emotions into flowing feelings, everyone can naturally find their way to One. We give the stress response its rightful name: the joy response.

Currently, 70 percent of US adults take one or more prescription medications, most of which are needed because we are not treating stress. The pills treat the symptoms of stress and disease and as we can now treat stress itself, fewer may be needed.

When Jessica started EBT, she was taking antidepressants. Kevin was on blood pressure medication, weight-loss drugs, and statins. Charlotte was on eight prescription drugs daily and four more as needed. None of their physicians had told them about EBT or prescribed a "dose of EBT" to switch off the Stress Triangle and boost the natural foundation of their health – a homeostatic set point. If EBT becomes more widely used, people may not need as many medications. Hopefully, someday all health professionals will check their patients' set point even before they check blood pressure or weight. The rationale is physiological: all other methods become more effective when your set point is in the homeostatic range.

More research is needed. However, many participants report that their quarterly visits to physicians while completing the EBT Program show improved chemistries and by six to 18 months, a significant decrease in need for medication. When I met Walt 10 years ago, he was taking eight medications. Within two years, he had lost 40 pounds and was down to two medications, needed for his long-term heart condition.

Celebrating the good news

If enough of us make that choice to use our natural emotional strength and resiliency to clear stress and unite around the seven spiritual rewards of a purposeful life, grand swaths of trauma circuits would be cleared, and not only might we save our nation and perhaps the world, but we would save ourselves. As Rabbi Hillel said, "If not now, when?"

The good news is that EBT brings optimism about our future. Our nature is joy, and each person has the hardware to create that joy instead of seeing all that is wrong with the world today and feeling divided on so many levels that we suffer in silence, shut down entirely, or find ourselves in such rage that we cannot speak.

Instead, we start right where we are and enjoy this moment, and the next, and the next. Our only adversary is not a person, group, country, or cause – but stress. Stress disrupts our joy, and that is the problem.

It's time to do a lot of rejoicing. When I realized that the most sophisticated fMRI could not activate and unlock a wire that made me crave sweets or dare to judge my body, I laughed out loud. Why doesn't everyone know this?

When I realized that our homeostatic Joy Circuits spew healing chemicals on demand allowing everyone to be their own natural pharmacist just by spiraling up, I jumped for joy. One day, Igor Mitrovic announced to medical students in our EBT elective: "We *are* our circuits. Whatever circuit is activated controls our reality." I was in awe. So were the students.

We have enormous, untapped power. The resiliency pathways in the emotional brain are encoded in our genes. There are times when we prefer to be miserable, as stress activates endorphins, and it is familiar. Other times, we need that 5 State, because it unlocks old, outdated wires and primes them for rewiring. Yet it is revolutionary to base our life on that ability and takes a while to adjust to how powerful we can be.

I just led the participants in my daily intensive telegroup through a guided visualization, an "Imagine." The group does not meet on Saturdays or Sundays, so I guided them through seeing themselves awakening each morning through the weekend and saying to themselves, "I am creating joy in my life" and then spiraling up throughout the day. One of the participants, Dena, said, "I keep forgetting that. It's so basic. I am joy and I am here to create joy. That's what I am doing with my life."

I realized that she had just said it all.

Making a paradigm shift

One of my early attempts to publish a book was when I pitched an idea to Esther Newburg at International Creative Management, one of the top agencies in the world. My working title was *Isolation: The True Cause of the Rise in Childhood Obesity.*

She was very kind but did not see this as a "good fit" for her, although she agreed that the book's point was well-taken. Children were bottled up with their emotions, unknowingly amid their own emotional bypass. What options did they have if they could not get the sweetness of love? They could get the concretization of that love: a sweet.

Homo sapiens, as are all mammals, are love bugs. Recognizing that makes paradise easier to find. We spiral up. We connect to the boundless love we have inside, on-demand and calorie-free. That gives us a secure base so we can radiate out our love in ways that give back and make the world a better place. Doing so makes our day – and our life – complete.

That is nirvana, and it is not for just the disadvantaged or the super-advantaged, the sick or the well, the black or the white, or the rich or the poor. It is for everyone.

At the EBT Annual Meeting on June 4, 2021, Igor Mitrovic commented, "I am surprised that EBT has not caught on yet."

I wasn't sure either, but an interesting incident that fall gave me a clue. I went with Walt to his class reunion at Yale, which was exciting. He took me to the library, with cubbies of chairs and long wooden tables. I told him that if I had been a student there, I would have camped out in the library and never left.

There were many talks and events, and I didn't know anyone but Walt. At one of the buffet lunches, I went through the serving line and piled up my plate with some tasty food. Then I walked out to the large, covered lawn area with hundreds of round tables, all with alums and spouses chatting and feasting. All the chairs seemed to be taken.

Then I spotted one empty chair. It was at a table that was populated with Black men, all from the first class at Yale that enrolled people of color. I asked if the seat was taken, and a large man, who turned out to be approachable and friendly, said it was not. Happily, I sat down, and we began chatting. I asked him what he did.

He said he was a researcher. He had just retired. I asked him about his research and his discoveries.

He chuckled and said, "I discovered nothing. Researchers don't discover anything. Research builds on one small aspect of another person's discovery."

I asked, "What if all those small aspects of research lead to a new paradigm?"

He let out a boisterous laugh. "They kill you. The system won't allow that much change."

At that moment, he had found a friend for life. He had put into words the problem we were facing. What we needed was empathy! Whether we are researchers, professors, or clinicians, we all have an amygdala encrusted with wires from a different paradigm.

EBT is an assault on the amygdala! It's hard for clinicians to change paradigms, just like it is for all of us. Instead of diagnoses, EBT asks us to think about set points, brain states, and circuits. The wires in our amygdala typically inform us to seek medications, but EBT tells us first to spiral up and unleash our own natural healing chemicals.

It asks us to rely on our natural chemical resilience first. Instead of asking what drug is needed, we say, "I've got this!" and question how many spiral ups we need. How many beautiful Joy Points do we need to collect? Only then, if our health still stops short of optimal, bring on the medication. It's a change.

The risks of apathy

Change takes time, but time is running short. When 70 percent of Americans are overweight, you know the problem is not the individual. Obesity causes people to suffer. Although there is more emphasis on not shaming us for carrying extra weight, perhaps the ultimate neglect is that the brain that causes the problem, our "stress brain," has been ignored in treatments, perhaps another consequence of disrespect of people struggling with obesity.

If you had cancer and your oncologist did not target and treat the tumor, you would be in an uproar. However, the "tumor" for obesity is the stress-induced circuits in the emotional brain. When EBT was shown to produce lasting weight loss after treatment ended, UCSF Public Affairs distributed a press release on the method entitled, "Obesity Program Keeps Pounds Off without

Diets or Drugs." Virtually nobody listened. As EBT is educational, not the profit center of drugs or surgery, there are no windfall profits to rocket the method forward. It would take 27 more years and the generosity of two grateful patients to bring the method into center stage.

As a believer that "everything is perfect" and the fruit ripens at just the right time, I do not question what has gone on up until now. The science supporting stress as the root cause of obesity is overwhelming. UCLA professor Janet Tomiyama wrote a scientific review the relationship between stress and obesity, concluding that overeating and obesity are rooted in stress and that current methods were not effective. She concluded, "The most logical intervention target would be stress itself."

Even though three meta-analyses have shown that cognitive behavioral therapy is largely ineffective, the professional community continues to apply it as the foundation of their treatments, and, when they do not work, they default to using drugs or surgery. Weight Watchers CEO Sima Sistani apologized for her company, saying "We got it wrong." I don't think they got it wrong, but they did not provide a complete program. Any intervention that does not treat stress when it is careening out of control will fall short of delivering lasting weight loss. This puts people in the difficult position of being out of control of their eating and weight or surrendering to drug dependency or surgical manipulations. It's simply not fair.

Meanwhile, medical costs are going to break the country. The medical cost of adult obesity in the United States ranges from $147 billion to nearly $210 billion per year, mainly for treating obesity-related diseases such as diabetes and cardiovascular disease. With the addition of the cost of weight-loss drugs, Sigmund Freud was right. In a 2006 article in *Molecular Psychiatry*, the authors reflected on what Freud would think about the obesity crisis. They concluded that if they ignored the emotional brain, it would lead to an obesity epidemic, the breakdown of society, and the financial collapse of our healthcare system. Perhaps they were right.

Neuroscience gives us new options

The good news is that we can switch off toxic states to body states and mindsets of joy, which is revolutionary. In our stressed-out but still beautiful world, each person has the power not only to control a great deal of the variance in their biochemistry but to use their forcefield of love day by day. Just as the world appears to be spinning out of control and at risk of collapse, something new emerges on the horizon, born of neuroscience: the power to control our own brain.

Although this book has focused on the physiological nature of EBT and its role in turning around the obesity epidemic, what ails us more than health problems is what stress does to our spirit. Our larger goal in EBT is emotional health for all because that will give us the best chance of meeting our formidable challenges ahead. If, as a nation, more of us can process our stress, we can unite around the seven rewards of EBT rather than divide.

One day after the end of an EBT in my home, a small group of participants continued listening to each other spiral up. They huddled in my living room, and I went upstairs. When I came downstairs 30 minutes later, they were all still huddled in the living room. I had to pass through the center of their circle to get to the front door, and they didn't notice me at all. They were utterly engrossed in listening to one participant's Cycle.

I thought, "This is how EBT will get out." It is by people connecting with people and listening to each other do Cycles, not just online and by telephone, but in living rooms, church basements, and conference rooms. Whenever people gather to use these skills, magic happens as the connection is pure: people are helping people help themselves. That is the most organic way for us to prevent diseases of despair as well as decrease the prevalence and severity of chronic diseases. All those MRI orders may not be needed. Instead of the current 6.7 billion prescriptions written annually, there might be only 3 billion, not because the drugs aren't available but because they are not needed.

Our children are suffering from a broad range of "stress diseases." Imagine a new world in which they learned to spiral up from their parents. I remember teaching my children the method's "3 Tool" and watching their anxieties vanish. Children acquire these skills much faster than adults, and when they use them, they learn better, love more, and find their own deeper meanings in life.

What would it be like if adolescents traversed the "potholes" of growing up with the security of having instant access to a complete set of these tools? What if we prepared them to be skilled at facing the inner void and instead bypassing their emotional brain and reaching for maladaptive ways of coping? They could turn toxic emotions into flowing feelings. That would be life changing for them, and for the future of our nation.

Imagine emotional safety in the workplace. Employees could share their brain state with no discrimination between Brain States 1 and 5 and take spiral-up breaks as needed. At one point at EBT, we had a rule that if anyone was below Brain State 3, they needed to take a break. In our team meetings now, there is a lot of authenticity and laughter. If someone is 5ish, they say so, and we all accommodate, as we all have those moments! Organizations can destigmatize emotions and efficiently communicate by applying this neutral, scientific stress system.

EBT has long certified mental health professionals in the method, but what if all therapists were EBT-certified? They could teach their patients how to get to One. It is time that psychotherapy becomes more physiologically-based, and what could be more fundamental than teaching patients how to engage their emotional brain? In their work with couples, they could better heal their hurts, resolve conflicts, and foster a "relationship reset."

The words John Lennon left behind as his greatest legacy were: "Imagine all the people living life in peace. You may say I'm a dreamer, but I'm not the only one. I hope someday you'll join us, and the world will be as one." Perhaps we can each do our small but important part to make his dream come true.

The revolution begins with you

Where do we go from here? I hope your first priority is to use the method personally. Validate everything I have written in this book for yourself. The brain we inherited from our ancestors has always been perfect. Love your brain but give it a software upgrade with EBT.

Second, please share EBT with your friends and family. Who doesn't answer YES to the question, "Would you like to feel less stressed?" or "Would you like to try a natural way to self-medicate, something free?"

Ask all your health professionals if they are EBT Certified. Tell them that you are raising your set point with EBT, and It's working. They will see the glow of your skin, the smile on your face, the new energy you have, and the way your lab tests and exams show improved changes for which they cannot account – except for with EBT.

Most importantly, begin by saying to yourself: "I can have joy. In fact, my essence IS joy." Then join us and move through The EBT 1-2-3 JOY Program and learn how to spiral up in more and more sophisticated ways. Watch your set point rise and notice that eating and weight are no longer issues in your life. You have an abundance of all seven of the rewards of purpose. At that point, you will have immense pride in what you have accomplished – and boundless joy.

That is a solution for life.

ACKNOWLEDGMENTS

The idea that health is a function of our capacity to dismantle maladaptive wires and construct circuits that bring us love, joy, and purpose is at the nexus of spirituality and neuroscience. Developing this method has taken more than 40 years and is the product of many people's talents, devotion, and wisdom. Although we were aware that the stress pandemic made dissemination of the method more critical now than ever, we could not begin to realize the dream of bringing the tools to more people until six months ago when the generosity of Jaime and Vern Disney made this book, our enhanced technology, and a new wave of promotion possible. Their extraordinary devotion to the method and wise advice about how best to expand the impact of EBT on emotional health have guided our efforts. To both of them, I am eternally grateful.

My husband and EBT chief executive officer, Walt Rose, had conceptualized "people helping people help themselves" and "emotional health for all," as well as a plan for this expansion. The Disneys' gift inspired our core team to focus their efforts on preparation for an increase in EBT support services that coincided with the publication of this book.

Dev Singh, EBT Chief Technology Officer, and Andrea Singh, Senior Software Engineer, developed the improvements of our mobile app and website, with exceptional devotion and at huge personal cost to both of them. Michael McClure, Director of Member Support, has been highly sensitive and tireless in responding to the complex needs of our growing community during this time. He has boosted the impact of EBT significantly as the originator of the concept of Spiral Up Groups and the Spiral Up Lite mobile app. Frannie Wilson, consulting editor and Certified EBT Coach, brought her sensibilities and precision to editing this book, making this book possible and improving the manuscript significantly. Michele Welling, EBT Medical Director, and Master Trainer, both edited this book and provided a valuable content review of both the science and practice of EBT, all while delivering her ever-popular Spiral Up Groups. Her contributions in metabolic health and pain management were particularly important to the direction of this book.

Kelly McGrath has coordinated the method's infrastructure for more than 20 years and has offered her steadfast support during this transition as well as her wisdom about the nature of the human spirit. Cassidy McCorkle, Manager of Professional Training, has expanded certification training during this time in preparation for the need for more availability of EBT support. I am grateful for the incredible creativity, skill, and dedication of our core team and the good humor and sense of family pride that has come from staying the course during this challenging but exciting new phase of the development of EBT.

During the writing of this book, EBT Scientific Director Igor Mitrovic devoted time he did not have to discussions about modifications in the methods techniques, carefully balancing the need to be responsive to participants while staying true to the science upon which the method is based. Lynda Frassetto, Director of Clinical Research, guided the research forward, including articulating the Stress Triangle. Director of the EBT Mental Health Initiative, Master Trainer, and Provider of the Year for 2023, David Ingebritsen inspired the expansion of EBT professional training in behavioral health. His devotion to EBT and key contributions prepared us to make decisions about the next steps in professional training in EBT.

Judy Zehr, Director of Emotional Health, supported the provider community in understanding modifications in the method and brought her nurturing ways to the community. Bill Mory, Director of Relational Health, broke new ground in integrating EBT into couple's counseling, and Barbara Gabriel, EBT Clinical Director, continued her support of EBT intensives and deepened my understanding of applications of attachment theory to the method.

Arinn Testa, Director of Research, facilitated the EBT training of mental health professionals in public health. Our three directors in the areas of nutritional health, Deanne Hamilton, Robin Anderson, and Eve Lowry, all contributed their perspectives on obesity treatment, impacting this work. Deanne's profound understanding of EBT, Robin's ability to bring thoughtful kindness to her coaching, and Eve's care about healing disordered eating have guided me.

Angie Jackson spearheaded the development of Spiral Up Groups and Anna La Motte has overseen the growth of the forum boards. Edie Winters often magically appeared to lend needed support for the method and is breaking new ground in bringing EBT into schools. Sherry Rostosky, Shelby Killion, and Janet Christiansen launched new Spiral Up Groups upon publication of this book. Sherry launched EBT research at the University of Kentucky, as a new leader in EBT. Molly Reno, who has supported the method during challenging times, continued to hold the method in her heart and offer wise advice. Special thanks to Diedre Taylor for her contributions to the method as we transitioned into new levels of applying technology and to Robert Lustig and Michele Meitus-Snyder for conceptualizing the limbic triangle and sharing their understanding of obesity and metabolic health. The memory of psychologist Anne Brown and her love of EBT still inspire me and her devotion to EBT continues through her son Julian and his father Beau.

Working with the TVA Media Group team led to a new way of thinking about EBT. Jeffery Goddard, Bruce Somers, Jason Latshaw, Grace O'Hara, Mark Wilkinson, and Eric Stoft each brought to the project a great deal of enthusiasm about how to bring EBT to a larger audience. Mel Toltz conceived of the title of this book: 1-2-3 JOY!

The support of my family has brightened this time and inspired me. My husband, Walt Rose, has overseen the growth of EBT for nearly a decade now, and our connection has only deepened. From the start, this expansion of EBT was his vision, helping people connect with themselves and others and move forward in life. This book would never have been written without his loving support, day by day.

My son John and his wife, Ana, have given me so much love and joy during this time, sharing their adventures raising two toddlers. My son Joe and his wife Meg have been so generous with their caring and support, all while welcoming their second child at the time of the publication of this book. My grandchildren – Henry, Iris, and Orion – make my heart sing. This book is a testament to my parents, Jack and Rosabelle McClure, who taught me to love, work hard, and care. Walt's family in Texas, Tom, Caroline, and nearby, Pete, Erin, Paige, and Gwen, have given us so much support during the health challenges that came up at the launch of writing this book. The kindness of my long-time, dear friend Diana Dougherty always warms my heart. Kelly McGrath shared her wisdom and sense of the spiritual nature of life with me at important junctures in developing this work. Her ideas sparkle throughout this book. I am grateful to Bruce and Lynn McDermott who sent encouragement and spiritual messages and Bill and Gail Hutchinson for their tenderness and caring ways. My brother Steve and his wife Vivian are both grounding forces in my life, with all the goodness they bring to Walt and me. I am grateful to Sarah, Ethan, Lisa, Michael, and Colleen for being family to me. Beth Pawlick, whom I have known since age 15, shared her love and wisdom during these past months in ways that put my heart to rest. Jami Spittler, who created the designs for our advanced courses, has been so generous with her time and talents for two decades, and Colleen Mauro has shepherded the method along in important ways over the years. Both are dear friends.

Finally, I offer my warm thanks to the participants in my groups and coaching practice who have brought me joy and taught me as much or more than I have learned from science. To the extent that this book is helpful to people, I hope they take credit where credit is more than due.

Made in United States
North Haven, CT
13 June 2024